BEATING MULTIPLE SCLEROSIS

Empowering Stories of Self-Healing and Thriving

AGOTA NAWROTH
& PAIGE NEWSOME

To my loved ones,

This book reveals the transformative path of my
MS journey and daily dedication required for a healthy life.
I'm taking care of myself, so you don't have to.

To the multiple sclerosis community,

May our stories empower and inspire, fostering understanding,
compassion, and progress. Together, let's navigate the challenges
of this journey, knowing that we are never alone.

With love and deepest admiration,
Agota Nawroth

ACKNOWLEDGMENTS

I would like to express my deepest gratitude and appreciation to everyone who has contributed to the creation and completion of this book.

First and foremost, I extend my heartfelt thanks to Paige Newsome. Without you, this book wouldn't exist. Your belief in this project, constant motivation, and endless hours of work have been a driving force. You shaped this book in ways I couldn't have imagined.

I would like to extend my heartfelt gratitude to all the remarkable individuals who graciously shared their heartbreaking stories for this book. Your bravery in opening up about your journeys will undoubtedly resonate with others who find solace and strength in knowing they are not alone. I am honored to have had the opportunity to give voice to your stories and express my deepest appreciation for your invaluable contribution.

Lastly, I extend my gratitude to my followers, readers, and supporters. Your enthusiasm, feedback, and reviews inspire me to continue sharing my story and the knowledge I've acquired along the way with the world, raising awareness about diseases that can be prevented.

To all those mentioned above and the countless others who have contributed in various ways, your presence in my life has made this book a reality. Thank you for being a part of this remarkable journey.

With heartfelt appreciation,
Agota Nawroth

AUTHOR'S NOTE

Many individuals are searching for a diagnosis while struggling with various symptoms. For those of us already diagnosed, having answers can be a relief but also adds a lifelong burden. At times, this weight can feel overwhelming. I wish a book like this had been available when I was first diagnosed four years ago. It would have made a world of difference. Back then, I wouldn't have felt so alone and lost. I wouldn't have had to search through numerous books to connect the dots. My goal with this book is to provide you answers and give you practical guidance to regain control and steer your life back on track.

The stories in this book showcase the remarkable potential within us as human beings. We can heal our minds and bodies, making full recoveries from autoimmune diseases when we cultivate the right mindset and well-being practices. I haven't encountered anyone who thrives with a pessimistic outlook. Our minds are incredibly powerful. It's crucial to remember that the path to healing often begins there. While change can be a challenge, it's a necessary step for those seeking a healthier life.

So, who is this book for? It's not exclusively for people with MS. This book is filled with ideas to improve the lives of anyone, diagnosed or not, who is facing symptoms. Each chapter is a glimpse into someone's life, flourishing despite the diagnosis. My hope is that you'll discover a story or two that resonate with you. Please share this book, help us spread the message, and raise awareness about this complex condition. It doesn't have to lead to life in a wheelchair.

CONTENTS

Disclaimer

1 Agota N. - Diagnosed in 2019   1

2 Paige N. - Diagnosed in 2019   28

3 Katy - Diagnosed in 2020   44

4 Angie G. - Diagnosed in 2004   56

5 Elisa F. - Diagnosed in 2011   65

6 Kelly G. - Diagnosed in 2015   81

7 Bob C. - Diagnosed in 1999   89

8 Nassira - Diagnosed in 2018   100

9 Biljana - Diagnosed in 2013   107

10 Mohammed - Diagnosed in 2018   112

11 Kathryn - Diagnosed in 2018   117

12 Claudie - Diagnosed in 1996   120

13 Laila - Diagnosed in 2010   129

14 Adria H. - Diagnosed in 2020   133

15 Mara R. - Diagnosed in 2004   159

16 Kelly K. - Diagnosed in 2015   164

17 Michelle - Diagnosed in 1996   182

18 Joanne M. - Diagnosed in 2009   190

19 Helena K. - Diagnosed in 2000   205

20 Sam P. - Diagnosed in 2015   212

21 Alicia - Diagnosed in 2018   230

22 Dawnmarie D. - Diagnosed in 2012   240

23 Clare M. - Diagnosed in 2019   243

24 Sofia C. - Diagnosed in 2013   250

25 Andrea - Diagnosed in 2000   257

26 Meryl H. - Diagnosed in 1999   268

27 Conor K. - Diagnosed in 2003   274

28 Parmjit K. - Diagnosed in 2008   286

29 Kadesha R. - Diagnosed in 2012   298

30 Melody W. - Diagnosed in 2013   306

31 Lieza - Diagnosed in 2016   312

32 Jasmin D. - Diagnosed in 2008   321

33 Megan L. - Diagnosed in 2007   325

34 Gabriel - Diagnosed in 2018   339

35 Talia - Diagnosed in 2016   348

36 Alice S. - Diagnosed in 2007   357

37 Maria I. - Diagnosed in 2012   373

Final Note

"Wellness is the complete integration
of body, mind, and spirit – the realization
that everything we do, think, feel, and believe
has an effect on our state of well-being."
– *Greg Anderson*

DISCLAIMER

The stories shared in this book provide personal perspectives and experiences, reflecting individual accounts. These stories should not be construed as professional medical advice or recommendations.

The author and publisher have made reasonable efforts to ensure the accuracy and authenticity of the stories. However, due to the subjective nature of personal accounts and the uniqueness of each individual's circumstances, the stories may not apply to or accurately represent everyone's experiences. The information and opinions expressed in this book are not a substitute for professional medical advice, diagnosis, or treatment. It is essential to consult with a qualified healthcare professional before making any decisions or taking any actions based on the information or stories provided in this book.

The author and publisher are not liable for errors, omissions, or consequences, resulting from the use of the information or stories in this book, which are shared for informational purposes only and do not guarantee specific outcomes or results. Health conditions and treatments vary among individuals, and what worked for one person may not be suitable for another. Therefore, readers should exercise caution and use their discretion when interpreting and applying the information or stories presented.

The stories in this book do not serve as endorsements or advertisements for specific healthcare providers, products, or services. Any references made are solely for illustrative purposes and do not imply endorsement or recommendation. Readers are encouraged to consult with qualified healthcare professionals for personalized advice and guidance, regarding their health concerns. Reliance on the information or stories provided in this book is done at the reader's own risk.

By reading this book, you acknowledge and agree to the terms of this disclaimer.

1

Story by

AGOTA NAWROTH

Diagnosed in 2019
Currently 39 years old
Lives in New York, United States
Instagram/Youtube: @BeatingMyMS
www.BeatingMultipleSclerosis.com

My journey started long before I was diagnosed with multiple sclerosis (MS) in 2019. Looking back, it all began around 2008 when I was in a very stressful relationship, and I wasn't taking care of my mental and physical health. In 2013, my dad passed away suddenly. I kept my pain to myself while living 9,000 miles away from my family.

Before I continue sharing my story, let me ask you something: If we can make autoimmune disease symptoms better by changing our lifestyles and diets, why do we get these diseases in the first place? Could it be connected to our society, how we live, how we think, what we eat, and even the air we breathe? I really believe so. Instead of just trying to treat these diseases, why don't we focus more on preventing them from happening in the first place? Maybe when I share my honest story, it will help you see things from a different perspective.

Originally, this book was not meant to be my "autobiography". However, I don't think I will be publishing another book anytime soon, so I decided to write down my entire story, at least what I think is relevant for this chapter. My life from the beginning – where it started, and where it's going.

What I understand now is that my MS diagnosis wasn't a coincidence. It didn't happen because it runs in my family, nor was it something I was born with. Instead, I'm personally responsible for "opening the gate" and allowing MS to enter my life through my choices and decisions over the years. I know that this might not be the case for others, but this is my story. There's so much to share. Let's get started…

During my meditation sessions these days, I find myself on a large field, covered with flowers as I walk toward an old, rustic house. Even though it's spring, the sun warms my skin. The sky above is soothing blue, and the scent of freshly cut grass fills the air, bringing back cherished memories of my childhood home. Do I miss that place? Yes! Do I want to live there? Maybe, but not anytime soon. For now, my heart resides in New York, where I've been for the past eighteen years. It's where I have my family, my husband, and our two beautiful babies.

When you are twenty-one, you don't think much of the future, you think of the "now". You are wild and selfish. I know I was. Nothing scared me. When I wanted something, I went after it. My mother often wonders where I got this adventurous spirit from. She still can't believe that her only daughter packed up her luggage and decided to move to a different continent because she wanted a "better life". (I put "better life" in quotations because since then, I have reevaluated the meaning of these two words.) Did I accomplish it? In some ways, yes; in others, no. I managed to achieve my dreams and desires – married the love of my life, moved to my favorite Upper East Side neighborhood in Manhattan, explored numerous Caribbean islands, and beyond. Life was wonderful…until it wasn't.

Having a passion is something we should all strive for. In my case, it took many years to discover. When it comes to accomplishing things in life, I often refer to myself as a "late bloomer". However, I find comfort through telling myself that it's not entirely my fault. I was born in a small village in the heart of Transylvania, Romania, known as Csíkdánfalva. The era of communism came to an end when I was just five years old. During that period, I distinctly recall my parents acquiring a substantial rectangular box that they referred to as a television. The screen displayed black and white and had no remote control. It was still magical with only one channel to watch.

I remember winters being long and cozy. Our family would gather around the fireplace, which was essentially a tiled stove, while everyone else was doing their thing. My great aunt who lived with us was knitting, my mom was sewing up holes in old socks to make them new again, my dad was reading the newspaper, and my brother and I were playing on the floor close to the stove where it was warmer. The scent of pine from the crackling fire would mix with the aroma of our dinner: oven-baked potatoes and homemade yogurt. Potatoes were the cornerstone of our kitchen. We had a love-hate relationship. I loved them for their taste, but I also resented them because we spent most of spring, summer, and fall planting them, weeding them, praying for rain, praying for sun, then harvesting and storing them with the hope of selling most to produce income. This wasn't unique to just us; it was the way of life in our village.

As a young girl trying to make sense of the world around me, toiling in the potato field felt like the ultimate chore. Back then, I didn't know the benefits of vitamin D that we absorbed from the sun, nor the value of the exercise we were unknowingly getting. All I could think of was why I had to do this, and why I couldn't just stay home and read my book – a novel from my village library, filled with stories that took place in a city called Los Angeles. A place that sounded more like a dream than reality. It painted a picture of a world where nobody worked, and everyone was happy. I found myself dreaming of living there, and the hot days on the potato field seemed much shorter. But, of course, I had school to finish and a few more summers to "survive".

Life used to be pretty slow; the kind of slow that I like these days. But during my youth, I didn't really see it that way. Thinking about my village back then is like a blast from the past, reminding me of those "Blue Zones" you hear about. Those are the spots around the world where people live very long, healthy lives. When I was a kid, everyone in the village had animals – pigs, chickens, cows, sheep, you name it. And horses, too, with those old-school carriages. This is how my grandparents lived, and I'm pretty sure it's part of why they're still alive. They barely left the village and rarely needed to see a doctor – well, until they got older.

Then, my grandpa went and got himself a tractor, and things started changing. These days, it seems like everyone has a car, and you hardly see any horses around. Supermarkets popped up, making it so nobody needed to raise their own chickens and pigs anymore. I'm sharing this because I believe autoimmunity started with this shift. Back in the day, cancer was this rare thing, and nobody even knew what autoimmune diseases were. Thank goodness my mom still has her little garden. The fresh berries, salads made from crispy greens, juicy tomatoes, fresh carrots, and summer cabbage…I only recently understood what she means when she talks about finding peace there. Me? I'm still struggling sometimes to find that peace. But you know what they say, awareness is the first step to making changes, right?

Moving has always been easy for me. I think it's because I've practiced it since I was twelve. It all started when I moved to my aunt's place in the city during my high school years. That felt like a major upgrade at the time. Fast forward to when I turned eighteen, and I made a big leap from Romania to Budapest, Hungary. Life was good, but three years down the road, I felt the doors for me there closed. Getting my visa sorted or dealing with legal paperwork to stay became a real hassle, even though I had Hungarian roots and fully spoke the language. Hitting wall after wall, I made up my mind: it was time to explore America.

I always wanted something better, not just for myself, but for my family, too. I was convinced that once I moved to the US, I could achieve all of that. Initially, I had my heart set on Los Angeles, but life had other plans, leading me to New York instead – the city that never sleeps. Well, that's exactly what happened to me. I was clocking in twenty-hour workdays and managing only four hours of sleep. When my friend came to visit after five months, he told me I looked ten years older. Truth be told, I felt it, too, but I didn't care. Back in the day, I never had much money, but now, I was finally earning, saving up, and even sending some back home to the family. It was the greatest feeling ever. I was convinced that having more meant a better, happier life. That is, until you experience the loss of your health. When confronted with a lifelong diagnosis that has no cure, suddenly, nothing else seems to matter. I'd taken my health for granted and never really slowed down until I had no choice but to take a step back and reassess everything – how I lived and what I prioritized. The things I wanted no longer meant anything. All I wished for was to get my health back. But let's not jump ahead of things. There's a lot more to my story before we reach this point.

My life living in New York was full of adventures. I moved about seven times – starting in Queens, Astoria, then to Brooklyn. I even lived in Jersey for a few months, and I finally settled in Manhattan. How could I afford this? I couldn't! I was always hustling to make ends meet, and I had a roommate. But I loved every bit of it. I never second-guessed my choice of moving to this country. Sure, there were moments I wished I could share with my loved ones, like becoming the first in my family to graduate from college on the dean's list, no less in America, without much knowledge of the English language.

Of course, there were lots of heart breaks along the way. There were also times when I felt I couldn't cope with homesickness anymore. Being apart from my family was the most difficult, especially when my mom was diagnosed with cancer. When I was finally able to go home and see her in the hospital while she was receiving chemotherapy, it broke my heart. Despite her difficulty walking, she convinced me that she would be okay. Thanks to my aunt, she changed her diet and supplements, and I think deep down, despite the fear, she believed that she could beat cancer. And she did! Back then, I didn't know anything about the healing power of thoughts or food. Unfortunately, it wasn't a topic that interested me.

Four years later, my father passed away from brain cancer. I was living under an illusion, failing to fully comprehend the gravity of his condition. It wasn't until I received an urgent call from my aunt while I was vacationing in Aruba that reality struck. If I wanted to see my father one last time, I had to go home. I got on the plane and went straight to the hospital where the doctor told my mom and me that there was nothing they could do. The doctor prescribed morphine patches and sent him home. Three days later, my father passed away in his bed, suffering from excruciating pain. I was just one wall away, helpless, listening to the agonizing sounds of a man fighting his last battle. Even though a decade has gone by, my eyes still well up with tears as I write this. I'm still not fully healed from his loss. My brother and I had to be there for my mom, and we stood strong.

There's a reason I'm sharing this. You've probably heard those miraculous stories of people making overnight recoveries from illnesses, leaving doctors scratching their heads. On the other side, there are those heart-wrenching cases where someone's given a mere two-to-four years to live, only to pass away within a week. It's all about how your mind works and what you believe; how you process things and move forward. In my mom's case, she made some significant changes – altered her diet, prayed every single day, and incorporated new supplements. Yet, above all, she genuinely believed all these things were contributing to her healing, and they were. Of course, credit also goes to the doctors, but it was she who did the work.

Now, let's talk about my dad. After his eye surgery, his confidence plummeted, and I don't think he ever really bounced back from that. Changing his mindset was tough, and he just couldn't bring himself to believe that something as simple as a diet change would make a difference or that he had the strength to fight off cancer. Instead of seeking that inner peace or taking control of his own healing, he looked outward for help. And by the time he was ready to make that shift, it was too late. I have this fantastic book recommendation for you, *Cured* by Jeffrey Rediger. I wish I had read it back then.

Another reason I shared these stories is because, at some point in life, we all face trauma that leaves marks. My dad's passing was the biggest trauma of mine. I thought I had moved on, but even years later, I couldn't talk or even think about it. Then, thanks to my husband's suggestion, I finally decided to see a therapist. I needed to forgive myself for not being there for my dad. It took me years to shift my focus from his death to the good memories of him from when I was growing up. Now, he is my guardian angel, always with me and looking out for me.

Just before my dad passed away, I had finally ended a terrible relationship that mentally destroyed me. I had three jobs—one was my new business, and the other two were solely to pay my rent. I was determined to make things better because I was tired of working in restaurants. Being an immigrant, working in restaurants felt like a safe space. Nobody made fun of how I spoke, and people even liked my accent. Restaurant work is tough—long hours on your feet, a crazy schedule, and you have to smile no matter how you feel. It gets really tiring. I was always exhausted.

Once more, I pushed myself too hard and didn't pay attention to the warning signs. I can still remember those times when I'd be dozing off and unable to focus – a can of Red Bull to my left and a slice of one-dollar pizza to my right, fighting with a problem I couldn't solve at 1 AM. By the way, those dollar pizza places in New York City should seriously be banned. That kind of food doesn't belong in our bodies.

It's hard to think about that period of my life because the company I was trying to build didn't make it, and it ended up causing a break between me and my friend. I lost all the money I had saved up, and the feeling of failure hit hard. But I kept reminding myself that success often comes after failure. What matters isn't how many times you fall, but how many times you pick yourself up again. That gave me some comfort.

I really believe that everything in life has a reason behind it. Around this time, I met my husband. I just knew he was the ONE for me; I had this feeling that we were meant to be. It was as if the universe was making it happen. I turned thirty, and there he was – my rescuer. It felt like everything was falling into place. But what I didn't realize was how much I had pushed my body to the limit up until then, and I just kept going...

Being someone who believed sleep was overrated, I shouldn't be surprised that my body eventually crashed. Back then, I felt invincible – strong and blessed with good genes. After all, my grandparents were in their eighties, and my incredible mother had conquered cancer. If I fell sick, it would be a matter of a few days, at most. I genuinely thought my body was unbreakable. And as for a healthy diet? Well, I never had the time to cook or the interest in learning about food (I figured what I knew was sufficient!). To me, the word "diet" just meant shedding pounds – something I struggled with since I was twelve. I wasn't overweight, but like any teenager, I'd compare myself to others and see those extra five-to-ten pounds.

In my mind, "dieting" meant not eating. It was that simple. If you don't put it in, it won't show up, right? Well, turns out I was dead wrong! When I wanted to lose some weight, I just stopped eating. It worked like a charm. I'd shed five-to-ten pounds before each vacation, only to gain back ten-to-fifteen during and after. Yep, Brian and I discovered those all-inclusive places and had a blast. That was my life before MS. Sleep wasn't really a thing I worried about, stress management wasn't even on my radar, and I didn't pay much attention to what I ate. My lifestyle was all about embracing every moment to the fullest, even though I'm not a fan of the term "carpe diem".

That brings me to the next part of my story: MULTIPLE SCLEROSIS. These two words completely changed everything in my life. Imagine a sunny, warm day at the beach, listening to the waves, sipping a strawberry daiquiri, and trying to decide between Italian or sushi for dinner. Life was amazing. I felt so lucky, dreaming about my destination wedding, holding my fiancé's hand as we waited for the sunset. And it happened, just like a dream. Our destination wedding came true, with a little meltdown on my side – but hey, what bride doesn't feel the pressure, right? Let me remind you that at that time, I had no idea how to manage or deal with stress. Stress was something I believed I shouldn't experience because everything was perfect. The tricky thing about stress is that it can sneak up on you out of nowhere, and if you don't recognize it, it can get out of control. I learned this the hard way a few months later.

But our wedding was a fairytale. We were surrounded by family, friends, and unlimited food and drinks. Love was all around us.

For our honeymoon, Greece seemed like the perfect choice. It's also a great spot to drink all day and night – that's exactly what we did! Except for a little hiccup in Santorini, where I had my first experience with anxiety. However, that was overshadowed by Brian's fear after being at the World Trade Center when the towers collapsed. His anxiety had a clear cause, so I understood it. As for mine, I brushed it aside. After all, being afraid of heights isn't a big deal, right? Many of us have that fear, but I'd never felt something like this before. I should have paid more attention.

This feeling was similar to what I would experience during a miscarriage a few months later. I remember telling myself that maybe I wasn't quite ready for a baby, and perhaps the doctors were right in saying that it's something common, almost "normal". Many women start their pregnancy journey with a miscarriage. Looking back, I can't even recall how many pills were prescribed to me, but eventually, I had a procedure to end the pregnancy. The following months were a blur. Again, I was blaming myself for what happened, and my body for failing me. Due to the amount of stress and anxiety this brought me, I finally took my husband's advice to see a therapist. He wanted me to see one anyway because of my dad. I knew something was wrong but didn't know what or how to fix it. I understood that relying on alcohol and painkillers wasn't the solution. You know the saying: "What doesn't kill you makes you stronger"? Well, I came to realize it's not always true. That fifth drink at the end of the night doesn't make you stronger, nor do the toxins in your food or the toxic relationships you're in. Even staying up all night doesn't make you stronger - I'm speaking from my own experience here.

It was early 2019, and Brian decided to surprise me with a ski trip to lift my mood. New York was freezing, so we picked an even colder but more exciting spot: Vail, Colorado. It's a stunning place, with a high altitude that didn't bother me at first. A few days into our trip, we went snowmobiling. It was fun, but my anxiety started to kick in. The night we got back to New York, my forehead felt like it was on fire, but I shrugged it off as the start of a cold. I took some Nyquil and went to bed. Reading this now, I just shake my head. Nowadays, if I have a headache, I grab turmeric or electrolytes, along with two glasses of water. When I catch a cold, I spend the day sipping honey-infused tea. Things have certainly changed since then.

The next day arrived, and I realized I couldn't hear a thing in my left ear. By now, my face was also tingling. Initially, I figured it was probably a side effect of the high altitude and the flight. But something just didn't feel right, so I decided to schedule an appointment with my primary care doctor. She immediately sent me to an ear specialist, but they didn't find anything unusual either. I'd seen two doctors by this point, and both were telling me that everything seemed fine, but I didn't feel fine. As I left the specialist's office, I gathered the courage to ask for magnetic resonance imaging (MRI). My dad had passed away from brain cancer, and all my symptoms seemed to be pointing in that direction. Thankfully, the doctor handed me a referral, obliging my request.

I had never had an MRI before, so I wasn't sure what to expect. I brought my headphones, thinking I could listen to my book while I went through it. That hour in the tube felt incredibly long with the loud banging noises and no music or audio to distract me. It made me anxious, but strangely, I wasn't scared. I had this feeling that things would turn out okay. A few days later, my phone rang, and the doctor didn't sound very positive. He said my MRI results were back and suggested I see a neurologist because it could be MS – multiple sclerosis. "Can you spell that out for me?" I asked, wanting to write it down. I had never heard of multiple sclerosis. You can guess what happened when I looked it up online. Everything went downhill from there. My world (or so I thought) seemed to fall apart. The only silver lining I could find was telling myself that it's better than cancer. I might not live as long as I had thought, but at least I would have some time.

The wait for a neurologist's appointment felt like an eternity. Finally, I secured one on March 5th, just five days before my thirty-fifth birthday. And there, in that office, she diagnosed me with multiple sclerosis. It was a brief glance at the computer screen, a few seconds that changed everything. She noted a couple of old, faded lesions and three bright ones responsible for my symptoms. I remember silently hoping for a positive outcome, but there wasn't one. Nothing positive. In that room, my entire life, dreams, and future collapsed. Beside me, Brian held my hand, but I felt like I was floating. Countless questions raced through my mind, but I couldn't find my voice. Brian was asking questions, yet I couldn't hear them. The only thing I recall hearing is that unless I start medication immediately, I could end up in a wheelchair. "What about becoming pregnant?" I finally asked her. She shook her head. Medication had to come first; we could discuss pregnancy six months later, she explained.

The next hour was the slowest hour of my life. I sat with six others in the room, receiving steroid treatments. I tried to hold back tears, but they flowed despite my efforts. There was a woman beside me, her cheerful and comforting presence felt like a gift from above. She had been diagnosed nine years prior and was there for her monthly Tysabri infusion. That was the same medication the doctor had mentioned. The room was filled with a sense of darkness; I felt I didn't belong there. As I was leaving, they handed me the paperwork to sign up for Tysabri, but I held off. It was a lot to take in, and I needed time to process. I'm thankful I did, as a few days later, my bloodwork results revealed that I was JC virus positive. This meant Tysabri wasn't the right choice for me unless I wanted to risk a brain infection later in life.

I needed another opinion, hoping that maybe the first diagnosis was wrong. The steroids seemed to help, as my hearing had improved by the time I saw the second doctor. Only a slight numbness remained on my face. Unfortunately, he confirmed the initial diagnosis. Interestingly, he suggested a different medication called Ocrevus. He also mentioned Copaxone as an option if I wanted to become pregnant – something I'd have to inject myself with daily. That idea was quickly dismissed; I couldn't imagine doing that even if my life depended on it. Feeling even more lost, I wasn't comfortable with his approach. Moreover, I was curious about other potentially "perfect" medications for me, so I decided to schedule an appointment with a third doctor.

Between the span of those two appointments, I received the results of the MRI of my spine – no lesions. Finally, something positive! I remember leaving the radiology department and seeing a sign on the street that said, "Beating Cancer". I took it as a sign. I was determined to beat multiple sclerosis, or whatever was trying to take over my life. I didn't have all the answers yet, but I knew this was my new mission. On that day, I created my Instagram account @beatingmyms and came across Dr. Wahls's book on Amazon. If you're going to read just one book about MS, this is the one you need!

After ordering the book, I changed my mind and decided to listen to the audio version instead. I couldn't wait for the physical book to arrive. I wanted to learn more from her, to understand how she regained her health and left behind the wheelchair, so that maybe I could prevent myself from getting in one. In just a few chapters, I came to recognize how unhealthy my lifestyle had been in recent years, and how it might have contributed to my symptoms and diagnosis.

Later that year, during my visit with the third doctor, I was already three months pregnant and had completely changed my diet. This doctor was more understanding and didn't push medication. He congratulated me on my pregnancy, wished me luck, and told me to come back after giving birth. When I mentioned Dr. Wahls, he didn't seem fully on board but didn't say much. I think he realized that trying to sway my decision was probably pointless. He's still my neurologist, even though I haven't seen him in two years.

I soon learned that MS varies from person to person. It varies in how it feels, the symptoms it brings, and how it manifests. If not managed, it can spiral. The first few weeks after receiving the diagnosis was the hardest period to get through. Trying to understand the disease, unravel how it uniquely affects you, comparing your journey to others', and facing the uncertainty of the future. None of us really knows what lies ahead, but seeing someone in a wheelchair and realizing that could be you brings a new kind of fear that you never knew existed.

My research started at the doctor's office, where I gathered brochures and learned about upcoming MS events in Manhattan. Suddenly, I was part of a new community – the "MS Community" – where everyone is friendly, yet no one really wants to belong. The first and only event I attended was quite overwhelming. It was sponsored by drug companies, and the pressure was tangible. By then, I had memorized the names and side effects of each drug. But don't ask me to recall them—that information is tucked away in a corner of my brain I rarely visit. I need my brain for more important tasks! Anyway, the event was depressing. The message was that medication or a cure were the only sources of hope.

"Cure" is an intriguing word in the autoimmune world. You see, all autoimmune diseases share two commonalities: The underlying cause remains mysterious, and the immune system goes awry, targeting its own cells. As a result, a range of symptoms arises, with some individuals experiencing more severe symptoms, while others may have none at all. Why? It's often tied to the amount of inflammation present in the body. In cases of autoimmune diseases, the immune system, designed to shield the body from invaders like bacteria and viruses, mistakenly attacks its own healthy cells and tissues. In my opinion, if we strengthen our immune systems and diminish inflammation, we might uncover the "cure" within. More on this later.

At first, I wasn't sure about taking the holistic route. Like "autoimmune disease", "holistic" was also a new term for me, but I knew the diet change was a must. While listening to *The Wahls Protocol*, I took notes. I made two lists: one for "good" foods and another for foods to avoid (the "bad" ones). The list of things to avoid seemed endless: pasta, pizza, artificial sweeteners, sausages, ketchup, bread, fried foods, alcohol, milk, cheese, hot dogs, ice cream, potatoes – all the foods I loved and ate. It felt like my world was crashing down. I later discovered many alternatives to replace these foods in my diet. And yes, I still enjoy potatoes – yellow and organic when possible!

During that time, I got invited to a baby shower. I left the event early, tears filling my eyes. It wasn't just because I could only find one thing to eat out of the numerous dishes beautifully laid out on the buffet (a salad with dressing), it was more about the sudden feeling of being "different". I didn't know where I belonged anymore. Explaining why I was walking around with an empty plate, looking at food became hard. My brain was frozen, and I felt all alone. But deep down, I knew I wasn't alone, and this gave me some comfort.

In a few months, I turned into one of those people in restaurants who asks a lot of questions about the menu, wants substitutions, and claims to have gluten and dairy allergies. I used to smile when I saw others ordering like this. Now, I was the one doing it. It felt a bit awkward at first, but I quickly got used to it as I started feeling the results from eating healthier. The brain-fog lifted, my anxiety got better, and my mood improved. So, if you're reading this, don't hesitate to speak up in restaurants! Maybe if we do it together, we can encourage them to offer more healthy options on their menus. We can't change the whole system on our own; we need a collective effort.

On March 16th, just eleven days after my diagnosis, I shared this on my Instagram, "I feel angry. But I also feel motivated to do everything I can to #beatms...". I don't feel angry anymore. I feel thankful that I was diagnosed when I was, right before starting a family. This diagnosis led me to discover more about health – how to be healthy and keep my loved ones healthy. That same year, I gave birth to my son on Christmas Day. It was a wonderful pregnancy, and easy delivery.

MS taught me valuable lessons: the significance of family and to appreciate and enjoy each day. It also taught me to listen to my body and take care of myself, so I can take care of others. While I questioned every symptom during pregnancy, I felt great. I later realized most symptoms were pregnancy-related, not MS-related. Now, I see symptoms as signals from my body, guiding me to slow down, eat well, avoid certain foods, and rest. I've become adept at listening and responding to these cues. Paying attention to my brain is a different story; that's much harder.

Before MS, I might have chosen formula over breastfeeding for many silly reasons. After reading the book *The Vaccine-Friendly Plan* by Paul Thomas and talking to my neurologist, my decision changed. When the time came, I was panicking because I couldn't "exclusively" nurse and needed to substitute with formula. I kept thinking about what the neurologist had said: "Exclusive breastfeeding prevents relapses." It was a challenging time. Looking back, I now see that stress and inexperience played a part. It's strange how I had prepared so much, yet brain fog hit when I needed clarity most. Brain fog led to frustration, which turned to anger, and then fear. I've traveled this road before, not knowing why or what's happening. Now I understand, but it's tough to navigate in the moment of confusion.

I waited for that relapse, questioning everything that was happening in my body. I struggled to sleep and find time to eat. Strangely, the relapse never occurred, though I experienced six months of numbness in my left leg, possibly from the epidural. My only other symptom during postpartum was eye twitching, lasting a few weeks. I'm unsure if it was a flare or my body was going through detox.

During my first pregnancy, I became really sensitive to smells, so I started using essential oils. Now, I keep the humidifier running day and night. My favorite oils to use include lavender, lemon, eucalyptus, peppermint, wild orange, On Guard (by doTERRA), and grapefruit. Once I learned about the harmful ingredients in our household and beauty products, I decided to make my own to avoid toxins and save money. The recipes are easy, and nothing is more effective than vinegar for cleaning. For an all-purpose cleaner, I mix 1/4 cup of vinegar, 2 cups of water, and 20 drops of peppermint oil. For the bathroom, I combine 3/4 cup water, 1/4 cup vinegar, 1 tablespoon of soap, and 20 drops of grapefruit essential oil in a large bottle. I even make my own eye makeup remover, using 2 tablespoons of witch hazel, 2 tablespoons of coconut oil, 2 tablespoons of distilled water, and 2 drops of tea tree oil. I also use an app called Think Dirty to rate all my beauty products. Yes, it takes time to implement everything, but it's so worth it.

My Instagram account truly made a difference in my life. It kept me on track and motivated me since the beginning. At first, I had questions, and then, I started receiving them from others. One question that sticks out the most is, "Where should I start when changing my diet?" For me the easiest way to start was in my pantry. I knew that if I didn't have certain foods at home, I wouldn't be tempted to eat them. I was fully committed.

I spent about five hours sorting through my kitchen cabinets. I had a simple rule: anything that contained gluten or dairy had to go. By the time I was done, I had five bags of food to donate, and I had emptied out many shelves. My goal was to eliminate gluten, dairy, refined sugar, and soy from my diet. Additionally, I wanted to minimize processed foods and increase my intake of vegetables, fruits, meat, and fish. At that time, I didn't know much about reading nutrition labels. When I went grocery shopping, I mostly paid attention to the front of the packaging, which often featured appealing marketing claims, like "fat-free," "low-fat," "zero calories," and "all-natural". I fell for those labels every time. It was easier to just trust the system, meaning that if a product was on the shelf, approved by the Food and Drug Administration, it must be safe.

After watching the Netflix documentary *Fed Up*, I realized it was time to make better choices. I decided to dig deeper and started learning about food labels. To keep it simple, these days I focus on one thing on the label: the ingredient list. If the list is long, I put it back on the shelf. If it's short (less than eight items) and I recognize all of them, then I'm willing to give the product a try. The first ingredient listed is the one that the product contains the most of. For example, if the ingredients are dates, mango, almonds, and chia seeds, then the product has more dates than mango. While all these ingredients are healthy, finding such products isn't easy. That's why you need to become a bit of a detective when grocery shopping. It's challenging and time-consuming, but it's necessary. I highly recommend following @thefoodbabe on Instagram. She shares fantastic tips on healthy options. If you're in the United States, I also suggest downloading the Bobby Approved app. You can use it to scan items in certain supermarkets, like Costco, Trader Joe's, Whole Foods, and ShopRite. The app will tell you which ingredients to avoid and why. The list of ingredients can be long and confusing. You don't have to memorize all the names, but you should be aware of how many different things are in your food that your gut can't process. In the U.S. alone, around 3,000 new "ingredients" are approved each year. These chemicals aren't tested on humans, and we don't know how they'll affect our bodies. What we do know is that the number of people being diagnosed with autoimmune diseases is steadily increasing.

Until you become familiar with what's truly healthy and what's not, the simplest way to transition your diet is by incorporating more vegetables. This could mean adding an extra serving of broccoli or enjoying a blend of root vegetables or cauliflower rice. I'd also suggest refraining from purchasing your go-to snacks. This helps you gain better control over your cravings, and you won't have tempting chips staring at you all day long. In my case, I took a more drastic approach and completely emptied out my pantry. However, this left me with limited food choices, which can be quite discouraging.

If you've seen the documentary mentioned above, you might be wondering about the types of sugar you can consume or how to eliminate sugar from your diet altogether. Sugar is widespread and can be found in various foods (even in items like bread, processed foods, and salad dressings). The more sugar you consume, the more your body craves it. Cutting down on sugar was a challenge for me in the beginning. It took about two weeks to gradually reduce my cravings. During that period, I opted for natural sources of sweetness, like dates, figs, bananas, raspberries with almond butter, and 90% dark chocolate. These options are not only nutritious but also offer a natural sweetness. I replaced artificial sweeteners with healthier alternatives, such as honey, maple syrup, stevia, and coconut sugar. While not all sugars are harmful, I've chosen to eliminate refined sugar from my diet entirely.

What I found fascinating is that the food we consume has a direct influence on the physical structure and well-being of our brains. The fats, carbohydrates, and proteins we incorporate into our diet serve as the fundamental building blocks that nourish our brain's health. Moreover, micronutrients like vitamins (such as B12) and minerals (like magnesium) also play essential roles in supporting our brain's functionality. The connection between our diet and our brain's performance is robust. Another thing to consider is the close correlation between gut health and brain health – they maintain ongoing communication. Opting for organic whole foods whenever possible and avoiding pesticides and herbicides can greatly contribute to a healthy gut microbiome. Making small adjustments to our diet, even during grocery shopping, can have a profound impact on both our general health and brain health. Ultimately, it all begins with the choices we consciously make. Things started to change when I embraced this power and began to make thoughtful decisions.

By this time, I had listened to numerous books about autoimmune diseases and had discovered many references to functional medicine and how it can help in understanding and addressing the root causes of my condition. Again, I asked my Instagram followers and soon, someone recommended Parsley Health (www.parsleyhealth.com). Although my insurance didn't provide full coverage for them, it did cover the bloodwork, which was huge, so I decided to enroll in their program. Holistic practitioners emphasize that the foundation of both healing and illness begins in the gut. A healthy digestive system and robust microbiome are two of the most important factors for sustaining overall wellness. We're all familiar with the saying, "You are what you eat." It's true. The microorganisms within our gut serve various critical roles, including regulating our immune, metabolic, and nervous systems. The microbiome continues to change due to an array of factors, such as our environment, diet, social interactions, medication use, chemical exposure, and more.

When I first went to Parsley's office in Midtown Manhattan, I knew I'd found the right place. Dr. McConnell made me feel valued, listened to my story, and asked questions that my previous doctors hadn't. We talked about my diet, lifestyle, and I mentioned my pregnancy. Unfortunately, due to my pregnancy, we couldn't delve deeply into extensive testing (as hormonal levels could alter the results). What stood out the most from my bloodwork was the hsCRP level, which is the inflammation marker in the body. The normal range is 1.0-3.0, but mine was high at 12.2 H in September 2019. By April 2020, it dropped to 5.2, and in my most recent bloodwork in February 2023, it reached a much better level at 2.0. However, it's important to note that this is just one piece of the puzzle. I wish it were that simple.

I was also curious about my vitamin D level. We all know how important it is to take vitamin D with K2 (K2 helps absorption), right? Well, I didn't. My primary care doctor never checked my vitamin D level. My neurologist did when I was diagnosed, and my level was 23, way below the normal range of 32-100. Did you know that vitamin D is actually a hormone? And that during the COVID-19 pandemic, those with higher vitamin D levels recovered faster and had fewer symptoms? There are many articles that discuss this. Now, my level is above 80. You can find my interview with Dr. Wahls about this on my YouTube channel. I had the amazing opportunity to interview her twice this year!

From my perspective, diagnoses can simplify treatment and medication for doctors. For me, it was about digging deeper to find the root cause and prevent future relapses. A friend pointed me to her acupuncturist, Lida Ahmady, L.Ac. at De'Qi Health in Soho, Manhattan. Our first appointment was two hours long; this was the second time I felt heard. She knew right away what I needed. Even though I'm afraid of needles, my weekly appointments were something that I looked forward to for eight months during my first pregnancy. Every time I left her practice, I felt "healed" in a sense. Sadly, I stopped seeing her because of COVID and relocating, but I still take the magnesium citrate she recommended. It solved the mystery surrounding my lifelong battle with constipation.

My second pregnancy also went smoothly. Lily, my beautiful daughter, was born in October 2021. After going through two pregnancies in three years, I've come to understand why relapses are more likely to happen during postpartum. The challenges of being a mom play a big role. The fatigue from lack of sleep, being exhausted all the time, not having enough time to eat nutritious meals, neglecting our own well-being, and the stress that comes with the unpredictability of motherhood – especially with your first baby. I remember I was constantly worrying. I consider myself fortunate that I had resources to turn to when I needed to overcome those moments of feeling down. I call it my "Emergency List", and it works most of the time. I'll share my list at the end of my chapter.

Having a baby is the most beautiful thing in the world, but motherhood is not easy. Mental preparation is key; you can't even entertain relapse thoughts. Not everyone experiences a relapse. Remember, our body hears our mind and responds to our thoughts. Positivity and optimism are vital. Your mindset shapes your future. *The Secret* by Rhonda Byrne explains this the best.

In the summer of 2020, right in the midst of COVID, my son Alec had just turned ten months old when I received my training materials from the Dr. Sears Wellness Institute. These marked the start of my journey as a health coach. While I may not actively practice health coaching, the training provided me with valuable insights into nutrition and highlighted the shortcomings of the Standard American Diet (SAD). By this time, I knew that food was medicine, and my body needed a "reset". The Autoimmune Protocol (AIP) diet seemed like a great choice for this. The diet involves a thirty-day elimination phase, followed by a reintroduction phase. Find more information on autoimmunewellness.com.

To this day, I mainly follow the AIP Protocol. I feel my best when I eat lots of vegetables, fruits, meat, and fish. I do eat gluten-free pasta and cauliflower pizza sometimes, but I stay away from dairy. The only dairy I might add is a little parmesan cheese. I like shopping at thrivemarket.com because I can easily find products based on my dietary needs. This is how I came across various healthy brands, like Siete, Simple Mill, Chomps, Kettle & Fire, Hu, Tolerant, and Bionaturae (just to mention a few).

Over time, I've realized a crucial truth about diet: There's no universal fit. Have you heard of bio-individuality? It's the concept that each person's unique makeup affects how they react to food, nutrients, lifestyle, and environment. This means no single diet or lifestyle works for everyone. Bio-individuality acknowledges our distinct nutritional needs and responses. What suits one might not suit another due to factors like genetics, metabolism, gut health, age, and lifestyle. We're all unique, and there's no one-size-fits-all approach. Experiment, find what suits you, and listen to your body. That being said, we all should keep in mind that eating whole foods just the way nature intended is best. Processed food that sits on the shelf at a supermarket contains minimal nutritional value and unhealthy additives. When you provide your body with what it needs, it has the ability to heal itself. Count nutrition not calories.

You know what the wonderful thing about eating healthily is? I no longer worry about how my clothes fit. Throughout my life, I tried various methods to lose weight. From extreme diets, like Nutrisystem, to even starving myself just to look good in swimwear. However, none of these approaches worked, and they likely exacerbated my health issues. I thought becoming pregnant meant saying goodbye to my clothes forever, as they'd never fit after. But guess what? I gained just a little weight during both pregnancies and lost it all within a few weeks. Some people say it's because of breastfeeding, but that's not the real reason. Now I eat three times more than before and still haven't gained weight. It's another small thing I can thank MS for. But how many of us struggle with weight gain? A healthy diet change is the solution. I wish I had known this sooner. By eliminating gluten and dairy, reducing refined sugar intake, and incorporating plenty of vegetables and protein into your diet, you can achieve remarkable results, not only in terms of mental well-being but also in terms of your weight. On a side note: I hope this book reaches those dealing with weight problems. I wish I had known back then that a simple paleo diet could have helped me lose weight, stay in shape, and possibly saved my health.

Instead of viewing diet and lifestyle changes as sacrifices or missing out, let's shift our perspective to a more positive one. Consider all the wonderful things you'll gain by making these adjustments. Envision enjoying delicious fruits and veggies that nourish your body and bring you joy. Picture the amazing experiences you'll have while running and feeling energized. It's about adding goodness to your life, not taking it away. Embrace these changes, and you'll set yourself up for a successful, fulfilling journey ahead! I like to keep this quote in mind: "The point is not to live longer but to live better, not just to add more years to your life but to add more life to your years." - Dr. Mark Hyman.

I'm not certain where I first heard this, but it's quite insightful: think of food like an amusement park. It can offer short-term entertainment or long-term nourishment. About 90% of the time, I opt for nourishment because I understand that's what my body needs to thrive and heal. While

I could write an entire book about diet, I've chosen to prioritize a more crucial message in my story: the incredible POWER OF OUR BRAINS, and the profound potential for change and healing that starts in our minds.

For a long time, I believed that diet was at the top of my list for healing. But about a year ago, something clicked when I listened to Dr. Joe Dispenza's book *Becoming Supernatural*. It made me realize I hadn't fully understood the power of the mind. Stress triggered my first relapse, and during stressful times, my body and mind seemed to shut down. We now recognize the importance of our thoughts and beliefs. Meditation has become a powerful tool for managing and reducing stress, bringing clarity and calmness to the mind. To me, meditation is like a form of prayer, offering inner peace. Some of us turn to God, a Higher Spirit, or the Universe for help. Regardless of our belief, practicing meditation is vital for self-love. It took me some time to forgive myself for feeling responsible for my mom's cancer and for not being there during my dad's surgeries. But through meditation, I have found peace and healing.

Just recently, I discovered that in 1872, Dr. Jean-Martin Charcot suggested that MS might result from prolonged grief and vexation. Another study by George L. Engel also found that a majority of patients had experienced psychologically stressful events before the onset of symptoms leading to a multiple sclerosis diagnosis. Dr. Gabor Maté, in his book, *The Myth of Normal*, discusses how stress-induced inflammation, triggered by nervous system discharges, is influenced by emotions. There's ample evidence supporting this connection. MS patients facing significant life stressors appear to be four times more likely to experience disease flare-ups. Stress and trauma worsen MS, which emphasizes the importance of meditation.

If you're looking for a beginner's guide to meditation, I recommend listening to *Stress Less, Accomplish More* by Emily Fletcher or taking the Silva Ultramind System course on www.mindvalley.com. As someone who skeptically dismissed meditation and sat on the couch four years ago, I now dedicate ten-to-twenty minutes of my mornings to practice it. Meditation is the best medication for the brain. I truly believe that if I'd practiced meditation all along, my life's path would have been remarkably different.

As we know, sleep is another important component of healing. I used to stay awake all night or get a maximum of five-to-six hours of sleep. Not anymore! I make sure to be in bed by 10 PM, after I take my magnesium and probiotics. I close my eyes, reflect on three things I'm grateful for, and peacefully fall asleep. If my mind starts to wander, I practice breathing exercises by Wim Hof (you can find them on YouTube: Wim Hof Method Guided Breathing for Beginners) or meditate for a few minutes. Of course, there are nights when my kids keep me up, but I try to compensate for those lost hours by napping with them the next day or going to bed earlier.

Getting enough sleep plays a significant role in how I feel. During sleep, our bodies have a chance to heal. Put simply, when you eat, your body focuses on digesting food rather than concentrating on healing. Even a small snack here and there can keep your digestive system engaged, diverting the attention of other essential organs. That's why I aim to avoid eating after 8 PM and before 8 AM.

I try to begin my mornings with gentle stretches to connect with myself. After that, I sit next to my red-light machine and meditate for ten-to-fifteen minutes. I'm not sure if it's the machine or the beauty in manifesting, but it helps me start my day with a smile. I try to drink two-to-three glasses of water as soon as I reach the kitchen. When we moved into our house, my only request was to have a reverse osmosis filter for drinking (and cooking) water under my sink. If I have time, I make celery juice or mixed fruit-and-veggie juice with my Omega Juicer. I picked this brand because it's quick to clean. Lily loves both; Alec is still experimenting. For the fruit-and-veggie juice, I add whatever I have in the fridge from this list: carrots, apples, lemon, mint, cucumber, cilantro, beets, pears, kiwi, orange, mango, pineapple, and spinach. Following my morning juice, I've made it a habit to sit down and eat a protein-rich breakfast. I've noticed that this change has led to fewer mood swings during the day compared to before. It turns out that the amino acids in protein play a role in balancing the nervous system. Who would have thought?

Intermittent fasting is huge, and you can learn more about it in other chapters. But for me, it was causing anxiety and mood swings. So, I adjusted my routine. I used to fast from 8 PM to 11 AM. It's easy when you have two young children and a household to run; sometimes you just completely forget to eat. Then, by noon, I would lose it. I literally needed to do breathing exercises to reset my mind and body. Not anymore. Don't get me wrong, intermittent fasting is very important as it gives the body a chance to repair itself. However, it's crucial to remember that everyone is unique, and you should experiment to find what works best for you and when to practice it. While I still fast for fourteen-to-sixteen hours, two days a week for the rest of the week, I opt for a protein-rich breakfast around 9 AM to start my day.

I like to take long walks with Lily in the morning, aiming to catch some sunlight. The sun is a powerful tool to boost mood and increase vitality. I also try to do some exercise in the morning. Why in the morning? Because it helps me sleep better. If I have babysitting help, I run to the gym. If not, I take out my yoga mat and turn on YouTube for yoga practice. Lily loves watching and practicing, which can be a fun distraction. When time is short, I do a quick ten-minute workout. This involves fifty squats (divided into sets of ten and fifteen), with two-minute planks in between, and then finishing with fifty sit-ups.

Cold showers are said to help with blood flow, lessen muscle aches, and boost the immune system. I end my showers with a twenty-to-forty second blast of cold water. I have tried to last as long as I can, but it's not as fun as it looks. Usually, my mood is elevated once I turn off the water. Give it a go and share your experience with me. Turns out, Dr. Wahls does it, too.

When it comes to lunch, I'm a big fan of using leftovers, having salads, or making smoothies. My smoothies aren't all about taste. They're about packing lots of nutrients into my body all at once. There's no strict recipe, but once you make enough smoothies, you'll know what to use and how to make them tasty. Here's a list of the main things we like (my kids are crazy about smoothies): protein powder, collagen powder, coconut milk, and a banana as the base. Then, depending on what I have, I choose five-to-ten items from the following (either frozen or fresh): blueberries, strawberries, raspberries, goji berries, mangos, pineapples, lemon, kiwi, ginger, apples, dates, figs, avocados (any kind of fruit), almond butter, walnuts, chia seeds, flaxseed, spinach, kale, carrots, cooked broccoli, cauliflower, sweet potatoes, and beets. You know the saying, "Eat the rainbow"? This is my way of doing just that. A tip: If you use enough frozen ingredients, you won't need to add ice to your smoothie.

I take my vitamins and supplements after lunch. These include vitamin D, K2, DHA, EPA, B12, magnesium malate, and a multivitamin from Seeking Health. This list and the dosage I take change based on the results of my bloodwork (twice a year) and microbiome test (once a year). In the United States, there are many options for microbiome tests. I used one called Viome, but I recently found another one in Hungary that I prefer. Feel free to reach out if you want to know more about it.

There's growing research connecting autoimmune issues to the health of our gut microbiome. Any imbalances in our gut, particularly leaky gut, can contribute to symptoms of autoimmune diseases, including multiple sclerosis. Ask your functional medicine doctor about this. The gut is where it all begins. What we put into our bodies reflects how we feel. I see this in action every day.

When it comes to staying hydrated, I aim for six-to-eight glasses of water daily. I focus on drinking more in the earlier part of the day to avoid waking up during the night. By incorporating lemon, sea salt, mint, apple cider vinegar, or electrolytes into my filtered water, I ensure that essential minerals are replenished. During colder months, I enjoy sipping on various teas throughout the day. I get my herbs and spices from herbco.com. I also like to have bone or veggie broth a few times a week and use it when I cook to boost the nutrients. Making my own broth is simple with a slow cooker. Collagen powder and bone broth are known for their potential benefits, including aiding digestion, supporting heart health, preventing bone loss, and increasing muscle mass. Additionally, they promote skin health and can reduce joint pain. Consider adding a spoonful of collagen powder to your bone broth before drinking.

Throughout the week, I try to incorporate one hot bath (with Epsom salt and essential oils) and one ice plunge or cryotherapy session. The first time I tried cryotherapy was right after my MS diagnosis. I'm not entirely sure how I discovered it, but what I learned back then was that cryotherapy causes anti-inflammatory effects for various conditions, including MS, and it did help with my symptoms at that time.

The idea of the ice plunge came from Wim Hof, also known as "The Iceman". He is a Dutch extreme athlete and advocate for cold exposure, breathwork, and meditation techniques. He believes that regular exposure to cold helps activate the body's natural mechanisms, boosts circulation, and has positive effects on the immune system, pain perception, and stress response. The first time I did an ice plunge for two minutes was in my bathtub. Without my husband routing for me by counting down the time, I wouldn't have lasted for more than ten seconds in the icy water. Again, the benefit of this overruled the "pain", just like my daily cold showers.

Cooking starts around 5 PM almost every day. I'm eagerly awaiting the day when the kids are a bit older and can help with cleaning and chopping veggies. The actual cooking part doesn't take much time; it's the preparation that's more time-consuming. I wish I could find four-to-five hours on the weekends for batch-cooking and to cook most of our meals for the week. To simplify things, I made a monthly chart listing all the foods we enjoy eating. This helps me plan meals and know what I need to buy at the supermarket. Now the entire cooking process, including grocery shopping, is more enjoyable. I love making blended soups and freezing leftovers. Believe it or not, lasagna and pasta dishes are still on the menu—just with gluten-free pasta. For healthiest cooking, I use my air-fryer three-to-four times a week for almost everything, from steak and chicken to meatballs and veggies. It's hassle-free to clean, and there is no need to "supervise" it. I love teaching Alec and Lily about food. That will be my gift that I know will help them the most throughout life. Alec is already searching for organic labels in the supermarket and scanning items with the Bobby Approved app. My only wish is that schools would focus more on healthy eating. It would prevent so many diseases and give children a healthy start in life.

As I'm close to finishing my chapter, I'm wondering whether I should share my new discovery. As you can see from my story, I'm using myself as a guinea pig before I recommend anything. I would also like to state here, just like we did in the beginning of this book, that none of this information is medical advice. Before you consider trying anything, you should do so at your own risk. But it's best if you consult your doctor. Have you heard about the book called *The Mood Cure* by Julia Ross? According to the book: "Serotonin deficiency is a factor in many seemingly unrelated psychological and physical symptoms, ranging from panic and irritability to insomnia, PMS, and muscle pain." Serotonin is made from essential amino acids, and all my symptoms, such as anxiety, mood swings, and sadness, were probably caused by inadequate levels of serotonin. While you can obtain amino acids from food, I found that supplementing with 5HTP, a natural serotonin precursor, was an effective method for improving my mood. I'll let you explore the book and learn more about this because you might end up trying another natural option to manage stress.

I solely believe that seeing a therapist was one of the reasons that I was able to put my life back on track and move forward so quickly after the diagnosis. These days finding a therapist is easier than you might think. Two sites that I highly recommend checking out are www.helloalma.com and www.headway.co. Your insurance might cover them. Another piece of advice is to begin journaling, as I've found keeping a journal to be an invaluable tool. If you're looking for one that allows you to track your supplements, mood, and diet all in one place, check out the one I created for people with MS. It's available on Etsy.

It takes time to process a diagnosis like this. There were lots of "why me's?" What did I do to deserve this? I don't ask questions like this anymore. Instead, I ask, "What was the purpose for this happening to me?" It helps so much. With time and a deeper understanding, I realized that my MS diagnosis gave me the purpose I had been searching for all my life. I'd always known I wanted to help others, and now, here I am, publishing a book that I believe will profoundly impact many lives. MS is awful, but there are awful things happening around us all the time. It all depends on our perspectives and how we process things that will ultimately move us forward.

I haven't had any major relapses since my diagnosis. My brain fog is rare. I used to struggle with memory problems and anxiety but "fixed" both. I used to struggle with slurring speech. It was the most annoying and embarrassing thing I have ever experienced. Thankfully, it's no longer present. I only feel fatigued after eating gluten. I did have some leg pain a few months ago that lasted a couple of weeks, but after some cryotherapy sessions, daily workouts, and stretching, the pain disappeared. My latest MRI (last year) showed no new lesions. I was a little surprised because the stress alone from getting an MRI is major, and last year, during 2022, I hit my lowest point during my postpartum. At that time, because of fear of the unknown, I decided to fill out the paperwork for the medication Aubagio. I received my first month's prescription; a year later—it's still sitting in my kitchen cabinet. I couldn't take it; I wasn't ready, and I don't know if I ever will be. Instead, I made a promise to myself that when I get my next MRI in 2025, it will be lesion-free. If you can reverse an autoimmune disease, you can reverse MS, too. Acceptance, being positive, willing to change, and ultimately believing that healing is possible are my secrets. I hate when I hear, "Don't get your hopes up." Why on earth not? If we have no hope, what else do we have?

Some of my friends are still unaware that I have MS. They don't know the challenges I face, and I understand they might not fully grasp what it means. Even if you just met me, you probably wouldn't guess that I have MS. Sometimes, I find it hard to believe it myself. As odd as it may sound, I feel grateful for the early diagnosis because it's like I got a second chance. It gave me the opportunity to reverse the damage from my twenties and early thirties. My ultimate goal is to live until I'm 120 years old, or even longer, and to keep my family healthy. This wouldn't have been possible if I hadn't uncovered ways to stay energetic and resilient. This brings to mind Dr. Mark Hyman's latest book called *Young Forever*, which I found to be truly insightful and relevant. In life, we must strive to find the positive in every challenging situation. It's essential to focus on the good and continue moving forward. With a positive mindset and determination, we can overcome obstacles and embrace a fulfilling life.

It's time to circle back to the beginning of my story where I discussed how we lived as human beings fifty-plus years ago. There were less cancers, less autoimmune diseases, less supermarkets, less processed foods, and less stress. If we look at the dramatic changes in the food supply over the past twenty years with the huge number of processed foods and artificial substances that infiltrated the food supplies, it's not shocking why our bodies haven't fully adapted. Stressful life adds just more to this mix. Our body's fight or flight response isn't triggered by the lion (or in my case, a bear–since there were plenty where I grew up) chasing us. Instead, it's set off by the onflow of caffeine, pressure, and urgency. There was a time when I believed that if I remained in Transylvania, Romania, my birthplace, I may not have developed an autoimmune disease. Now, after my recent visit this summer, I see that things have also drastically changed there, and that statement is no longer valid.

It's vital to check in with yourself a few times a day, paying attention to how you feel. If you're tired, give yourself permission to rest. If you're hungry, nourish your body with food. When stress creeps in, take a moment to breathe and find calm. Remember to acknowledge your emotions and listen to what your body is trying to communicate. I went through a period of learning how to "manage" everything, but then came a profound "aha" moment. Instead of merely "managing" or "fighting", I wanted to THRIVE, despite having MS. It was a simple shift in mindset, but it made an immense difference in how I approached life. By prioritizing self-awareness and embracing a positive perspective, I found the strength to thrive beyond MS. I hope this small change in mindset can also make a significant impact on your journey. Remember, the power is in your mind.

If you're reading this without a diagnosis but feeling overwhelmed, take a moment to pause and breathe. The answers will come, but for now, focus on what you can change. You already know that your health is in your hands, and there are many things you can do right now to improve it. For those who have already been diagnosed and are reading this book seeking hope or a path to healing, my advice remains the same. Be kind to yourself, and remember, just like Dr. Wahls said: "Don't give too much credit to the diagnosis." Highlight some actionable tips from the book that you can try today. Whether you have MS or not, if you experience symptoms, your body might be inflamed, and you should explore ways to reduce inflammation. It may not be an easy process, but you are capable of doing it.

My chapter wouldn't be complete without mentioning Matt Embry and his incredible organization, mshope.com. If you're not sure where to begin, I highly recommend downloading his free cookbook. If you want to be truly inspired, watch his documentary *Living Proof*. It's eye-opening to witness how one person's unwavering determination and resilience inspired an entire community and brought hope to those facing challenges.

One thing is certain: continuing with the same lifestyle may not be the best approach. While medication can slow down progression, it doesn't guarantee protection from other potential illnesses. It's crucial to proactively manage your condition by embracing positive changes in your diet, mindset, and nurturing your body from within. I believe in the efficacy of food as medicine and the value of mindfulness in healing. Cultivating a wholesome lifestyle provides a solid foundation for supporting remission and complementing medication when necessary.

You might wonder why I took on this enormous project of publishing this book, and why now? The answer to the first part is quite straightforward. I envisioned a book that could serve as a practical guide for those newly diagnosed with MS. I wish this book was available when I got diagnosed; it would have made things much easier. Regarding the second question, it's a bit tricky. I might have considered waiting until my kids were older because raising a four-year-old and a two-year-old can be quite demanding. However, I've come to realize that people getting diagnosed today can't afford to wait. They need this guidance right now to know where to start. My purpose with this book is to raise awareness about how our lifestyle choices influence our health. It's about returning to fundamental principles, not necessarily living under trees (although that might be fun!), but rather focusing on aspects that genuinely impact our well-being.

These days, I balance being a stay-at-home mom, a certified health coach, and a graphic and web designer. I'm also an MS warrior and a friend here to support you on your journey. Looking back over the past four years, I take pride in my emotional, spiritual, and physical progress. My hope is that you too experience the same sense of accomplishment. For me, it all began with the creation of my Instagram account, @BeatingMyMS. Today, my aspiration is to launch a program where I can share the knowledge I've gained and organize retreats focused on inner healing. If you're ready to take the first step towards a brighter, more hopeful future, I invite you to join me by visiting **BeatingMultipleSclerosis.com**. Together, we can work towards regaining our health and explore thriving.

My "Emergency List" to Improve Mood and Symptoms

1. **Breathe:** Try the 4x4 breathing exercise - inhale for 4 seconds, hold for 4 seconds, exhale for 4 seconds, and pause for 4 seconds. Repeat this 8 times for immediate relaxation.
2. **Cold Shower:** Shift your mood and increase your energy with a cold-water shower. Start warm, then switch to cold for thirty seconds. Use this time to dance, sing, or take deep breaths.
3. **Meditation:** Download a 5-10 minute meditation on your phone, or simply close your eyes and envision yourself in your happy place, doing what brings you joy. Engage your senses—smell the air, feel the grass, touch the trees.
4. **Mindful Eating:** Have a quick protein smoothie or a colorful meal. Sit down, chew slowly, and fully savor the taste and textures of your food while avoiding distractions.
5. **Hydration:** Drink 1-2 glasses of water with electrolytes, a pinch of sea salt, or a slice of fresh lemon.
6. **Embrace Nature:** Step outside for fresh air. Sit under the sky or take a walk to connect with nature.
7. **Physical Activity:** Release emotions with exercise tailored to your preference - 10 burpees (works for me) or a gentle stretch. Listen to your body's needs.
8. **Read:** Always have a book or audiobook ready. Start something new or continue a favorite to shift your mood. Social media doesn't count.
9. **Journal:** Remind yourself that whatever you feel is temporary, and things will improve. Write it down in a journal or on paper. Be kind to yourself.
10. **Supplements:** Check if you've taken them for the day to support your overall well-being.

Recommended reads:
The Wahls Protocol by Terry Wahls
Cured by Jeffrey Rediger
The Mood Cure by Julia Ross
Becoming Supernatural by Joe Dispenza
Forever Young by Mark Hyman
Overcoming Multiple Sclerosis by George Jelinek
The Autoimmune Fix by Tom O'Bryan
The Microbiome Solution by Robynne Chutkan
Feeding You Lies by Vani Hari
Medical Medium by Anthony William

2

Story by

PAIGE NEWSOME

Diagnosed in 2019
Currently 36 years old
Lives in Denver, Colorado, United States
Instagram: @the.new.paige
www.paigenewsome.com

It's Thursday. I'm driving to my OBGYN's office for a check-up, again. Because the deep ache and throbbing like two unforgivably sharp objects wrestling in my uterus has become unmanageable…again. Three months prior, during my last visit, my doctor (who delivered my daughter, giving her a front row seat to all the horrific complications of my pregnancy) gave me disheartening news. She told me that the only solution she had for the unknown cause of my invisible, impossible pain was to perform a partial hysterectomy.

A partial hysterectomy? That seemed a little extreme. Not that I had any more babies planned for my future, but still. Can't your body be thrown into early menopause because of that? I'm only thirty.

Thoughts rushed through my head, like a violent waterfall, drowning out the noise around me.

I'm at a stoplight. I reach over to adjust my seat belt. I despise seat belts that lock on their own—mini straightjackets. As I reach, the belt tightens over my right hip, and a lightning bolt of electric pain shoots like a bullet from my hip down to my toes. A snapping, like a rope being pulled too hard in opposite directions in a game of tug-of-war, occurred simultaneously. Then came the fire. The scathing, hot pain of flames engulfed my right hip.

How is this possible? This can't be happening...AGAIN.

During the first trimester of my pregnancy, I experienced this same pain while getting off the couch one day. Three doctor visits later, with nothing but the option of narcotic pain medication to help me move, my primary care physician (PCP) decided it was shingles.

"Shingles? Isn't that a rash?"

"No, sometimes it can manifest as severe pain without the rash, or vice versa."

I had never heard of this before. It felt weird. I always listen to my "feeling". But she's the doctor. She knows more than me...right?

I agreed to put the antiviral medication into my pregnant body, exposing my daughter's undeveloped immune system to God knows what. But this pain—this fiery hot pain from the seat belt—while it felt similar, this was heavier. Relentless. Unforgiving.

This was not shingles.

As the day progresses, so does the pain. It is alive—with a mind of its own, wandering into the caverns of my sciatica, and quickly tangling up my spine. I call my trusted physical therapist (PT), a man I had been seeing weekly since an unexplained infection waged war on my intestines a year prior. The "infection" that changed everything, causing my intestines to contract over and over, mimicking labor pains. After an emergency colonoscopy, the only conclusion the doctor could cough up was irritable bowel syndrome (IBS). I have later come to know that this is a common diagnosis, fed to complicated patients with complicated cases. IBS is the last house at the end of the street; the place they store people they don't know what to do with. As soon as I was stamped with the label, they handed me a pamphlet about the Low FODMAP diet—without any explanation of what IBS was—and threw me out the door. The pain lingered around me like a shadow, studying my every move. No matter how hard you try, you can't outrun your shadow.

I was bed-ridden for months. If I was able to get out for a short walk or do a small round of stretching, I felt I deserved a gold medal. After pleading with my physical therapist for help, he told me that one day of lying in bed is like one week of bedrest on your body. The toll was deafening. Somehow, I had to get up.

I followed the Low FODMAP diet, as best I could from a bed. I cleaned the library out of all their information and cookbooks pertaining to the diet. Initially, it helped the pain immensely! One of the most insightful things it showed me was my intestine's aversion to garlic and onion. But what the gastroenterologist forgot to tell me is that it is not meant to be a long-term diet. It's impossible for your body to receive all the nutrients it needs from this diet alone. Eventually, you are supposed to start adding foods back in. It's an elimination diet—not a way of life. A shiny, golden nugget of wisdom that oh-so-caring doctor forgot to impart on me. I lost thirty pounds in three months.

After hearing my sobs on the phone, describing in between gasps of fire that the hip pain had returned with a vengeance and was accelerating at an alarming rate, my PT says he will stay late to have me in for dry needling. I'll take dry needling over a massage any day. My body likes to fight pain with pain— "if it doesn't hurt, it's not working" mentality. Dry needling has helped me countless times in the past, taking the edge off the pain that was enveloping my body and imprisoning me to my bed. My husband helps me hobble to the car. He opens the door like a gentleman for my daughter. I can't hide the tears anymore. I feel horrible for him. Watching the person you love writhe in pain, and not being able to do a damn thing about it, is pure agony.

We arrive at my PT's office quickly. He and my husband manage to get me on the table, face down. He inserts the needles into my sciatic area and my hip flexors, per usual.

Ouch! That's not normal. This doesn't normally sting.

I don't complain, I just keep going. I don't listen to my "feeling". He's the doctor. He knows more than me, right? He connects the stem units to each needle (there are around twelve), and BOOM! Fireworks of pain shoot up my back and down my legs. This is new. This has never happened before. I'm screaming. I can hear myself screaming, but I am not in my body. Everything goes black.

We arrive home, and my walking is worse. PAIN; it's the only thing I can think, feel, see, hear, touch, or smell. I try to go to bed, but I can't sleep. If I talk, I will scream, so I stay silent. My husband wakes up and asks how I'm feeling. I open my mouth to tell him and only stutters fall out. I can't release the words. Once they reach my tongue, they get stuck, bouncing around. My right shoulder begins jolting up and down, like I'm unsuccessfully trying to match the beat of a song. This is no song. My husband laughs because he thinks I'm joking. I don't return the gesture.

This is not a drill.

We drop my daughter off at my sister's house. My husband speeds me to the emergency room, like he's playing a game of *Grand Theft Auto*. He's just scored the car, and we're on the run from the cops. I love him for that. My caretaker. My hero. My sweet, sweet ride or die.

I can't walk in. He leaves the car running as he jumps out and runs inside to get me a wheelchair. I attempt to tell the nurse at the check-in station my symptoms. Again, stutters and spasms are all I can muster. She picks up her phone, and I'm catapulted to the back. She says the word "code", but that's all I can pick up. The pain is so loud, making the rest of the world inaudible. I am wheeled to a room, packed with computers and one pretentious neurologist. He does a few "follow my finger" tests and takes my vitals, showing zero empathy or compassion as he does so. He asks me to explain my symptoms to him. Haven't they gotten the memo that I'm here because I physically can't explain my symptoms? I try, again, and he thankfully sees I cannot help him understand. My sweet husband steps in and takes over.

Thank you.

I'm beginning to understand what it means when people say you need to advocate for yourself. It's not fair, and it's excruciatingly exhausting, constantly beating people over the head with your information. But in the end, you can truly only rely on yourself.

My husband explains to me, as I'm being wheeled down the hall, that they need to take emergency magnetic resonance imaging (MRI) of my brain to ensure that I am not having a stroke. I am an MRI virgin. I am wheeled into a room with a tall, narrow table, surrounded by what looks like a massive innertube. The radiology tech and my husband help me onto the table, lying me back. The tech secures a cage over my face and snaps it shut.

"Don't move, or we'll have to start over. This will take around forty-five minutes."

The whites of my eyes fly open, and my chest tightens and recoils, like a sea anemone that has been unwantedly poked. I'm claustrophobic. He doesn't know that. I can't tell him. I start to panic as the table slowly slides me backward, head-first into the innertube. I feel my husband's warm hand wrap around my foot.

"I've got you," his touch signals, "I'm not going anywhere."

After an eternity in the face cage prison, the intensely sharp noises swirling around my head during the MRI, attempting to hold still for forty-five minutes while spasming, and the endless amounts of breaths while waiting for results, a group of three doctors finally walks in. They introduce themselves as the neurological team assigned to my case. One is holding a manilla folder in his hands, their faces void. The man in the middle steps forward, announcing his authority.

"We have your MRI results. We found one, possibly two, lesions in your brain." No pause for reaction. He quickly pulls the scans out of the folder, places them on a lit-up white board, and turns off the overhead lights. He points to a black spot on the scan and proceeds to explain.

"This lesion is in the white matter in the frontal lobe of your brain. The other possible lesion is in the back."

"So, this is the reason she can't talk?" My husband asks, his face contorted in concern, mixed with frustration and anger at the lack of explanation.

"We aren't positive the lesion is affecting her cognitive function, but it's our best guess. We think she may have multiple sclerosis (MS)." He turns to me. "You didn't have a stroke, and you aren't dying. That's where our job in the emergency room ends. We suggest you see a neurologist as soon as possible." He returns the scans back to the manilla folder and hands it to my husband. Stuck to the top is a blue post-it with a name and phone number. They leave the room as swiftly as they came. I did not have a stroke. I am not dying. Thank you, please leave.

To them, I am just a number.

For the next year, I was bound to a wheelchair and/or crutches. My mom had to be with me every day because I couldn't drive, take care of my daughter, make dinner—I couldn't even get to the toilet without help. I also needed her to be my mouthpiece at appointments because the stuttering and spasming continued to get only worse.

Overnight the world had become loud. I was sensitive to everything. A thick fog constantly cloaked my brain, making a thought process impossible. My daughter's adorable laugh was overshadowed by my constant shushing. Overstimulation became the word of the day, every day. I spent the duration of my days during that time (2018-2019), when not at PT or a doctor's appointment, with headphones in my ears, playing white noise to shut out the intrusive noises the world was using to attack me. Over time, as one can imagine, I became seriously depressed. I am an editor. My degree is in English Writing. I live to read and help others write. The plan my husband and I made when we decided to have our daughter was that he would work full-time, and I would stay home with her and freelance. I could no longer read without becoming confused or nauseous. The lesions in my brain were stealing from me, and each thing they took was a little closer to my core.

I've just met with my fourth MS specialist, and I'm still no closer to an actual solution. Everything I know about this horrific disease came from desperate midnight Google searches, and the tidbits of information the doctors are willing to spill. The first specialist took a personal phone call, regarding his upcoming golf game, while my husband and I were sitting directly in front of him, waiting to hear my fate. Bedside manner should be a requirement to graduate medical school. The MRI in the emergency room doesn't capture the scans as thoroughly as a freestanding clinic, so he reordered them. I had to call his office every day for two weeks just to get the orders for the scans sent to the imaging clinic, which takes them less than five minutes to complete. Like I said before, I was learning how to advocate for myself, and it became a full-time job. Then came two more specialists. One sent me for a spinal tap that came back negative. The hangover headache from a spinal tap is by far the most excruciating pain I have experienced to this day. I was literally screaming in the emergency room, waiting to receive my blood patch, the only remedy for this symptom. The specialist had told me not to worry, reassuring me that only five percent of people experience the skull-crushing headache.

I am the five percent.

Her diagnosis was that my symptoms were presenting as MS, but the frontal lobe lesion had wrapped itself around something in my brain, which is why she wouldn't officially diagnose and treat me for MS without further confirmation of more lesions. (A blessing in disguise that would come to fruition two years later.) This fourth specialist was the highlight. He is well-known at the University of Colorado Hospital for his work in multiple sclerosis. I was referred to him by a friend of mine with MS, who had seen him and spoke very highly of his bedside manner (cue laughter).

I waited two months for my appointment, which isn't bad when you're working with neurologists in high demand. But when you can't talk, walk, smile, breathe, or participate in your life, two months is hellishly long. The relief I felt when walking into his office and checking-in was palpable. I was desperate for a firm diagnosis and a course of treatment. I was desperate to be me again.

Someone is finally going to care.

My husband wheeled me back when they called my name. My shoulder bounced up and down as I waited excitedly in my wheelchair. The doctor barged in but seemed to have left his impeccable bedside manner at the door. He refused to meet my eyeline, speaking only to my husband. When bound to a wheelchair, you already feel low to the ground. This made me feel even lower, like an annoying piece of gum stuck to the bottom of his shoe. He asked me to walk down the hall and back as best I could. His one and only test. By the time I returned to my wheelchair, tears from the scorching hip pain were streaming down my face. He didn't care. I'm not even sure he watched me walk or what he was looking for, but he met me with, "You don't have MS. You have anxiety. I'm going to call you in a prescription for Zoloft." I was dumbfounded. My husband tried to ask how he could tell that from a simple walk, but the doctor briskly (and rudely) left the room. He was supposed to be my saving grace—the one who wasn't going to give up on me because I wasn't a cut and dry case.

Case closed. Fairytale officially over. To them, I would never be a life—only a number.

My fifth neurologist was my final neurological stop. He was recommended to me by another doctor in my queue. He was a general neurologist, meaning he did not specialize in MS. I figured I'd give it a try since the specialists were failing me, one after the other. He took a long look at my scans, performed a thorough examination of my entire body, and escorted my husband and I back to his office. He was different from the other neurologists. He smiled when he talked, listened to my painful journey without interrupting, and showed empathy. A neurologist with impeccable bedside manner—I could get used to this. We sat in his cozy, light blue office, overlooking the snow-capped Rocky Mountains. He took one more look at my file, put it aside, and looked at me instead. I held my breath.

"From what I can see, you have what is known as clinically isolated syndrome (CIS). This is the first level of multiple sclerosis."

I exhaled. A diagnosis. Finally.

"You are classified in this area because we are certain you have the one lesion. I can see you are clearly in distress and struggling. I like you, and I want to help you best I can."

He wanted to help me. Another exhale.

"I would like to start you on a medication called Tysabri, but if your insurance won't cover it, we will go with another called Gilenya. It won't help with your symptoms, but it will hopefully stop your brain from forming more lesions. We need to order another MRI of your brain before you start. Then, a registered nurse will come to your house to administer your first dose and monitor your vitals for eight hours to ensure your body doesn't react negatively."

That sounded scary, but hey, my life was already a horror show. I was desperate and willing to take whatever he was offering. I would have stood on my head for eight hours a day if it would have healed me. Desperation brings people to dark caves they never thought they'd be forced to mine. With my diagnosis in one hand and a prescription in the other, I wheeled out of his office, and onto my next phase: solution, or so I thought…

While I was waiting to be seen by these specialists, my PCP, Dr. Judd, was working side-by-side with me, who, as luck would have it, is also a Doctor of Osteopathy (D.O.). He tried endlessly to help me, from injections to adjustments to pain medications—they were simply Band-Aids. Nothing improved my brain function. The witty, funny, snarky, kind, feisty, fiercely loving parts that make-up me had been sucked into the lesion like a blackhole. Every possible "solution" made it worse. I was stagnant. I could feel the "me" I loved slipping away. Depressed does not describe the heaviness of what I felt. I spent months, from sunup to sundown, drenched in tears, my mood constantly swinging. Dr. Judd also realized, through trial and error, that I am what they call "selective serotonin reuptake inhibitor (SSRI) resistant", which means that antidepressants do not work effectively on my brain.

I am the five percent.

I saw myself as a burden to everyone in my life. One day, I had been fine, and the next, I was falling to my demise, literally. To say I was hopeless would be a laughable understatement. I wanted to kill myself, kill the pain, kill the burden I was becoming…

During one of my routine check-up appointments, Dr. Judd wheeled in a large, gray machine with eight gigantic, round electrodes, along with their cords, dangling from the sides. "SANEXAS" was written in bold, green letters across the front. A tall glass beaker sat on top, filled with water and yellowish-brown circular sponges. He looked at me, eyes brimming with hope. "I have an idea. Are you ready to get better?"

I mustered "yes" through a broken smile. He held his hand out to me, offering me grace, knowing how beaten down I had become from wrestling with hope. After boosting me on the table, he began attaching the electrodes to my hips, hip flexors, and surrounding areas. He grabbed one sponge at a time, wet it in the beaker, put it on my skin, and sealed it tight with the electrode.

"This is called an E-Stim machine, and it costs more than my car," he says. I give a little chuckle. He always tries to make me laugh. "It uses electrical pulses in three different ten-minute intervals to activate the muscles and nerves in your legs that aren't working properly. I've seen this machine work miracles. It's time you get yours."

And a miracle it was! Initially, it was mildly painful—more so jarring, like hundreds of bees buzzing around under my skin. During my first few visits, my legs flopped around on the table, like a fish stuck on dry land. My mom captured videos of my hilarious leg dance. Laughter is always my best medicine. After my third visit, I crutched myself into his office versus my normal route of being wheeled in. This was the first sign of ANY progress I had seen in an entire year!

On my eighth visit, I crutch into the waiting room, and sit down.

"Paige, you can come on back," the medical assistant says with a smile. They are, and always have been, so kind to me here. My hands instinctively reach out toward my crutches, but I pull back. I can do this. I hand my crutches to my mom.

"Are you sure?" she asks, hesitantly. I nod. I grab hold of the wooden arm rests on the chair with my shaky hands and push myself up. And then, it happens. One shaky foot in front of the other, I walk myself into his office.

Look, ma, no hands!

After my miracle, I began to get my life back, one shaky footstep at a time. Dr. Judd continued to do research on my behalf. I knew he cared because he never, ever gave up on me. He believed me. He saw my pain. That was all the validation I needed. I received E-Stim therapy weekly. During one of my sessions, he asked me if I had seen the documentary *Living Proof* on Amazon Prime. I shook my head no, and he continued. "It's about a man named Mathew Embry. He was diagnosed with MS over twenty years ago. He was told he would be in a wheelchair within six months. He and his father refused to accept that answer. They researched his disease themselves, and he's been living symptom and medication-free ever since. He's cured himself with intense diet change, vitamins, and exercise. The wheelchair never got him. He even runs marathons!"

I nodded along as he spoke. I've heard countless success stories like this. And to be honest, they always make me feel worse because it's not me running those marathons. The wheelchair got me. It's not me driving my daughter to school every day, listening to her sing. I am not the person people are looking at, thinking, "But she doesn't look sick." It's etched on the bones sticking out of my face from lack of nutrition and sunlight.

Yes, I was walking again, but the pain was still screaming at me daily. Forget running marathons, I craved a simple day of walking the dogs with my husband and daughter, the warmth of the hot sun on my face. I couldn't handle the sun anymore. It stole my breath—not in a good way. After my session, I told him I would watch the documentary before I came back the following week.

"What have you got to lose?"

Nothing. I've lost it all.

I went home and watched. As the final credits rolled up the screen, I picked my jaw up off the floor and wiped my tears. He had a firm diagnosis, with lesions trailing up and down his spine. He had the prison sentence of the chair waiting for him...but he ran the other way. For the first time in a year, I was inspired. If Mathew, riddled with spinal lesions, could do it, then certainly I—with one or possibly two lesions—could do it...right?

I shuffled into my next appointment with Dr. Judd, notes in hand. He was elated to see my hope had returned, this time with wings. Mathew Embry created a webpage called *MShope.com* for people newly diagnosed with MS. He offers advice, success stories, AND a free cookbook. When you've flushed thousands of dollars down the toilet attempting to heal yourself from a chronic illness, the word "free" is like finding a golden ticket, wrapped around a simple bar of chocolate, opening a world of pure imagination. And I was here for it! I reached out once to Mathew on Instagram for advice about clogged jugular veins, a common symptom he uncovered in his documentary that plagues many people with MS. He responded promptly and was very kind and helpful. Someone else cared.

At this point, I decided to ditch the western medicine route I had been trudging tiredly down for so long and give the holistic approach the old college try. I spoke with my neurologist about quitting Gilenya. He was supportive of my goal but made me promise to undergo an MRI first to ensure the lesions were doing as they were told. They were. The funny, and not so funny, thing about Gilenya is the warning about quitting. The pamphlet cautions that if a patient decides to stop taking Gilenya, their risk of developing new lesions becomes 75% higher within the first three months. This terrifying warning kept me tied to the medication much longer than I would like to admit. Gilenya was only meant to stop more lesions from forming, not to reduce any that were already there. After ingesting it for six months, I felt worse. It took me another six months to gather my bravery and take the giant leap off the cliff. I took one final look at the pamphlet as I was disposing of my Gilenya literature, and saw in fine print, the last warning:

"May make multiple sclerosis symptoms worse."

I threw it in the trash, and never looked back.

After I made the leap, the universe began falling into perfect placement. I met a lady who had been plagued with Lyme disease. The symptoms forced her into her bed full-time, as well. The western medical system had failed her, just as it had me. While researching the holistic route, she came across a woman who owned a holistic nutritional consulting company. Within one year of seeing her, my friend with Lyme disease was symptom-free and bed-free. I scheduled with her immediately.

During my first appointment, she strapped her biofeedback machine around my head and extremities, placed a circular red-light directly over my forehead (which I now know is a low-wavelength red light, used to help inflammation and pain), and began explaining her line of work. The biofeedback came back with mind-blowing results. She was able to tell me what my body was lacking so in depth, it made a blood allergy test look like child's play. I knew she was the real deal when she asked me if I had been in close contact with a pig recently. Apparently, my toxin level in that area was shockingly high, but she had no way of knowing that my sister has a pet pig that lives indoors. I was officially intrigued.

On the Low FODMAP diet, you are allowed to consume dairy if it's declared lactose-free. The biofeedback results showed that I was having severe reactions to dairy, corn, soy, red meat—all of the ingredients I had been consuming daily for years on my doctor-suggested diet. She also informed me of the vitamins, minerals, and supplements my body was lacking. I learned about the benefits of red-light therapy and how it is more effective on my inflammation pain than a narcotic. It also helps immensely with mood and brain fog. Another technique she used was Bemer Therapy, which increases blood circulation, mobilizes the immune system, improves energy, and decreases inflammation. She gave me a list of vitamins and minerals to start taking immediately and scheduled me for my next visit. And...sent me home with a free cookbook. Score!

Two days after removing all dairy products (and byproducts) from my diet, my skin pain vanished. The pain that felt like a thousand little needles attacking my dermis every second of every day, the pain that no medication could take the edge off, had been thrown out with the dairy.

It's working. I'm not broken.

I took the vitamins and minerals suggested by my nutritionist religiously. After every appointment, the levels of toxicity in my body were down, along with my pain, while my nutrient levels were up. I bought my own red-light box for my face (Bestqool), a panel for my body (Mito Red), and began exposing my brain and body to red-light therapy for fifteen minutes a day. The results were unmatched. I was finally able to step into my life again. The gut-wrenching intestinal pain faded into the background. The true miracle—my brain peaked its head out of the fog. I started driving again. I tried yoga, and my muscles thanked me instead of screaming. Music and reading danced back into my life. My daughter's magical laughter brought joy to my ears instead of pain bombs. I was healing from the inside out. I was becoming a success story. The pain still existed, along with the fog, but it was manageable. It was in the background this time, not me.

One area I was still struggling to find my footing was on the mountain of mood swings and depression I was climbing that were untreatable with SSRIs. I was becoming happier, but that emptiness lingered. It didn't make sense how my life could be returning to me so beautifully, while my mental health was suffocating. I was doing everything suggested to me—exercise, meditation, my diet was on point, surrounding myself with positive things—still, the sadness came. I felt like MS had come into my brain and stolen my pause button. You know, the pause you experience before you react? The pause that blesses you with time to decide if you want to get mad or let it go? My pause was gone. There was no time between feeling and action, and my family was receiving the brunt of it. After an intense meditation session, the strongest urge to get online and do a little more research crept up on me. After minutes of researching SSRI resistant depression, something called ketamine therapy popped up.

Ketamine? The horse tranquilizer?

I'd heard of people using it recreationally when I was younger. I also knew someone with a severe chronic pain illness who would fly to Stanford University hospital every few months to receive ketamine infusions for her pain management. That's where my knowledge of ketamine ended. As I sat reading about it, I heard Dr. Judd's voice whisper in my head, "What have you got to lose?"

Nothing. I dove headfirst.

After an induction reset round of ketamine intramuscular injection therapy (consisting of six appointments, spread over three weeks), I felt the darkness begin to lift. Several booster sessions later (you can return every three weeks), my pause returned. An added bonus—it also helps with chronic pain and resetting the pain receptors in the brain. It's a journey, but it worked! I went every six-to-eight weeks for over a year, and the results have been life-changing. The first time I noticed it truly working was the day I found a note from my seven-year-old daughter on my nightstand, reading, "You are a really fun mommy when you are happy. I love to be with you." Those two sentences gave me the validation to keep going, to keep pushing, to keep trying, to keep falling, and to never give up because I am a fun mommy when I'm happy. I love to be with me, too—I deserve to be happy.

I didn't realize until a few years after that initial emergency room visit the importance of the words "we found" to a patient with an invisible disease. So often we are left in the dark, being told repeatedly that it's not real or we're making it up. It's this feeling of desperation that led me to beg my neurologist for medication—a very harmful medication I did not need. Thankfully, I took it for only a year before an actual solution found me. Through a strict diet that is tailored to my body to keep me away from inflammatory foods (gluten, garlic, onion, dairy, corn, oats, soy, broccoli, cauliflower, red meat—to name a few), I keep my digestive system flowing naturally. I never cheat on my diet; the consequences are too substantial. Sometimes, I unknowingly consume something I shouldn't, and I feel the consequence within minutes. The company Seed makes a great probiotic+prebiotic supplement called DS-01© Daily Synbiotic that I take morning and night, which also helps with my intestinal pain and digestion. Omega-3 by Nordic Naturals plays a huge roll in keeping my intestines happy, as well.

I now know food is truly medicine. I eat triple the amount of green vegetables I did in my previous life. SUJA green juice is a staple in my refrigerator. Consuming vitamin D daily has also proven vital to my health. During a minor flare-up of symptoms while editing this book, Agota, the publisher, kindly informed me that vitamin D cannot be properly absorbed in the body without K2. I did some research and came across a well-reviewed brand called Bronson and immediately ordered their D3+K2. I have noticed a difference in my energy since making the switch. The flare-up I experienced was my own fault. I wasn't taking care of my stress management, and it pummeled me. Function and feeling comes and goes throughout my extremities when I'm experiencing a stress flare. Thankfully, the universe sent me only warnings. I spent a week in my house, red-lighting and meditating—doing anything I could think of to heal (and taking every suggestion). I emerged symptom-free two weeks later.

When I first began this journey, I was taking all sorts of vitamins and supplements (recommended to me by my holistic nutritionist) to lower the toxicity levels in my body. Now that they've balanced out, I've been able to scale back to only a few. I take digestive enzymes three times daily (Digest Gold by Enzymedica), along with a fermented women's multivitamin twice daily (CodeAge). I start my day with DS-01© (Seed), followed by a warm mug of lemon water. When I'm finished, I take methyl B12 (Jarrow) and magnesium malate chewable (Seeking Health). I prefer to take my Omega-3 in the evening. I like to wake up much earlier than the rest of my family, so I can complete my routine quietly in the dark before the stimulation of the day begins. It also helps cultivate a positive mindset and set my daily intentions, enabling me to be the wife and mother I aspire to be for my family. After my vitamins, I do fifteen minutes of red-light therapy while listening to self-hypnosis meditations. I've tried several apps, and I've settled on one I really enjoy called *Breethe*.

During one of my meditations, I came to the realization that I needed to eliminate unnecessary stressors from my life (like caffeine) over which I had control. Apparently, my nervous system is hypersensitive to any type of stimulant. Once removed, I noticed my strength returning, my energy-levels rising, and my stress-level reducing. I am so grateful I was given that warning; it's something I don't take lightly. I now have a schedule set for my workday to keep me up and moving hourly. My sweet husband suggested setting an alarm every fifty minutes while I'm working at my computer. The purpose is to prompt me to take a break, stretch, enjoy a song, or engage in something that brings me joy (unrelated to work) for about ten minutes. After that, I return to my computer. I highly recommend giving this approach a try; your body and mind will thank you. I emphasize the idea of finding joy because I've recently grasped the significance of genuine joy in my own life. This entails activities that you enjoy doing without a specific end goal—activities that transcend daily routines. Your soul thrives on joy. I owe this valuable insight to Glennon Doyle's podcast *We Can Do Hard Things*; another life-changing tool for me.

Through daily exercise of light stretching, yoga, and walking, my muscles have regained their strength. My bed is now a place I sleep at night, compared to the prison it was before. I've collected a remarkable team of physicians who actually listen and care about me as a human being. They don't waste time on the basics. I tell them what I need, and they help me. Always. I see my more recent PT, Dr. Luke Harmon, on a regular basis for dry needling and adjustments to keep my muscles mobile and my ribs in place. They like to wander off sometimes. He is truly phenomenal, and the doctor-patient relationship of trust we've established is incredibly encouraging for my healing journey. When the MS hug found me, I found the kindest pelvic floor physical therapist, Katherine Koch. I see her regularly to keep my breathing muscles in check through dry needling and trigger point massage. What makes these two medical professionals different, and of course, Dr. Judd, as well, is that they truly see and care about ME. And they have never given up on me. I feel incredibly blessed to have crossed paths with all of them.

I am happy to announce that I am back in the editing game, helping people share their stories while preserving their unique voices. This is a genuine passion of mine and one that I do not take lightly. Everyone has a story inside them, and I'm here to illuminate those narratives. You can reach me at www.paigenewsome.com.

I've learned things through this journey that are imperative to my health that I was blind to before. For example, when it comes to my body, I'm the professional. When it's speaking to me, or sending intuitive feelings, I need to listen and speak up. I thank my body daily during morning meditation for allowing me to move, to stretch, to speak, to dance—to be free. I still get brain fog, I still experience pain, but it no longer controls me. I am the conductor on this train, not multiple sclerosis. I also surround myself with people who, even though they may not understand, validate my journey, walking alongside me. As helpful as western medicine can be, it did not help me. I now choose my doctors very wisely; they don't choose me. I keep the ones who show me they care and discard the rest.

To them, I am just a number.
But to me, I'm everything.
I'm worth it…and so are you.

3

Story by
KATY

Diagnosed in 2020
Currently 35 years old
Lives in Chicago, Illinois, United States
Instagram: @katemay26

Hi! I'm Katy. Nice to "meet" you! I'm a thirty-five-year-old, busy mom of four from Chicagoland, and this is my story. I grew up in a small town in southern Illinois, the oldest of four kids. My mom was a stay-at-home mom while my dad made a living as a pastor. We spent countless hours digging outside in the dirt and playing Apple Derby with dad. We were really just dodging smashed pieces of apples from our apple tree that dad hit toward us with a baseball bat—don't knock it until you try it! There was never a lack of baked goods in our house growing up. In 2003, our family moved to northern Illinois, just northwest of Chicago. I met my husband, finished high school, started college, got married, and graduated college all within a span of four years. In 2011, we welcomed our first baby, Calvin. In 2013, Norah was born, followed quickly by Caroline in 2015. Nothing like cranking out all the big milestones, one after another!

My story really started on September 28th, 2017, with the birth of my fourth baby—an 8 lb.19 in. beautiful baby girl named Hattie Paige. Her delivery was normal. The beginning of my recovery was normal. Even adding a fourth baby into our crazy family was normal. Little did we know, what we knew as normal wasn't going to be normal much longer. I've never been a big fan of rides, but I didn't choose to ride this rollercoaster. It was starting, and I was on it—whether I liked it or not.

When Hattie was born, my other kids were six, four, and two. As you can imagine, I was no stranger to living in a permanent state of exhaustion. This wasn't my first experience with a newborn. I had already been through three deliveries and recoveries, three rounds of long days and sleepless nights, and three breastfeeding journeys. I knew what to expect. But as the days and weeks went on, I quickly learned that my expectations for this postpartum experience weren't going to be met in the same way.

A few months after Hattie was born, I started to feel some strange dizziness. Not necessarily like spinning or vertigo, but more so unbalanced. I noticed I reached for the wall more often as I walked for a safety net. I sat down throughout the day far more than I ever had in the previous six years of my mothering journey combined. I just felt "off". After a few months of this feeling, I decided it was time to reach out to my midwife for a checkup. She checked my iron levels, which were normal, and assured me she didn't see anything alarming. She sent me on my way with the "prescription" to rest more (haha) and eat more calories to make up for those lost with breastfeeding. In the back of my mind, I think I knew this wasn't the answer, but I was willing to try it.

Thankfully, I lived in the same town as my parents. My mom took the midwife's advice and ran with it. She tucked me into bed at her house, watched my older kids while I napped during the day, brought the baby to me to nurse, along with plates and plates of food to bump up my calorie consumption. Remember those baked goods I mentioned earlier? I vividly recall a plate of warm blueberry muffins, slathered in butter. Even after I left my parents' house, my mom made sure I was eating and resting as much as possible.

After a few months of trying this new plan, I knew it wasn't working. The dizziness persisted, and it was time to reach out to my primary care doctor for more answers. She started by running all my labs. Within a week, she called to let me know my vitamin D levels were extremely low (not surprising, knowing what I know now). I was thrilled —a simple problem with an easily fixable answer. She prescribed a mega dose of vitamin D, 50,00 IU per week, and said that should "fix the problem". For a few months, I pretended it did. I so badly wanted the vitamin deficiency to be the problem, and the supplement to be the answer.

Unfortunately, it wasn't. I finally admitted to my husband that I wasn't really feeling better. The dizziness was lingering, and I just couldn't keep going with the way I was feeling. So, back to my primary care doctor I went. This time, she diagnosed me with an ear infection and prescribed an antibiotic—my poor gut! I left with another prescription and a prayer that this would be the answer. It became clear very quickly that it wasn't. By this time, new symptoms were slowly being added into the mix. Tingling, twitching, and numbness in my legs, along with bladder issues and extreme exhaustion were the most troubling, on top of the continued dizziness.

At the risk of sounding like a broken record, I went back to my primary care doctor. I didn't have any other options. When I went for my third visit, I remember sitting on her table in tears, trying to get her to understand how I was feeling—that I knew there was something wrong with my body. I had recently experienced a new symptom that seemed like it might be the key to solving the puzzle in her eyes. I struggled finding my footing in a dark room. Darkness made me feel very unbalanced, like I didn't know where my foot was in relation to the ground for my next step. This made nursing a baby in the middle of the night very difficult. When I shared this, her ears perked up. She thought she'd figured it out. I didn't even care what it was: I just wanted an answer. Vestibular migraine. An answer that came with no solution. I asked what it meant, what it looked like long-term, and what treatment was. It was a "wait and see" approach. Another "answer" with a dead-end fix. I left her office feeling so scared and alone.

It was clear at this point in the journey I was going to have to medically advocate for myself in ways I'd never done before. I'd heard others share how important it was to them and their families in countless stories, but never in my own life. Thankfully, I had a friend who worked for a functional neurologist, Dr. Matthew Imber. I reached out and asked if he worked with vestibular conditions. The answer was yes! We scheduled a phone consultation for early February 2020, two and a half years after the onset of symptoms. We were finally off to the races!

I remember the phone consultation like it was yesterday. I sat on the floor of my bedroom closet, hiding from the kids and the noise. My heart pounded as I waited for the phone to ring. What if he didn't understand?

What if he couldn't help me? What if there were no answers? I was prepared for that, but hopeful I would be met with a different outcome. From the beginning of the phone consultation, I could tell this was the start of something new.

Dr. Imber took the time to listen to all my symptoms together, not just a snippet here or there of what I'd been experiencing. He asked amazing questions about my balance—things no one else had ever considered, as far as I knew. I'd always used the term "dizzy", but he described it as a catchall. He asked me to explain my sensations without using the word dizzy. As I did, he listened, continuing to ask detailed questions. Before we wrapped up the phone consultation, I remember him asking me, "Is there anything else that you feel like you need to tell me that might be helpful in understanding your story?" That's where I got a chance to be completely honest with him…and myself.

I'd been experiencing some weird twitching and tingling in my legs for a few months. Since it was dismissed by so many other people, I talked myself into believing it was nothing. It didn't deserve attention. Before the phone consultation with Dr. Imber, I prayed that if I was supposed to share that piece with him, that God would provide a clear open door, and I'd feel comfortable sharing it. When he asked me that last question, I saw the open door and decided to walk through it. I told him about the weird feelings and sensations I'd been experiencing, but I wasn't met with invalidation. Instead, he said how important it was that he knew this piece of the puzzle. It made sense to him, fitting into the grand scheme of things he was seeing. In that one moment, I felt so seen and so validated.

I scheduled my first in-person appointment with him while we were on the phone. On February 17, 2020, my husband and I made the hour-long drive to his office for a two-hour appointment. It was filled with neurological tests, eye exams, sensory tests, balance, and walking. I did so many strange things in those two hours. I didn't understand how we were going make any progress, but since this was my only option, I (mostly) trusted the process. We followed up a few weeks later. He showed me a "brain map" and had marked the areas of my brain showing weakness. We immediately started neurotherapy to work on strengthening those areas. Neurotherapy is a drug-free treatment that uses real-time displays of brain activity to help improve brain function.

It felt like we were finally moving in the right direction. Even without an actual diagnosis, someone listened and took me seriously. I believe that finally having that also gave me the internal motivation to do what I needed to feel better. Despite COVID, I continued to see him weekly for neurotherapy, which made a huge difference in how I felt. But the biggest noticeable difference came as I implemented dietary changes.

At Dr. Imber's recommendation, I dove head-first into the Autoimmune Protocol (AIP) diet. This diet is not for the faint of heart. But, as a friend reminded me, "nothing tastes as good as feeling good feels." I found that to be absolutely true. I can't even begin to describe the changes I felt in my physical body within a matter of weeks. By removing the inflammatory foods and giving my body a chance to heal itself, I began functioning again. Slowly at first, but it was enough to help me keep going.

At the same time as implementing AIP, we ran the Cyrex food sensitivity test, which gave a clearer picture of the foods I was reacting to personally. Not only were we working with the eliminations of AIP, but also a list of other foods that were causing inflammation in my body. I genuinely think that by eliminating the foods on these two lists, my body finally got the break it so desperately needed. It got a chance to rest, repair, and reset from the damage the inflammation had caused for years.

Unlike a lot of stories, mine doesn't start the diagnosis process with magnetic resonance imaging (MRI). Because of COVID, it was difficult to get in for one. Dr. Imber felt confident we were dealing with multiple sclerosis (MS), based on history and symptoms. In June 2020, I finally received an MRI, confirming the diagnosis of multiple sclerosis. While patiently waiting felt difficult at the time, I'm actually thankful for the order in which things took place. I was able to work on healing with therapies, diet, and supplements before the diagnosis. When it finally came, I had some successes under my belt. I think that was a big part of why I chose to continue my journey on a holistic path. It was the only thing I'd done over the two-and-a-half-year journey that provided any help.

It's been nearly three years since my diagnosis. As cliché as it sounds, I can honestly say I'm not just surviving with MS—I'm thriving! But it hasn't been easy. While I've had great support from family, friends, and my doctor, it's not the same as hearing personal experiences from people who have chosen to walk the same path. I wish so badly there had been a resource like this available when I started this journey. It would have saved me countless hours, scouring Google and Instagram with the hashtag #thisisms for people with similar stories.

But that's just it: they're similar, not the same. I've heard it said that MS is the snowflake disease. No two people are alike. Just as frequency, severity, and location of symptoms vary from person to person, so do the many ways of treating and managing them. I love being on a journey of learning what works for my body and what doesn't. I'm excited to share them with you here.

If you've been around the MS world for any amount of time, especially on the holistic side of things, there's no doubt that you've heard of the huge impact that the right diet can have on symptoms. With my doctor's recommendation, I started with the Autoimmune Protocol. For the first several months, I did the elimination phase of the diet. It was tough! During this time, I paid close attention to how my body was feeling. I felt great. Symptoms were lessened, and I felt better than I had in a long time. I knew it was attributed to diet, but at the time, I didn't realize the full extent.

A few months into the diet, my husband brought me home a Strawberry Cheesecake Blizzard from Dairy Queen. Having not had treats in a while on the AIP elimination, I was so excited to enjoy it. I genuinely didn't think that a little bit of ice cream was going to impact me in a big way. I was so wrong! The next day, my dizziness and balance issues were back in full force. I remember being outside with my family on a spring day, sitting in a chair, curled up with a blanket because I didn't feel well enough to join in on the playing. At that point, I knew my dietary choices were going to be a big piece of the puzzle going forward.

Since then, I've stayed strict on AIP, working my way through the reintroductions. I've found things I can add back into my diet (eggs and nuts) and things that will likely always be a no-go for my body (nightshade vegetables). This varies widely from person to person but so worth the time, effort, and intention it takes to narrow down what makes you feel well. While it's easy to get caught up in what you're eliminating, I was given great advice early on to focus on what you're adding like nutrient density, more vegetables, and high quality ingredients instead.

Managing a strict diet like this long-term can be daunting. I imagine it's a pretty big reason that people don't start in the first place. It's not a good feeling when you're starving and open the fridge, only to realize there's nothing prepared for you to easily grab. Been there, done that. Having a meal prep plan saved my life in this area, quite literally. There are plenty of ways you can go about this, but I'll share what's worked for me personally. Maybe it'll be a jumping off point for you in figuring out your own plan.

As I'm writing this, I'm eating lunch made of my "cheater" meal prep. One of my favorite meal prep hacks is to not make meals at all. Instead, I prepare a protein while roasting a huge variety of vegetables for the week. Throughout the week, I combine them in different ways, depending on what sounds good, adding different spices or sauces for more flavor. For example, on a Sunday afternoon, I throw several chicken breasts in a crockpot, along with roasted brussels sprouts, broccoli, carrots, parsnips, sweet potatoes, and onion. That usually gets me through a week of lunches. Then, I include AIP dinners during the week, utilizing the "cook once, eat twice" rule.

Another thing that has made it easier for me to stick to AIP so well is having variety in my meals. While I do my "cheater" prep once a week, I also love including new recipes for dinner. This keeps it interesting and forces me to try new foods, varieties, and flavors. At the end of this chapter, I've listed some of my favorite AIP blogs and recipe websites. There are so many available! Hands down, my favorite AIP friendly blog is "Unbound Wellness" [unboundwellness.com]. I haven't found a single recipe there that wasn't wonderful.

All in all, I feel like adjusting my diet and being intentional about what foods I put in my body has made the single biggest difference for me. Removing inflammatory foods and replacing them with nutrient dense foods would be beneficial for anybody. But for someone with MS, I can say from personal experience, the benefits of an anti-inflammatory diet outweigh the difficulty of giving up familiarity and comfort. If you love to cook and bake like me, it's really a fun challenge to learn how to do things differently with new ingredients.

After implementing dietary changes, supplements came next on the list. I've said it before, and I'll say it again—there is no "one size fits all" approach. This rings true for supplements, as well. Over the years, I've tweaked and changed what I take to find the best fit. I think I've finally settled on a good routine that works well for my body.
My first step was to work on repairing my gut lining. There's so much research available that explains the connection between a leaky gut and the development of an autoimmune disease. At my doctor's direction, I tackled this right away with a few products by Apex Energetics Nutritional Complexes called RepairVite and ClearVite. Both are formulated to support immune and gastrointestinal health. I currently take one scoop a day of each blended into unsweetened coconut milk and drink it quickly. It's not my favorite, but if it's doing its job—it's worth it!

As we all know, inflammation plays a huge role in MS symptoms, so it's important to keep it under control. When I feel like my symptoms are beginning to flare up for any reason, I take two supplements that help calm down inflammation. The first is called Turmero, made from turmeric extract; the second is Resvero, both also from Apex Energetics Nutritional Complexes. Typically, I take 10 ml/day of each while symptoms persist. I also take two capsules of EnteroVite daily which delivers short-chain fatty acids and butyric acid to replenish what my body needs due to the elimination of grains and dairy products.

In addition to the Apex supplements, I take 4,000 IU of vitamin D and omega 3 with dha/epa daily. Currently, I'm taking Nordic Naturals ProOmega 650 EPA/450 DHA. When I get sick with cold or flu symptoms (or my double run-ins with COVID) my MS symptoms always flare up alongside. When that happens, I add 50 mg of zinc, 1000 mg of vitamin C, and 500 mg of lysine into the mix.

Admittedly, I've always been an old lady when it comes to sleep. I like to go to bed early to ensure lots of rest. When faced with the decision between going out for an evening activity or staying in and going to bed, it's always been an easy choice for me. With the exception of the years tending to little babies, I've always been able to prioritize sleep. When it came to making lifestyle changes after my diagnosis, this one wasn't as challenging for me. Even though it's easier, it's still something I have to make a conscious effort to keep as a priority.

Falling asleep isn't typically an issue for me (hello, four kids) but middle of the night wakeups are a completely different story (hello, MS bladder). I've found that when I use calming scents, I sleep better overall and have an easier time falling back to sleep in the middle of the night. A few scented things I like to incorporate into my bedtime routine when I have the chance (time doesn't always allow for all of them) are a bath bomb in a warm bath, lavender scented lotion, and my full skincare routine. I currently use organic natural skin care products from a company called Be Well [bewellcompany.com] and they're amazing! The founder, Natalie, was diagnosed with MS many years ago and changed her lifestyle to manage her symptoms. I love supporting their business and mission to bring clean skincare products to people.

Another thing that has really helped with falling back asleep is not checking my phone or watch for the time. When I do check the time, my mind starts to spiral with how much time is left to possibly fall asleep. The fear that I won't get any more sleep that night gets very loud, usually preventing me from falling back asleep. When I just roll over and take some deep breaths (and ask my husband to stop snoring) it's much easier for me to fall back asleep!

A physical therapist friend of mine once used the phrase "motion is lotion". I'd never heard it before, and I love it! I love the reminder that movement and motion is so soothing for our physical bodies. I'm a firm believer in the concept of "move it or lose it" for anyone, but even more so for those of us living with MS. I've seen the benefits of this in my own life, along with the drawbacks of not making movement a priority.

While I've never been much of an actual athlete, for the past ten years I've been very active. I love to hike, lift weights, bike, run, and swim. Leading up to my diagnosis, my fitness had to take a backseat to survival. I knew I had to figure out how to get back on track. Last year, when my ironman brother-in-law encouraged me to attempt a sprint triathlon, I figured it was worth a shot. I absolutely didn't feel ready, but I knew the challenge would keep me focused on making movement and fitness a priority. So, I did the unthinkable. And I loved it! I was so proud of what my body was able to accomplish in that race.

I've also had a front row seat to what happens when I allow movement to be pushed to the back burner which is different from listening to your body and resting when needed. Right after the triathlon, we decided to get a puppy for our family. I knew bringing her home would shake things up a bit, but I wasn't prepared for how scared I'd be to wake the sleeping puppy by sneaking into my basement gym! For several months after getting her, I just didn't. It was clear it was impacting me in more ways than one. I was exhausted, which seems counterintuitive, but all the research points to movement reducing fatigue. I didn't sleep nearly as well. The pain, tingling, and discomfort in my legs was noticeably more during this time.

I'm currently working toward running my first half marathon. It's terrifying, but I know it's helpful for me to have a goal to work toward. As I do this, one thing I've learned is that it's so crucial for me to listen to my body. I have pushed it too hard before, only to be met with a cranky body afterward, forced to spend the next day in bed recovering. If your body needs rest, then rest! Amid prioritizing movement, it's also important to pay attention to the cues that your body is giving you. The more you learn to listen to those little cues, the easier life will be, and the better off you'll be long-term when it comes to movement.

It's no secret that stress impacts MS symptoms. Ask anyone, and I have a feeling they'd agree that stressful situations are a prime opportunity for symptoms to flare. At the time of diagnosis, I had been dealing with several years of intense family stress. I have no doubt it played a role in my symptoms becoming full blown when they did. Stressful situations are an open door to increased inflammatory activity; something someone with an autoimmune disease should steer clear of.

I've never been one to regularly live at low levels of stress. In fact, I've always prided myself on how well I've handled stress over the years, typically by pushing through on my own, not accepting extra help, and not admitting there's a stressor in my life. I continued this pattern for a few years after my diagnosis. It worked for me, up until the moment it didn't anymore. I was exhausted, frazzled, and completely overwhelmed. I reached out to a friend who suggested counseling. I was in such a rough place that I was willing to give it a try.

In our first session, my counselor asked, "What made you decide to seek out counseling now?" I told him I realized I couldn't keep going like I was anymore. I finally admitted that the stressful lifestyle I was living wasn't serving me well, and I needed to make a change. I have been seeing my counselor now for nearly two years, and it has helped with my stress levels immensely. I have more strategies for coping with being overwhelmed, and I've learned to use my voice more in hard situations. I've tackled challenging things from other stages of my life that had been causing extra layers of stress. I recently, with a few extra nudges, joined group counseling. Having the extra safe space for my hard work has helped calm down my stress in huge ways.

In addition to counseling, having a strong faith in God has also really helped me keep my stress levels in check. This comes in many different forms: bible reading, books, attending church, worship music, prayer, and journaling. In times of stress, I can pick a few from this list and put them into practice. Different times call for different options, but I have a variety of tools available to me. Overall, knowing that I don't have to know the whole plan to trust the God who made the plan is a stress reliever in itself. Whether or not I always remember this part is a totally different story.

The final thing that is huge for my stress management personally is friendship—true, encouraging, connected friendship. For the most part, I don't share a lot of MS related things with my friends. The reality is that I have stress from all different areas of life, MS just happens to be one of them. Having a group of friends to be able to share and process with when the stress and feelings become too much is vital. They help me stay calm and rational amidst what could often spiral into extra stressful situations. Having support from people around me has been pivotal in helping to keep stress in check.

The final piece to managing my MS holistically and with lifestyle changes are my biweekly doctor's appointments with my functional neurologist. When I was sharing my story aloud in preparation for this chapter, it really struck me how fortunate I am to have this resource available to me. I know not everyone has access to a doctor who is one hundred percent in their corner. He not only supports my lifestyle choices but also has a wealth of knowledge to encourage changes that actually make a difference. On top of that, his experience with neurological disorders allows him to treat the root causes of my symptoms in very specific ways.

He explained it to me like this. Imagine MS like a city on fire. The initial goal is to put out the fire which is a metaphor for calming the immune system. This is done through prioritizing nutrition, supplements, stress management, etc. After the fire is out, he comes in with neuro rehab and therapy. Essentially, his job is to rebuild the buildings (or the parts of the brain) that are damaged from inflammation. For example, when I flare up, I tend to notice left-side symptoms like tingling and sensory issues. That's tied to the right parietal lobe. When I go to my appointments, we focus on exercises that stimulate that area of the brain to encourage healthy pathways.

As thankful as I am for his support, he once told me that neurotherapy is actually the third or fourth line of defense in managing my MS. He wholeheartedly agrees that diet, stress management, and supplements are huge in symptom management and should be the first steps on an autoimmune journey. Thankfully, I had his support and encouragement figuring those pieces out in the very beginning because it was extremely overwhelming deciding where to start.

Early on in my MS journey, as I was listening to podcasts to sort through all the available information, I remember hearing someone use the phrase "control the controllables". Over the past three years, I've made that my MS mantra. If I have learned anything about this disease, it's that it's unpredictable. A flare can come on without warning. Any new twinge, pain, or sensation sends my mind wandering to possibilities and worst case scenarios. There are so many things about my body that are outside of the realm of my control. But there are also so many areas where I get to maintain control. Focusing on those has made the journey, while still terrifying at times, more manageable.

To those newly diagnosed or (impatiently) awaiting a diagnosis, I would say be kind to yourself. Go slow in taking in information. It's overwhelming, even on a good day. Try not to jump straight to applying every bit of information you hear and read to your specific situation. The possibilities of how this disease will progress are endless. It's important to allow yourself to feel the fear, sadness, grief, and the rollercoaster of emotions as you walk into the unknown.

While you can count on the hard days to come, you can also count on being able to find joy in the midst of them, if you're willing. Contrary to most conventional doctors, I believe that not all people need medication to manage their MS symptoms. I absolutely believe that anyone, regardless of medication choices, can benefit from lifestyle changes. Only good can come from fueling, moving, and caring for your body in such practical ways. It's so possible to live a full, active, wonderful life after an MS diagnosis. Is it easy? Nope. Does it take extra focus and effort? Yep. But is it worth it? Absolutely!

Resources:
Diet
AIP Blogs- Just a few of my favorites!
> unboundwellness.com
> autoimmunewellness.com
> healyeatsreal.com
> healmedelicious.com
> gohealthywithbea.com
> thepaleomom.com

Supplements
Apex Energetics Nutritional Complexes: Repair-Vite, Clear-Vite, Enterovite, Turmero, Resvero

Vitamin D
Omega 3 with DHA/EPA
Zinc
Lysine
Vitamin C

Sleep
bewellcompany.com

Dr. Visits
Dr. Matthew Imber - Interactive Neurology
www.interactiveneurology.com (630) 637-8887

4

Story by
ANGIE GENSLER

Diagnosed in 2004
Lives in New York, United States
Instagram: @Angie_msstrength
"19 years on my chart, ZERO in my heart"- Angie G. 23'

As a mom, wife, and business owner, I have always prided myself on juggling my busy life. I lived on coffee, diet soda, and adrenaline.

I was diagnosed with multiple sclerosis (MS) in December 2004 on Christmas Eve. I had been suffering from blurred vision, pain, and numbness for a few months. Before my diagnosis, I had brain and spine magnetic resonance imaging (MRI) with contrast, did the typical neurological exams with evoked potential testing, and a neurological eye exam.

The doctors said: "Your brain lit up like a Christmas tree with lesions." I believe five were located in my brain, but my spine was clear. "You have multiple sclerosis. You should rest and prepare for a wheelchair." Followed by, "You need to begin a drug modifying therapy (DMT) immediately to prevent further progression."

Life, as I knew it, PAUSED.

That Christmas, I forced myself to put on a smile. It was our first Christmas in our new home. The children were excited. We had a surprise trip to Disney World planned, and I powered through like I always do. I honestly don't remember much of the trip because I lost a lot of memories due to my head trauma from a car accident in 2017.

My sister has had MS five years longer than me. My mom was broken by the news when her second daughter received the same diagnosis. She felt like a failure. It was awful. My brothers were shocked. Witnessing my sister already living with MS (struggling with dosing/side effects of her many DMTs) scared the crap out of me. As I looked at my two young daughters, I knew medications were not going to be an option for me.

Looking back now, I believe I have had MS since my early twenties. I experienced severe symptoms, and I now see the correlation with MS. I was a partner in a landscape construction company with my brother for a few years. During the hot summer months, I would experience severe vertigo, blurred vision, and numbness of my legs. One day on a job, I became temporarily paralyzed with severe shooting pains in my legs and was hospitalized. I was misdiagnosed with Lyme disease. They gave me high doses of antibiotics and eventually sent me home. I remember missing a few weeks of work.

There were also several weeks where I spent days just bedridden from exhaustion. Not the typical exhaustion, but one where my body was so heavy that it felt impossible to lift. During these years, I did not stop. I would blame my issues on heat exhaustion and overworking. I lived on caffeine and stress. I pushed my body to the limit most days with twelve-hour workdays and labor-intensive work. It wasn't until I was in my thirties and a mom of two beautiful young daughters that the diagnosis came. Our daughters were four and six years old at the time.

When we returned from Disney, the diagnosis started to sink in. I looked my husband in the eyes and said, "You can divorce me—you didn't sign up for this." He married a strong, vibrant, full-of-life woman. One who could manage every physical and mental challenge that she faced, but this was so unknown. In my younger years, I watched an uncle deteriorate with progressive MS and eventually die. Upon my diagnosis, the doctors marked my future with fear and debilitation. I gave my husband an out, and he wouldn't have it. He said he would support me in whatever I needed to do, and that he would be at my side.

I had been seeing a holistic chiropractor for many years prior to my MS diagnosis for regular spinal adjustment and care. She always took the time to ask about my overall health and wellbeing. Along with my adjustment, she would question me on my water intake, my nutrition, sleep, and stress, and she would apply different essential oils to improve my function. She was always there to provide me with professional advice on certain issues when I needed it. During the first visit to her office following my MS diagnosis, I shared the news and burst into tears. She looked at me and said, "Ang, you need to drop the artificial sweeteners", then printed out a list of anti-inflammatory foods I should eat, and what to avoid. She xeroxed a page from a book and handed it to me. The list of foods to AVOID was basically what I lived on daily.

This was the first positive advice from a doctor, post diagnosis. I quickly learned that the haphazard way I was living, without regard for my health, would no longer serve me well. I am forever thankful to Dr. Diane Zemba. I continue to see her monthly as part of my self-care regimen. She keeps my spine aligned, does atlas adjustments, and has helped me build my own essential oil collection to use daily. I still use the chlorophyll drops she recommended years ago to help with digestive health.

The first thirteen years, I quietly navigated my MS with alternative care and nutrition. This approach wasn't discussed or accepted back then. I made a drastic change to my nutrition, removing artificial sweeteners and quick-to-go food. Within weeks, symptoms began to quell. Over the years, I've dabbled in different therapies, nutrition, supplements, and exercise, but nothing sustained as I lacked true knowledge, consistency, and support. I would have times of good function, and times of struggle.

Our home was where the neighborhood kids gathered for pool parties, bonfires, snowmageddon sleepovers, disco parties—you name it. I strived to be the ultimate cheer mom, stay-at-home mom, and track and field mom, who traveled back-to-back weekends with my children. My husband was carrying the weight of working and unable to accompany me most of the time. I prided myself on being the class mom and involved in the Parent-Teacher Association (PTA). I was at every concert, event, party, and fundraiser. I needed to make every moment a memory for my daughters that their mom was present and capable, but then I would over-do it and become bedridden. I would drop my kids off at school and spend the day in bed. I prided myself on cooking dinner every night, packing healthy lunches, and having a perfect home, but my self-care would fall short, causing me to suffer with derailing issues. During those times, I suffered major setbacks, including mini optic neuritis flares, bowel dysfunction, MS "hugs", complete numbness of left leg/ foot, months of "bugs crawling on my body", and internal itching. I received different durations of steroid infusions, for different flares, which helped. I mainly leaned on my chiropractor, essential oils, acupuncturist, nutrition, and rest to get through.

The most profound MS relapse was my optic neuritis. It lasted months, and it was terrifying. My daughters were All Star Cheerleaders and competed nationally. I was that mom that drove to every competition, even the ones out of state. The optic neuritis attack came as we were in New Jersey. After a six-hour drive, my eyes were in pain and a touch blurry. I chalked it up to the long, stressful drive, and we settled into the hotel. One mom wrapped my head with toilet paper, creating a patch to calm the pain and stress. I laughed about it, and she helped my daughters with their hair and makeup. I took my place in the stands, alongside hundreds of other spectators, and waited for the competition to begin. As my daughter tumbled across the stage, I jumped up, screaming with pride, and my eyesight went black in my left eye. I was terrified, thinking I'd had a stroke. I couldn't balance due to the loss of sight and was disoriented. We made it through the crowd, and I saw the paramedics. They said it wasn't a stroke, but I should get to a hospital. Another mom drove my kids and me home in my car. Upon getting home, my husband drove me straight to the hospital where I spent ten days getting steroid infusions. With no improvement, I was devastated and broken, unable to fulfill my daily responsibilities with our children, home, and business. It was such an emotional blow. Thankfully, I had amazing friends that drove my kids to school, practice, and religion. They also helped me around the house and with cooking. I promised myself if I ever got my eyesight back, I would never miss a sunrise. God heard my prayers, and five months later, it returned to almost 20/20.

Through the years, "personal accountability" has been the motto to which I strive. I found when I had inconsistencies in my diet, symptoms flared. When stress arose, I'd have setbacks. When I lacked sleep, my cognitive function declined. If I didn't exercise, I'd be more fatigued. As a busy mom, I found my excuses crept in, and my self-care got derailed, time and time again.

For many years, I kept my diagnosis secret as I felt shame and fear that people wouldn't understand or feel sorry for me. There were a few people I did share my diagnosis with because they supported me during my times of struggle and helped with my family, but for the most part, it was very private.

Then, life took a major turn. As mentioned above, I was in a horrific car accident in February 2017. The head trauma I sustained mimicked multiple sclerosis. It was a year-long, painful recovery. My eyesight was affected as I was seeing orbs and suffering from crippling migraines. I had severe vertigo, memory loss, loss of coordination and balance, I had numbness of my left side, severe tingling of the hands, feet, and patches on my back. I was unable to drive because shadows cast on the road while the car moved would create strobe light visuals, making me throw up. I had to cover my eyes in moving vehicles. I had major panic attacks in cars and was crippled with fear. My life consisted of being driven to occupational therapy, physical therapy, neuropsychologist, neuro-ophthalmologist, chiropractor, acupuncturist, orthopedics, and neurologists. These endless appointments and therapies were part of my healing process and necessary in rebuilding my health. I will never forget a conversation I had with the acupuncturist.

I said, "My life is over—I will never be the same".

She responded with, "You are right, you will never be the same. This can be your restart. Start where you are and move forward with each day."

That hit my soul.

I spent weeks lying in a darkened room to quell my brain, with no television or computer usage. I missed weddings, funerals, celebrations, family time, and just everyday life. I gained forty pounds from depression due to inactivity.

Life was an unbearable PAUSE that I couldn't see past. I wanted my life to end… I didn't realize the Lexapro the doctors prescribed me after my accident began making me suicidal. One evening, I waved goodbye to my husband and children as they climbed in the truck and backed out the driveway, heading to dinner without me, once again. I sat on the porch of our beautiful home, sobbing uncontrollably, with bottles of pills in hand, watching the setting sun change the sky into brilliant colors. I was done. I faintly heard my cell phone ring, and in a brief moment of clarity, I answered. It was my mom. She immediately came over, and through that act, saved me. We called the doctor and stopped the medication. As spring began to show its renewal, I finally turned a page in my recovery.

March 2018 is the month my purpose and passion was ignited. After watching *Living Proof* by Mathew Embry, the story of his journey living with MS, I felt compelled to reach out to him and another gentleman in his movie, David Lyons. I quickly learned my inconsistencies, lack of knowledge, and lack of support kept me from my optimal health.

Support is KEY! I started to implement the Best Bet Diet and followed the MS Fitness Challenge free eight-week workout that was available at the time. I joined the Multiple Sclerosis Fitness Challenge (MSFC) Facebook support group.
https://www.facebook.com/groups/674667742732961

I scrolled through inspiration from the members at that time who were talking about their strengths and achievements. It was a positive, inspiring page with support and information to live your best life with MS. I joined a monthly challenge and began to post daily. As I began to share my diagnosis, support started to build. After about a year, I began to pivot from receiving support to giving support, and I saw my purpose begin to grow. David Lyons saw something in me and suggested I get certified to become an MSFC Coach. I was humbled and honored.

In 2019, I decided to go back to school and become a certified personal trainer (CPT), an additional certification in Multiple Sclerosis Fitness. I wanted to learn how to properly train the brain/muscle connection, and with proper training, develop neuroplasticity. This certification was important to me as I wanted to build my greatest function, overcome my brain trauma, and stay ahead of MS. With these certifications, I began coaching for OptimalBody Training Program, optimalbodyfitness.com, and became a trainer for MSFC Virtual Training Camp, hosted during COVID. This is the fitness I'm doing these days. It is an online program —the culmination of David Lyons training methods. I implement these training methods at home with my RBS4 system and when I train at the gym. The training methods are focused on challenging your muscles and brain connection. It's purposeful movement versus throwing weights and jumping around sweating. I love to balance it out with yoga and meditation.

I have been on several podcasts, sharing my story and mission of hope. I have grown passionate about fitness and planned on opening my own gym, focused on women. I was all set to start construction when I was derailed with other health issues unrelated to MS. I was suffering from severe abdominal pains. Through testing, I was informed that I needed to immediately schedule an open abdominal hysterectomy to remove abnormalities and precancerous uterine cells that were aggressively growing. Another PAUSE.

The surgery was a success, and with removal, all fears of cancer were suppressed. However, two days after surgery, I went into a postoperative crisis. I began internally bleeding, which required four blood transfusions on my forty-ninth birthday to survive. Another PAUSE with a long, grueling recovery ahead. I decided to make good with my down time and completed my Health Coach Certification.

Although my goal to open my gym has been delayed, I have moved toward a positive personal PAUSE. Pausing for me means taking time to truly focus on my health, fitness, and to connect with newly diagnosed MSers through social media, podcasts, and zoom calls. I'm very active with the MS Fitness Challenge support group and hope to continue to be that positive influence of change for others. Having this community is so powerful.

My last MRIs were two years ago, and they showed an improvement in my lesions. I saw my neurologist several months back, and she informed me she was leaving the traditional practice. When she said that I, Angie Gensler, had inspired her to incorporate holistic care along with traditional neurology, we literally hugged and cried! I'm waiting until she opens her new private practice, Integrative Neurology, Dr. Tal Mednick, MD, in summer 2023 to have my new evaluation and MRIs.

Over the past five years, my daily commitment to self-care has yielded me my greatest function in life. My daily routine includes sunrise walks to the beach for meditation and prayer, fitness/training, and supplements. The Best Bet Diet is the foundation of my nutrition, and I make sure to get seven-to-nine hours of sleep a night.
I have come up with an additional personal motto: "TODAY I CAN, SO I DO." I had it screened on shirts, hats, and recently got it tattooed on my arm as a reminder of my purpose. With all the pauses and setbacks through life, I don't ever want to waste a good day. On good days, I challenge my strength and look for ways to improve. On tough days, I rest, focusing on mindfulness and recovery. It's truly about finding balance between grit and grace within yourself.

In the early years, I was duped by dozens of supplement companies with promises of "healing", "improved brain function", "gut health", etc. I had a cabinet full of half-used bottles and expired promises. I found myself choking down fifty-to-sixty capsules a day at one point–it was awful.

Four years ago, I was introduced to Previnex, and I love their entire line of products, including their brain health, probiotic, omegas, joint health, and multivitamin. Their plant-based, vegan protein meal replacement shakes are a staple in my everyday health. I never realized how the quick-to-go whey protein shakes I drank daily were so inflammatory and kept me from my optimal health. I have had tremendous success with this brand and will never use another. They have an amazing giveback program. I encourage you to look at it.

I have been micro dosing CON-CRĒT® Creatine HCL daily for four years and have given away countless bottles to other MSers around the country. My sister has also been micro dosing for two years. It is amazing how important creatine is for brain health, mood, lean muscle, and recovery. Creatine is being more and more understood as not just important for muscle health, but also as one of the most important supplements you can take for overall health. All our cells crave it, and our diets often don't give us enough. And very importantly, all creatines are not created equal. Many absorb poorly in the body and are a waste, while others contain ingredients that aren't healthy. I have had several conversations with the Founder and President of the company about the profound health benefits we MSers are experiencing with supplements like his. His company is currently doing research on creatine's key role in brain health, and I hope there will be in-depth research specifically on the positive impact of creatine on the MS brain. I encourage you to look at it.

Regarding my diet, I always have organic turkey meat on hand. I love to sauté it with veggies and spices and put it in lettuce wraps or on roasted spaghetti squash. I avoid dairy, gluten, and sugar. If it's grown, I enjoy it. If it's packaged and has a shelf life, I avoid it. Alcohol is very rare. I love chlorophyll water. It's a wonderful digestive aid. I encourage you to try.

During the pandemic, social media became an incredible platform to connect with MSers worldwide. I truly feel blessed to be a positive influence of change within our MS community, and beyond. I never want anyone to carry the burden of this diagnosis alone like I did back in 2004.

Finding support from people like Mathew Embry at *MSHope.com* and David Lyons at MSFitnessChallenge.org has been life changing. I admire their mission of educating others on the profound impact that optimal nutrition, proper fitness, and faith have in overcoming multiple sclerosis. Personal accountability is my motto, faith is my foundation, and sharing my passion and knowledge with those newly diagnosed is my mission.

My greatest advice to a newly diagnosed person is to PAUSE. PAUSE, and do a full assessment of your daily life up to your diagnosis. Do a full, honest review of your nutrition, stress levels, previous illnesses, sleep patterns, environment, etc. Then, commit yourself to a "detox" of your previous life. Start implementing anti-inflammatory nutrition, stress reduction and sleep regulation, learn to properly train your body, and please don't expend all your energy trying to be that "ultimate" mom, father, spouse, business owner, or student; it will only derail you from building your life post-diagnosis. Pause and acknowledge your feelings, your shock, your fear, and then pivot towards people like me in the community–and in this book. Learn from our mistakes, borrow from our tools, be inspired by our resilience, and create your own path moving forward —a path of hope, discipline, resilience, and community. Don't focus on an end result but grow through the process, one day at a time.

We are truly stronger together.

GOD BLESS!
xo Angie Gensler

5

Story by
ELISA FERGUSON

Diagnosed in 2011
Currently 48 years old
Lives in Oxford, United Kingdom
Instagram: @elisaferguson_msnutrition
www.elisaferguson.co.uk

I was diagnosed with multiple sclerosis (MS) on May 9, 2011.

I remember calling my close friends to let them know. Some of them were speechless, others burst into tears, and one, whose birthday is on May 9, was worried that I'd always associate the day my life flipped upside down with her.

The prelude to my diagnosis was indistinct. My main symptoms were a little numbness in my left arm, and when I bent my head forward, there was a tightness in my neck like pulling on an old scar. Which, as I later found out, is exactly what it was. Other "episodes" seemed so banal—they weren't even worth considering. For example, I was wobbling a bit more than usual in advanced balancing yoga postures that were only discernible to me as a yoga teacher. My left leg also felt a little weaker after walking long distances. During the last mile of a ten-mile hike with my husband, my left leg became more tired and a little heavier than my right. I also vaguely remember my left eye going blurry as I was skiing down a mountain the year before, but that easily could have been caused by the cold weather.

I assumed I'd trapped a nerve in my neck. When physiotherapy didn't resolve the numbness, my friend, who is a doctor, advised me to ask for a referral to a neurologist to undergo magnetic resonance imaging (MRI). Maybe she knew. I certainly didn't, even when the neurologist advised that I come back to get the results of the scan with my husband.

On the morning of the appointment to review our results, I had this strange feeling that life was about to irreversibly change. Our four-year-old daughter had gone to school, and my mum was on her way to look after our one-year-old, while we went to the hospital. As I sat waiting with my daughter on my knee, I remember fixing my gaze on her big eyes, rocking her back and forth, firmly repeating that everything was going to be okay.

At the hospital, my husband and I were called into the consulting room, and the nurse who had come to meet us in the corridor, closed the door and sat behind us. I was oblivious, but my husband later said that he knew it was going to be bad news when she stayed. The neurologist opened the scans of my brain on his computer, and I remember seeing lots of white blobs everywhere that I thought were brain tumors. I vaguely remember his lips moving as he pointed to the screen, but the only words I heard were "99% sure" and "MS". I vividly remember my husband putting his head in his hands next to me.

I felt surreally calm and did my best to ask lots of intelligent questions without hearing any of the answers. I remember feeling ever so proud that the doctor praised me for the quality of my questions. Forever the people pleaser in the direst of circumstances. I left with a prescription for some steroids and a heavy feeling in the pit of my stomach when I thought about telling my mum the news when we returned home.

Nothing prepared me for this. It felt like someone had lobbed a hand grenade into my seemingly perfect life. I was married to a man who was the love of my life and best friend; we had two beautiful daughters together. I was a yoga teacher running a busy, successful yoga studio in a pretty village in Cheshire, spending more time with my mum since we moved from London, and my childhood friends lived a short walk away. Life was good...on the outside.

The truth is I was struggling. The aftermath of a stressful, soul-sucking career; the divorce of my parents; the death of my father; an ugly probate situation with his girlfriend of less than two years; the estrangement of half my family; a traumatic birth story, subsequently followed by post-natal depression. I was nursing an internal cocktail of self-loathing, insecurity, negative self-talk, and anxiety. By creating this illusion of perfectionism on the outside that was at complete odds with how I felt on the inside, I was living in a state of perpetual tension.

Following a lumbar puncture, which confirmed the MS diagnosis, and a second MRI scan to see if it was as active as he suspected (it wasn't), the neurologist was very negative about my prognosis. He said I would undoubtedly be in a wheelchair within a couple of years, and I needed to start potent, high-strength, high-risk disease modifying therapy (DMT) straight away to give myself a little more time before the inevitable happened. Quite uncharacteristically at the time, I said no (politely, of course) and that I wanted a couple of weeks to think before deciding. I don't know why I did this. Perhaps it was because my symptoms were quite mild, or the medication's long list of side effects (including cancer risk and brain infection) scared me more than MS, or because the way the neurologist spoke to me made me feel like a passive recipient rather than an active participant in my healthcare. I was already feeling uneasy in the hospital environment because it was the same place where I had been visiting my dad a few years earlier before he died. I'd also just had two overly medicalized births. The pressure to decide quickly made me feel stressed and out of control. It further compounded my decision when the neurologist called my husband a few days later to have a man-to-man talk with him about how important it was for me to start a high-strength DMT. He urged him to talk sense into me.

Two weeks turned into two months. While my husband was supportive, he was also very scared as I didn't have any firm evidence to show that the "wait-and-see" tactic was a good idea. I had no-one else in a similar situation to discuss it with. At the time, social media was non-existent, the online forums I read seemed overwhelmingly negative, and googling "MS prognosis" was terrifying. There were hardly any positive stories out there. I kept on returning to the question: Why? I was completely dumbfounded—there had to be a reason. I was probably one of the healthiest people in my family and social circle. Nobody knew of anyone in my family who had been diagnosed with MS. Why this? Why now? Why me?

I found some books on Amazon which, although didn't provide specific answers to my "why me" questions, turned out to be transformative and pivotal—providing me with a roadmap going forward. These were *Overcoming Multiple Sclerosis: The Evidence Based 7 Step Recovery Program* by George Jelinek; *The Wahls Protocol* by Dr Terry Wahls; *Minding my Mitochondria* by Dr Terry Wahls; and *Managing Multiple Sclerosis Naturally: A Self-Help Guide to Living with MS* by Judy Graham.

These books, although sometimes contradictory with each other in places, gave me some conviction that there were things I could do to help myself through diet and lifestyle. I thought I knew what healthy eating and living looked like as I had been a yoga teacher for five years at that point, but in truth, I was miles off.

Looking back, I now realize how overwhelmed I felt. The books provided a lifeline but without anyone or a community around me to talk with and make sense of them, it was just more information going into an already overloaded brain. For example, I quickly learned from my research that I needed to go gluten and dairy-free, so I bought the entire contents of the "free from" aisle in the supermarket every week. I begrudgingly made my way through the tasteless cereals, breads, and vegan cheeses, blissfully unaware that they were filled with sugar, sweeteners, inflammatory vegetable oils, artificial flavors, preservatives, fillers, and emulsifiers. Annoyingly, everyone else around me continued to eat delicious fluffy bread and "proper" cheese. I just didn't have the bandwidth at the time to learn more about the difference between being healthy and unhealthy while gluten and dairy-free. The whole area of what I should and shouldn't be eating felt like a minefield.

I would cycle in and out of reading through the books carefully. Afterwards, I put them back on the bookshelf, so the spines were facing inwards and out of sight. When I think about why I did this, I realize I was in denial. I could not and would not identify myself as having MS, and I didn't want my husband to either. I thought he would find me less attractive or damaged in some way. Because of this, I rarely talked about having MS and acted as though everything was normal on the outside.

Apart from being gluten and dairy-free at home (I didn't really check labels or worry too much if I was out of the house), nothing else really changed. Being a chronic people pleaser, I didn't want to cause problems or draw too much attention to myself. If family or friends had cooked for me, I felt it was rude not to eat it. I was embarrassed to be "that" person in restaurants. I also still drank the same amounts of alcohol as I did in my early twenties, satisfied my addiction to chocolate on a daily basis, placed little importance on sleep, and still used an array of chemically laden beauty products.

MS paranoia began to creep in. I became aware of aches, pains, numbness, and muscle tightness that I hadn't felt before. I started convincing myself it was the beginning of another relapse. The more stressed I became, the worse the symptoms got. Luckily, I'd been referred to an amazing neuro physio, who quickly dispelled my fears. The muscle tightness turned out to be just that; there was no weakness or spasticity in my body. She helped me see the connection between my thoughts and my physical experience. What you think literally becomes your reality. Being a yoga and meditation teacher, the impact of stress on my MS symptoms interested me the most as it was so familiar to me, but I didn't really do much at this stage to address it.

Two months turned into six, which turned into a year. I never went back to the neurologist. We moved to Oxfordshire, and I didn't reinstate myself with a new consultant. I saw it as a clean slate. Nobody knew I had MS in the village we moved to, and I lived the next few years without thinking about it too much.

I added more books to my "healthy eating and living" collection. Inspired, I started training to be a Nutritional Therapist in 2013. I completed a year of biochemistry before studying Nutritional Therapy for three years at the Institute for Optimum Nutrition in London. During this time, I learned about the different systems of the body and how they were all connected. Not only did I learn about the health and disease promoting properties of different foods and lifestyles, but I was also understanding the importance of personalized nutrition. There is no "one size fits all". We all have genetic predispositions, but our genes are not our destiny; in fact, it is our diet and lifestyle that determine how those genes are expressed.

During my studies, I started to become more discerning about the quality of food my family and I were eating. I began reading labels and ditched a lot of the gluten and dairy-free products I had previously bought and sought out healthier alternatives, or just did without if I couldn't find a good substitution. I cooked most of our food from scratch, made my own nut milk in a blender, signed up for a huge weekly organic vegetable box, and sought out grass-fed meat and wild fish. I also swapped my self-care and household products for more natural options to avoid the toxins and endocrine-disrupting chemicals found in the majority of beauty and cleaning products on the shelves.

Where I had previously felt overwhelmed, I started to see that healthy eating was actually very simple. By focusing on unprocessed whole foods, mainly vegetables, good quality proteins, and the right type of fats, I noticed how it was actually more about unlearning a lot of the marketing hype that we have been spoon-fed by the food industry. I started buying most of my produce from the first two aisles of the supermarket instead of the middle sections, and eventually found that ordering boxes from an independent local organic farm ensured better prices, in-season, sustainable produce, and quality of food that I could trust.

I was introduced to the concept of functional medicine, addressing the underlying causes of disease rather than just the symptoms. It was like a light had been turned on. At last, I had found an approach that really resonated with me, focusing on root cause medicine and promoting health rather than disease management. It was a framework in which to address the big burning question I had about my MS diagnosis—why?

I was learning about different body systems and pathways, and it felt like solving a jigsaw puzzle. Gathering important pieces made me excited. However, I was unable to find the right practitioner to work with. At the time, I couldn't find a nutritional therapist who worked within a functional medicine framework, that specialized in autoimmunity, never mind MS. So, I became my own practitioner, ordering and analyzing my own functional tests, speaking with experts at the labs, learning on the job, and making a few costly mistakes along the way. I wouldn't recommend it—I lacked an independent critical eye to look over my timeline and results, but I had no other options available. I was both the jigsaw puzzle and the person trying to solve it. As I now know, you ideally need to have a bit of distance and perspective to be able to see the whole picture.

I also discovered that while diet and supplements (where appropriate) are key areas of the jigsaw puzzle; equal weight needs to be given to other aspects of health, such as sleep, movement, mindset, connection (with self and others), and a big one for me that I was about to fully discover—stress management.

I think of my MS journey as a tale of two halves. The first half spans from 2011-2018. The second half is from 2018 onwards. This is when I learned that you could eat all the organic broccoli in the world, but if you are still living under chronic stress and negative thought patterns, you can't be in a healing state.

In 2018, my husband and I were going through a very intense period of financial stress, which was having a detrimental impact on both of us. To protect each other and our children, we were both suppressing our fear, putting a brave face on things, pretending everything was okay to the outside world. This, of course, was a well-worn path and very familiar territory to me. I began experiencing a slight decline in my gait; however, I was still practicing yoga daily, teaching yoga classes, running after my children, and eating fairly healthily. It wasn't until my daughter's teacher asked me if I had hurt my knee while I was walking across the playground that I noticed the weakness in my left leg was becoming visible to others. One day, I was out shopping for a birthday card. Without looking where I was going, I tripped over a paving stone. I still don't know whether it was inherent clumsiness, which I am well known for, or foot drop that caused me to trip, but I landed badly on my left knee. There was a sharp pain in my knee joint, and it was tender to touch. Rather than getting it checked out, I hobbled home in pain and had a few sleepless nights. I thought that would be it. Little did I know, it was the prelude to months of disrupted sleep, chronic neuropathic pain, muscle spasms, muscle spasticity, and a lot of distress.

The inflammation caused by the acute injury to my knee, a normal and important immune process, did not switch off, unfortunately. This physical stress, combined with the financial stressors of our day-to-day life, as well as my own personal stress rucksack that I carried on my back, created the perfect storm. There was no resolution to the inflammation; it became chronic and continued to escalate. In his book *The Survival Paradox*, Isaac Eliaz likens a healthy inflammatory response to turning on a single light to illuminate the need for repair. However, when the light is switched on and can't be switched off, it's like a circuit malfunction. More lights are switched on, eventually pushing the body into crisis mode. I started to experience painful muscle spasms in my left leg, relentless neuropathic pain, and a tightening of the muscles in my abdomen, hips, and thighs; walking became more and more difficult. I found myself in a whirlwind of self-perpetuating stress, inflammation, and pain.

Reading my journal from this time is a hard thing to do. There were some very dark moments where I felt I was in a downward spiral. I just wanted the pain to end, whatever that meant. It was a disorienting time when the days merged into nights; I didn't know what to do with myself. I would dread going to bed because I knew I had a night of waking up every thirty minutes or spending hours awake in the dark in excruciating pain. Sometimes I would wake my husband because it was so unbearable, but most times, I would sob silently into my pillow because he had to be up

71

early for work the next day. When the light broke in the morning, I would roll out of bed onto my hands and knees, puffy-faced, and rock back and forth on my yoga mat in an attempt to bring movement to my stiff body. I would splash my face with cold water and slowly make my way downstairs, one painful step at a time, to make a cheery-faced breakfast for my daughters before they went to school. I canceled all the plans I had made, didn't want to see anyone, didn't even want to speak to my closest friends because I simply didn't have the energy to call them. I had completely lost myself. I couldn't practice yoga, I was in too much pain to sit and meditate, and I couldn't stay still long enough to read. I had to keep moving, but I was utterly exhausted. I couldn't sit at my desk to work. I was no longer able to watch my girls play sports, go shopping with them, have fun in the garden, go out for dinner with my husband, or meet my friends for lunch. The pain was occupying all the spaces in my head where my identity and joy had previously resided.

Even though it's difficult to read now, journaling became an important process for me. By writing negative thoughts down, it helped me to offload things from my head onto paper, often multiple things, which overall helped lighten the load. Reading my scribbles now has enabled me to look back and see how far I have come, as well as what worked for me and what didn't. No matter how relentless or dark you are finding your days or nights, by journaling and looking back over the years, you realize that nothing remains the same. We are more resourceful than we ever give ourselves credit for. Patterns will start to emerge that will become our greatest guides. I recommend journaling to everyone with MS—especially during the dark times.

I booked an appointment with a doctor to get something to help with the pain. I tried gabapentin and baclofen (both made me feel nauseous), as well as tizanidine, which made me even more drowsy and disoriented. I tried clonazepam to help me sleep. For the first time in months, I slept for a few hours. It was really effective, and I started to sleep for longer periods each night. However, it is only meant to be taken short-term as it is a benzodiazepine, which increases risk for addiction. Plus, not only has long-term use been linked with cognitive decline, but sleep deficiency has also shown similar associations. Therefore, I found myself caught between a rock and a hard place, as sleeping provided immense comfort despite the potential risks involved. I decided to stay on it for a while longer.

The doctor also referred me to a new neurologist. This time when I went to see him, I didn't feel pressured to take immunosuppressant medication. He was a lot more relaxed during the appointments about what he thought were my next steps. We agreed that I should have an MRI to see if there had been any further activity since 2013. Unfortunately, the scan was inconclusive, probably because, after an hour of being in the cylinder, the muscles in my legs were spasming. The movement blurred the images. However, without the scan and just considering the progressive worsening of symptoms in my left leg, the neurologist re-diagnosed me with Primary Progressive MS (PPMS). He believed that the fall and subsequent inflammation had been a catalyst, catapulting me forward to a place where I probably would have been in my MS journey if I hadn't done so much work on my diet and lifestyle. I would need another MRI to qualify for Ocrevus—the only DMT suitable for PPMS.

This was hard to hear. In truth, it sent me into a depressed state for quite a while. However, as I replayed the conversation over and over again in my head, two things began to stand out. Firstly, the neurologist's acknowledgement that it was likely diet and lifestyle that had significantly slowed the progression of the disease. Secondly, if I did have PPMS, the potent medication that had been strongly recommended to me in 2013 after my diagnosis would not have made a lot of difference.

With the help of the clonazepam at night, I was able to cope better during the day. I started to double down on my efforts. I went back to my original resources and read *The Wahls Protocol®* cover to cover. I followed the elimination diet for 100 days to see if anything I was eating was adding to the inflammation. When I started to systematically add different foods back into my diet over time, I discovered that my symptoms worsened when I added most grains and legumes back in. I started following The Wahls Paleo Diet™ (level two): eating meat, liver, fish, eggs (I was fine with them), even more vegetables, berries, and soaked, activated nuts and seeds. Then, I tried The Wahls Paleo Plus Diet™, which is a ketogenic diet, focusing on a higher fat, lower carbohydrate macronutrient distribution to encourage more mitochondria production (the organelles which make energy in the cells). I switched between the paleo diet and the ketogenic diet to encourage metabolic flexibility (the ability to easily switch between fat and glucose metabolism). I also started going to bed earlier and invested in an Oura ring, so I could track my sleep and see what was disturbing it. Over the next six months, I was able to come off the clonazepam. My energy levels slowly began to improve. I was able to move more and started to practice some light yoga. As my brain fog also began to clear, I started researching the impact of stress on my health in more depth.

I conducted more tests. One that was pivotal was genetic testing with Lifecode GX. My training with them to become a Nutrigenomics Practitioner really helped me place quite a few of the jigsaw pieces around stress and its impact on me. Nutrigenomics looks at the role of nutrients in gene expression. The food you eat doesn't change the sequence of your DNA, but your diet and lifestyle can switch certain genes on or off, or change the way they are expressed, which plays a major role in health (and disease) outcomes. These genetic tests can pinpoint unique vulnerabilities and highlight areas that can benefit from additional diet and lifestyle support.

My own test results showed a lot of vulnerabilities in the nervous system report. They highlighted that I have a genetic susceptibility that makes cortisol, the stress hormone, upregulate inflammatory pathways more than necessary. This also creates "tryptophan steal", which means less tryptophan is available to produce serotonin and melatonin. The upshot of this is that high levels of cortisol, especially when produced over long periods of time, can be highly inflammatory for me. It can also have a detrimental impact on the quality of my mood and sleep. On top of this, I also found that I have a reduced ability to clear the stress hormones out of my body (via a slow COMT gene), which means that they circulate around my body for much longer, making the problem even worse. It began to dawn on me that the cascade of inflammation triggered by my fall did not subside, particularly due to my prolonged state of elevated cortisol. It highlighted just how important an anti-inflammatory diet and nutraceuticals were for me. Alongside all the anti-inflammatory foods I was eating more of on the Wahls Protocol ®, I further increased my dose of omega 3 (found in oily fish), curcumin (found in turmeric), ginger, and green tea. I also introduced cold water therapy and infra-red light to my daily practices, as well as limiting behaviors and avoiding people and situations that raised my cortisol levels as much as possible. By this point, it had been about eighteen months since my knee injury, but better late than never! I used to say that I wanted to be the practitioner I wish I had met when I was first diagnosed in 2013 and couldn't find anyone to support me. When I look back now, I want to be the practitioner I wish I had met in 2018! Hindsight is a wonderful thing.

I learned that while stress is not inherently bad (as we are equipped with a strong survival mechanism and have adapted as a species because of it), it is unrelenting chronic stress and the subsequent inflammation that is the driver for many of today's diseases, including MS, as it:

- Down regulates the immune system - when you are in a chronically stressed state, you are more susceptible to infections from opportunistic pathogens.
- Dysregulates blood sugar levels, which is a driver for inflammation.
- Has a negative impact on gut health - we can't digest or absorb nutrients from our food as effectively. It can lead to intestinal permeability or "leaky gut" and has a negative impact on the balance of our microbiome.
- Causes mitochondrial dysfunction - the inability of cells to produce energy effectively.
- Increases oxidative stress, which can cause damage to DNA and cell structure.
- Creates hormonal imbalance - the production of stress hormones is prioritized over sex hormones as a key survival mechanism.
- Creates nutritional deficiencies - the adrenal glands, which produce the stress hormones, adrenaline, and cortisol, use up a lot of B vitamins, vitamin C, magnesium, and zinc, draining resources from the rest of the body.

We are supposed to move with ease between the two arms of the autonomic nervous system: the sympathetic nervous system (SNS), known as "fight, flight, or freeze'", and the parasympathetic nervous system (PNS), known as "rest, digest, and restore". Yet in today's society, we are SNS dominant as we are inundated with constant pings from texts and emails, work deadlines, traffic jams, overexposure to blue light, alarming news stories, and social media 24/7, 365 days a year.

It is the PNS that holds the key to health. In this system, the body is shifted to a state of homeostasis. Our heart rate slows down, our breath is regulated, our digestion works effectively, and our hormones are in a state of balance. Our bodies are fully equipped with healing mechanisms while in the parasympathetic state to fight infections, clear damaged cells, improve cellular energy, repair and restore damaged tissue, and reduce inflammation.

When I shifted my perspective and conducted a "stress audit" of my life, I transitioned from asking "Why me?" to asking, "What is stressing me?" I saw that, even though I had done a lot of important and necessary work to reduce my physical stress through nutrition and functional medicine, my stress bucket was overflowing from psychological, spiritual, emotional, and perceived stress. The list below is what I run through now with my MS clients to see what is stressing them:

- Physical – injury, infections, sleep deprivation, blood sugar imbalance, gut microbiome imbalance, oxidative stress, nutrient deficiencies, environmental toxins, heavy metals, mold
- Psychological – relationship conflicts, financial strains, increased demands, loss of a loved one, exposure to traumatic incidents
- Spiritual – not connected to a higher purpose, not having a "big why", not having a supportive community or framework
- Emotional – not living in alignment with your values, not speaking your truth
- Perceived – mindset and positive/negative beliefs, ruminating over the past and worrying about the future

My upbringing hardwired my nervous system for a fight, flight, or freeze sympathetic dominant state. I was in a constant state of second guessing what the mood at home would be, so compliance and anxiety became second nature to me as I tried to make everyone happy. As a child, I remember feeling different from everyone else. I felt disconnected from myself and those around me and was desperate to be seen and heard, so I developed people-pleasing as a survival mechanism really young. As a young adult, not feeling like I fit in made me say yes when I meant no. I was hyper vigilant about what everyone else was doing, so I could know how to feel and act. I was a born introvert who, for most of my life, had been acting like an extravert to fit in and be liked.

Part of my life audit included reducing my alcohol intake considerably. This helped me to see how stressful and exhausting I found larger social groups. The fact that I used to do tequila shots to relax before I went into larger social situations probably should have been a clue! I also discovered that I really needed a lot of time alone regularly to re-energize. I'm an only child, so I don't know if this is nature or nurture, but I start to feel untethered if I'm around too many people for too long. Feelings of anxiety allowed me to reflect on whether it was the person or situation I was in that was wrong for me rather than thinking something was always wrong with me. Removing myself allowed me to define my acceptable boundaries. In doing so, I was able to start carving a life that is now bringing me much more joy.

Despite being a yoga teacher for quite a few years, when I did some honest self-reflection, I could see that I had been good at talking the talk —but not so good at walking the walk. When I initially practiced yoga, it was as a panacea to my stressful job in London. It gave me a strong, flexible body which I liked. Then, when I did my yoga teacher training, I was honestly more focused on producing perfect lesson plans and being the best yoga teacher rather than teaching from a place of practice and authenticity. When I opened a yoga studio and therapy center, yoga became more of a business for me—another source of stress. I think this caused quite a bit of internal tension. I was practicing from my head rather than my heart while teaching others to do the opposite. Consequently, I felt inauthentic and out of alignment with my own values.

When I had to stop my yoga practice after I fell, it felt like a large part of my identity had been taken away. I was devastated that I could no longer practice at the advanced level I had once been at. Eventually, when the pain and muscle stiffness eased a little, I was able to slowly introduce some yoga movements and a seated meditation practice. I was forced to practice as a beginner, learning what my body could and couldn't do. As infuriating as this was at the beginning, approaching my practice with a "beginner's mind" helped to deepen my mind-body connection; I felt a state of flow and ease that no amount of advanced yoga postures had ever given me before. This was a profound shift for me, and I started to rebuild my yoga and meditation practice with complete integrity and authenticity. My meditation practice became consistent because I wanted to keep returning to it rather than always feeling like I should do it because it was on my to-do list. The more I practiced, the calmer my nervous system became, and the more spacious my mind felt—settling back into a place of awareness and observation rather than anxiously jumping between every thought and emotion.

As well as building on my yoga and meditation practice, I intentionally found lots of other ways to signal to my brain that I was safe and relaxed in order to move into the parasympathetic state. These included:

- Waking up and going to bed earlier, so I could follow my morning meditation practice with journaling, writing, breathwork, or just sitting listening to the birds with a cup of tea. I kept my phone out of sight as allowing the outside world in straight away by checking our emails, reading the news, or social media is never a good idea for nervous system regulation. The book *Miracle Morning* by Hal Elrod really inspired me.
- Directly activating the main component of the PNS—the vagus nerve. This is a long nerve, reaching from the brain into the gut and is activated through deep diaphragmatic breathing, gargling, chanting, humming, and singing. I love yoga chanting, so I also started incorporating this into my day at the beginning and end of my yoga practice.
- Becoming much more aware of people and situations around me that provoked a fight-or-flight response for me, I would either avoid them

or, if I couldn't, then I would make sure I spent time afterwards calming my nervous system down.
- Spending more time in nature
- Doing more things that brought me joy, such as reading (I have listed my favorite inspirational books at the end of this chapter), cooking new recipes, and designing our garden. This meant a lot of enjoyable time spent observing the seasonal cycles of the garden, the wildlife, and birds in it, as well as searching for new plants in nurseries, planting them, and of course, weeding.
- Cryotherapy (cold water therapy)
- Infra-red light exposure
- Improving my circadian rhythm by morning light exposure, wearing blue light-blocking glasses, and using blue light-blocking light bulbs in the evening.
- Social connection – spending more time with a few close friends and less time in larger social settings. I also started to connect with others in the MS community and other practitioners involved in supporting people with MS.
- I began having appointments with a Clinical Psychologist, which has been tremendously helpful in processing a lot of my past experiences. We have been using Eye Movement Desensitization and Reprocessing (EMDR), which uses side-to-side eye movements, combined with talk therapy in a specific and structured format to process and help me recover from some of the traumatic experiences in my past.

The progression of my symptoms in 2018 forced me to strip away the inessential; rock bottom became the solid foundation on which I started to rebuild my life. I had been trying to fit into perfectly wrapped boxes my whole life. Trying to be the perfect daughter, the perfect friend, the perfect girlfriend, the perfect wife, the perfect mum, the perfect yoga teacher—I had completely lost any sense of who I was at my core. It was a wake-up call to face and embrace my MS diagnosis, and it forced me to stop, slow down, and look within. I had thrown myself into learning about nutrition and eating well but neglected some of the other fundamental pillars of health, such as prioritizing rest and stress management, as well as connection to myself and the wider community. I had been isolating myself from the MS community when I had needed to be around others who understood how I was feeling. In this way, MS has been a guide, showing me how to live a fuller, more purposeful life that is more in alignment with my values. I now see my MS diagnosis, not as a jigsaw puzzle to be solved, but as a lesson that has taught me that the way I was living my life before was completely misaligned.

My experience has also given me true empathy for others with MS who are suffering from their symptoms. Without those three years, I wouldn't have the same depth of understanding what it's like when symptoms progress. I struggled to feel authentic as a nutritional therapist specializing in MS because I hadn't really experienced any suffering, so how could I relate with anyone who had? When I faced true suffering, I felt inauthentic discussing health in the context of MS, as I was personally going through the challenges myself. It wasn't until I subsequently felt improvements in my health, contrary to everything that I had been told and read about what to expect with PPMS, that I felt I could truly help others. This is when I decided to complete the remaining modules with the Institute for Functional Medicine and become certified as a Wahls Protocol® Health Practitioner, so I could start making a difference in others' lives who were living with MS, too. I am also enrolled in a "Compassionate Inquiry" training with Dr. Gabor Maté and Sat Dharam Kaur, starting in September 2023. This psychotherapy approach will further support my clients by helping them safely uncover and release trauma and suppressed emotions, enabling them to access deeper healing and transformation.

So, where am I now? As I write this in 2023, five years after my "MS awakening", I have seen improvements in my physical and mental health. I feel more energized; I am sleeping well again; the pain, muscle spasms, and frequency of muscle spasticity have vastly reduced; my brain fog has completely vanished; and my moods are much better. I am also feeling more at ease in myself and more aligned to my purpose—what brings me joy. I am aware of the boundaries I have set up. However, I still have minor balance issues, and some of the nerve pathways in my left leg are disrupted or dysfunctional. This means that I am not able to bend my left knee fully or kick my heel back completely, which has an impact on the quality of my walking. This is where my journey with electrical stimulation (E-Stim) began.

In April, my husband and I traveled to Austin, Texas, so I could attend an "MS Bootcamp" at the Neufit headquarters to try their Neubie device. This is the same technology that Dr. Wahls has used to help restore her health, alongside functional medicine. It uses direct current, working at the level of the nervous system, to accelerate rehabilitation, restore function, and increase mobility by using neuromuscular re-education (neuroplasticity). We were so impressed with the Neubie that we made the investment and brought the device back for me to use at home, alongside a personalized training program. It's still early, but if you want to follow my progress on Instagram, you can find me at www.instagram.com/elisaferguson_msnutrition.

As I write this chapter, I have two teenage daughters who I am aware have been watching me face this adversity over the last few years. From my own experience, I know how important it is to give them the space to speak their truth and feel their feelings, for them to live in alignment with who they are, and to find joy in what they do. They have been the main driver for me to keep going, to keep getting back up when I have felt utterly defeated, and to be a role model to show them how to cope when life sometimes gives you lemons. So far, my MS story has been a tale of two halves, yet I feel there is a lot more to come. I feel positive about it. Maybe it's going to be a tale of three thirds or four quarters? After telling my daughter when she was one year old that everything was going to be okay, I now know that it is.

Some of my favorite inspirational books:

- *Cured* by Jeff Redriger
- *The Biology of Belief* by Bruce Lipton
- *The Survival Paradox* by Isaac Eliaz
- *Spontaneous Healing* by Andrew Weil
- *Mind over Medicine* by Dr Lissa Rankin
- *Why Zebras Don't Get Ulcers* by Robert M. Sapolsky
- *Atomic Habits* by James Clear
- *The Miracle Morning* by Hal Elrod
- *When the Body Says No* by Dr. Gabor Maté
- *The Myth of Normal* by Dr. Gabor Maté
- *Molecules of Emotion* by Candace Pert
- *Radical Acceptance* by Tara Brach
- *A New Earth: Awakening to Your Life's Purpose* by Eckhart Tolle
- *The Diamond Heart: Book One* by A. H. Almaas
- *The Presence Process* by Michael Brown
- *The Body Keeps the Score* by Bessel Van Der Kolk
- *Waking the Tiger* by Peter Levine
- *The Drama of the Gifted Child* by Alice Miller
- *My Grandmother's Hand* by Resmaa Menakem

6

Story by
KELLY GEORGE

Diagnosed in 2015
Currently 40 years old
Lives in Winchester, United Kingdom
Instagram: @thekellygeorge
Youtube: @kellygeorgetv

During May of 2015, while on a family holiday in Texas and Las Vegas, the feeling in my left cheek began slipping away. As the holiday continued, the loss of feeling traveled up toward my eye. Fortunately, my vision was not affected. The facial numbness and its effects were invisible to the naked eye. By the end of the trip, I had zero feeling in the left side of my face. Talking was a struggle, as I couldn't feel the muscles pulling my regular facial expressions during conversations. We returned home: I knew something was seriously wrong. My words turned into slurs as they left my mouth. I walked into an accident and emergency (A & E) department, hoping to be seen. Due to my appearance being visibly healthy and tan from my recent holiday, they insisted I was fine and sent me home, giving zero consideration to the loss of feeling consuming my face.

My concern grew as the lack of feeling climbed higher with each passing day. I worried it would eventually affect my vision. Unsatisfied with the first round of results, I rushed myself to a different hospital, miles away from the last. This time, I was pushing for testing, despite their opinion on my outward appearance. By this point, my speech was so heavily affected by the slurring, I was becoming inaudible. After three days in the hospital and numerous tests later, we finally convinced them to perform a magnetic resonance imaging (MRI) on my brain. The results came immediately. They told me "white matter" had been found in my brain, but refused to share anymore information without a neurologist present. It was four in the afternoon when they asked me to stay *another* night as the neurologist couldn't see me until the following day. They relocated me to the "brain tumor" ward. Thoughts raced through my mind. What did they find —a tumor? What was happening to me? How serious was this? As you can imagine, sleep did not come easily.

At noon the following day, a neurologist and his students came to my bedside. They made me wait in the brain tumor ward without answers until after lunch. He opened his mouth and dropped the bomb. "Miss, I'm afraid you have something we call multiple sclerosis (MS)." He didn't say anything about a brain tumor or tell me how many weeks I had left to live. Relief quickly washed over me. I didn't know anything about multiple sclerosis, so I asked question after question—verbal diarrhea.

"What does this really mean? I can live with this and not die?"

"Yes, it's a condition you live with," he answered. He continued offering up information. I'll be honest: I heard none of it. I could have kissed him on the spot! Imminent death was not in my future. I could live with this, whatever it was. That is all I cared about. My one-year-old daughter wasn't going to lose her mummy! I was over the moon.

The following days brought regular morning headaches. They administered a course of steroids specifically for the face. In the United Kingdom, you are appointed a multiple sclerosis nurse, along with a neurologist. The nurse is the main point of contact. She informed me she was able to do home visits in case my mobility became affected in the future.

And so begins the endless onslaught of MS information. From lesions to scans, relapse to flare-ups, relapse-remitting to progressive—this was a world I knew nothing about. I didn't know anyone afflicted with this complicated disease who could offer me advice either. I guessed I would be wheelchair bound by the age of fifty. A huge misconception, but the only bit of knowledge I'd gathered.

The large amounts of information uploaded into my brain in quite a small span of time left me emotionally drained. Bear in mind, I began the month of May on holiday with a fully functioning face. By the end, I'd lost feeling and function, leading to a heavy diagnosis. This massive event unfolded in only three weeks. I was left with an assigned MS nurse (whom I was extremely grateful for) to answer all my questions and to help me "carry on" after receiving my diagnosis. I felt confused.

How can I "carry on"? Is this a ticking time bomb? Will I die young? When I finish the steroids, will I suffer another relapse? Do I have to take daily meds for the rest of my life? Can I have more children? I want another child! Will they inherit my condition? Do I need to change my diet?

The questions were endless, plaguing me day and night. I began writing them down, readying myself for the nurse's next visit. I also had my husband to consider. He, too, had burning questions, conducting his own endless research to find answers.

The next factor to consider was how to tell my nearest and dearest that I've been diagnosed with a serious health condition I'll carry around like baggage for the rest of my life. I'd be bombarded with questions I simply didn't have the answers to. This was depressing, to say the least. I kept the news to myself for quite some time. I did tell my closest family and friends but had to end it there. I didn't have the brain capacity or emotional strength to continually repeat myself, answering the same questions over and over: how I knew, how I got diagnosed, what to do next.... Retelling the story depressed me further, which I could not afford.

The type of multiple sclerosis I was diagnosed with is called relapsing-remitting. This means I am prone to relapses. But, with a quick fix of steroids, my symptoms will die down and subside after a few months. This did happen in my case. A win I gladly took! The steroids slowly brought feeling back to my face, and the headaches diminished. Luckily, my speech returned to its normal state.

I was slowly regaining physical freedom, yet I was also struggling with these feelings of guilt. I am an only child, and what if my illness causes my mum to an early grave? Or worse—me! She was questioning herself, too. She worried she had done something to cause this while she was pregnant. "Why doesn't she have MS, but I do?" This thought ran daily circles on a hamster wheel in her mind. Seeing her so distraught ate me alive. Not to mention the guilt I felt for my husband and daughter. Unknowingly, he married and had a child with a woman he would probably outlive. Taking care of our daughter would fall on his shoulders in the case I became heavily disabled in later years. The dream of one day retiring in the sun while our carefree daughter went to college or traveled the world was becoming just that—a dream. The nightmare of him having to take care of me instead encroached on my sun-soaked fantasy. He deserved an "opt-out" clause in this marriage. In sickness and in health never felt so real as it did right now at the age of thirty-two.

In reflection, keeping my MS hidden for months was a mistake. Now, I'm an open book. I'm happy to bore anyone with my story. It feels like therapy, honestly. It's no longer a dirty secret everyone feels awkward addressing. If it means I can laugh, cry, or even help others, I am more than happy to overshare.

After many chats with my MS nurse over the following six months, it became apparent how important vitamin D is to a body living with this condition. She informed me that some of her other patients use sunbeds to deal with the deficiency. Others choose relocation to more vitamin D-friendly climates. At this time, I was offered multiple sclerosis medication to slow down the possible recurrent relapses. Neither sunbeds nor medication were appropriate for me as we wanted another baby. A healthy pregnancy and MS preventative treatment do not go hand in hand. Thankfully, I became pregnant with my second child, giving birth in August of 2016. A turmoil of emotions befell this pregnancy as we made the decision to move abroad once the baby was born. My husband expanded his research to include how multiple sclerosis could possibly affect children if one of their parents is afflicted. He discovered that exposing toddlers to all-body, high levels of vitamin D could dramatically lower their chances of developing MS as they grew. This was enough for us to take the scary plunge!

Three months after the birth of my second child, we packed up and jet set to sunny California. We settled our three-year-old, three-month-old, and our business in North County San Diego. We completely relocated there after being granted a work visa called an E2, lasting five years. I wrestled with fear for the future but was forced to trust the process. Over time, I realized stress is my trigger. Symptoms began flaring whilst preparing for the move. It was loads of stress selling our cars and belongings, all while setting up a life, a business, and a home across the ocean in a foreign place where everybody was a stranger. The stress triggered balance issues, dizziness, and numbness around my hands and feet. Once

I boarded the plane, I felt the worst bit was behind me. Most of our belongings had been sold or rehomed. The packing was complete. The teary family and friend goodbye's were done, and the dog was on our flight. Little did I know what was coming...

Stress of the life move led me to my worst relapse to date. After a month in sunny San Diego, I spent a week in the hospital away from my husband and babies. They administered a round of intravenous steroids for an attack on the left side of my face. This time, it was visible. My face appeared opposite of a stroke as the corner of my mouth was lifted up into a permanent smirk. This led to further treatment with steroids after being discharged from the hospital, followed by months of home visits from a nurse. A California neurologist urged me to consider a real treatment called Lemtrada. Lemtrada functions by killing bad white blood cells in the body, then regrowing healthy cells that won't attack themselves the way mine currently do. So, my Lemtrada journey begins. It's a two-year course. Year one consists of a five-day infusion process. During year two, whatever good cells grow back, they kill again to really ensure your body is growing healthy cells. This is a three-day infusion.

The five-day infusions during year one were tough. I was stuck in the hospital, linked-up to a drip, feeding my body Lemtrada. They also include a cocktail of other drugs to counterbalance any reactions one may have. It is not an easy ride. During those five days, I experienced headaches, heavy fatigue, and lumpy hives. I was also medically advised to follow a Lemtrada diet, similar to the guidelines of what you can and can't eat during pregnancy. For several months following the five-day infusion, I was forced to wear a mask. This was long before the COVID era where masks were accepted. I was given strict instructions to keep away from public places like swimming pools, crowded areas, and cafes/ restaurants. I was rebuilding my immune system, and I couldn't risk catching a common cold during recovery. A cold would no longer be "common" for me. It could cause serious damage.

The side effects of Lemtrada can be worrisome, requiring consistent monitoring. Precancerous cells, thyroid issues, and kidney problems can occur. To keep an eye out for these detrimental side effects, I gave monthly urine samples and blood tests for five years, beginning the first month of my Lemtrada journey. To ensure the Lemtrada was doing its job by stopping the progression of MS and to check that no new activity or lesions had grown, yearly MRIs were also scheduled. I found much needed comfort in the monthly testing. It felt like I was actually being cared for when my neurologist checked my blood work every month. It was a nice, new feeling.

I am now one year post the five-year window of monitoring, following my Lemtrada journey. I am no longer required to give monthly blood or urine samples. And, I'm thrilled to report I am medicine-free! I don't intend on taking any more medication. I can't say "never" because it depends on how bad the next relapse will be when/if it comes and what treatments are offered at the time.

Vitamin D is the only thing I take daily, and my body is thanking me. I feel great. I also exercise regularly to keep my body healthy and moving. I just completed another yearly MRI to check all is going well in this little old brain of mine. Yes, I occasionally experience odd flaring symptoms like balance issues or pins and needles in my foot, but they pass. I know stress is my main trigger. Getting a common illness like a tummy bug or a cold causes my body stress, bringing on MS symptoms. But, as I said before, nothing lasts longer than a few days.

I realized, from countless hours of research, how healthy eating and a balanced diet could aid the Lemtrada in helping my brain. During my diagnosis and flare ups, I researched food I could eat that fell under the anti-inflammatory category. I knew inflammatory foods could be the cause of the dizziness, numbness, and fatigue I was experiencing. After the start of my Lemtrada journey, I went gluten-free. And—WOW! This made an instant difference in my brain fog. I could now hold a conversation in a restaurant with a friend while reading the menu simultaneously. A task I simply could not complete before. It wasn't until the fog lifted that I realized how bad it had actually been living with it for all those years. Cutting gluten was the best food choice I made for my brain. I also reduced my dairy. I haven't seen an instant change the way I did with cutting gluten, but from my reading, I've determined it's best for me to reduce or cut it out completely.

I'm so happy with my Lemtrada journey. I do believe that having a positive mental attitude, along with supporting the medication by educating myself in nutritional health and general wellbeing is what led me to where I am today. I don't wake up everyday in fear that I have MS. Far from it! Instead, I wake up thinking, "I feel good today, so I'm going to work out!" I ride the good days so well, appreciating them to their fullest. When the odd bad day comes along, I know it won't last with the help of my daily diet. Well, it's not really a diet—it's a way of life. I see food as medicine. I know the power of a walnut and the benefits it brings to my brain. A handful of leafy greens a day keeps my neuro away.

I love going to restaurants but being gluten-free presents its own challenges, especially when eating out. These days, I find there are more and more options for gluten-free than when I first started. My favorite app that I use is called "Find Me Gluten Free". It shows restaurants where it's safe to dine, being gluten and/or dairy-free. I always check beforehand to make sure the menu has a great selection - —not just salad. Pre-planning is essential if you're eating gluten-free.

Finding food to eat on-the-go is hard, too. A banana and some nuts are always a strong, go-to option. Meal prep is a game changer when it comes to combating the food struggle. When I'm hungry and tired, it helps immensely to have premade food to choose from. I often turn to Instagram for gluten-free recipes.

I cook most evenings, especially having two young children to feed. I make sure we are always eating from multiple food groups. For example, we typically have meat/fish as our protein, potatoes or pasta, and a portion of fruits and vegetables. However, in our home we do "Fun Friday" where the children get pizza. Sometimes, we get takeaway.

During my nutritional research, I stumbled across Dr. Terry Wahls, a medical professional who herself was diagnosed with MS. After trying several MS treatments without success, she decided to take a close look into her diet and the impact of food. This was her game changer. She's very accessible on Instagram and other social platforms, giving daily updates. She is a huge inspiration for me. The power of food as medicine is quite the discovery.

My daily routine begins with exercise every morning. This includes the gym for dance classes and running, plus walking my dogs. I can't squeeze in time to meditate, so twenty minutes a day of being outside in the quiet with only my dogs is enough meditation for me. I'm very aware how important it is to keep my body moving. Some days, I have the strength to do weight training and cardio. I often do intermittent fasting in the morning, which means exercise first, followed by a late breakfast of either a homemade smoothie or gluten-free porridge with berries. I tend to drink one smoothie a day. Typically, I make them from scratch, but I'm also fond of ready-made smoothies if I'm rushing out the door. My favorite smoothie I make is pina colada flavored. It has pineapple, mango, spinach, coconut water, and banana. Frozen fruit is the best because it's icy cold. Adding chia seeds and a little fresh passion fruit on top gives it a nice crunch. I'm a strong believer that food is fuel for the body. Figuring out the correct fuel allows my body to function at its best.

A good night's sleep is important for everyone, especially if you have a chronic illness. Luckily, I've never had an issue sleeping. My top tip is a candle-lit, lavender salt bath before bed. A hug-in- mug works wonders, too. I have yet to try "golden milk", consisting of a warm milk of choice, turmeric, ginger, and cinnamon. I'm told it's the best. Any "sleepy" tea does the job for me.

My career is in the media. Sometimes, I fear my foggy brain will get in the way. I worry I'll have trouble holding down a job in front of the camera, receiving information through an earpiece, and talking all at the same time. I used to dream of taking the physical therapy or dance teacher route, but I've learned to be realistic with myself when it comes to my limits. On heavy fatigue days, there's no way I'd be able to show up to teach a class of gym enthusiasts. On a more positive note, I refuse to let MS define me or stop me. I am still working in the media, taking it day by day, giving everything my best. Today, my best is enough. My plan for the future consists of staying busy and career-driven, while being the most present, active parent I can be. Multiple sclerosis opened the door to a new career path I never would have considered prior to my diagnosis. I'm currently studying to become a nutritionist. The power of food is so remarkable. I'll be thrilled to help other chronic illness warriors on their journeys in reducing inflammation and flare-ups through food, once I become a qualified nutritionist.

Having an actual diagnosis is a blessing and a relief. From here, you can move forward, working to see which route is best for you and your MS. I found that having a diagnosis helped me to research and understand my condition more fully. I have a regular doctor, but I hardly need to see her. The only specialist I see is the MS support team that checks in with me every six months, along with my neurologist I'm currently seeing once a year. I also fully appreciate the multiple sclerosis community I've found online through Instagram. It's so inspiring seeing people live with their conditions, day in and day out, holding down their jobs, being full- time parents, and everything else in between. Multiple sclerosis does not define me. It makes me more thankful and appreciative for the good days I'm blessed with. I live for those days and no longer take anything for granted. I've become one badass warrior for my children to look up to!

7

Story by
BOB CAFARO

Diagnosed in 1999
Currently 64 years old
Lives in Haddon Township, New Jersey, United States
Email: BobCafaroLLC@gmail.com
www.bobcararo.com

Since my teen years, I have been in fairly good health, despite having allergies and asthma as a child. I discovered yoga while still in high school, and since then, I have exercised just about every day and lived on a relatively healthy diet. I have been a cellist with the Philadelphia Orchestra since 1985.

In December of 1998, I experienced symptoms of numbness and a limp in my right leg. Both my family doctor and my orthopedic surgeon surmised it was nothing but a pinched nerve—nothing to worry about. It cleared up on its own after a few weeks. But in February of 1999, I experienced optic neuritis in my left eye. My peripheral vision was affected as areas of sight were disappearing from view. I saw my first neurologist, and he ordered magnetic resonance imaging (MRI) of my brain. Despite there being no brain lesions, he diagnosed me with multiple sclerosis (MS). He immediately sent me to an esteemed neuro-ophthalmologist at Wills Eye Hospital in Philadelphia, who started me on three days of 1,000 mg of intravenous methylprednisolone per day. The symptoms subsided for several months, but I suffered slight permanent damage to my left optic nerve. The loss of some peripheral vision and brilliance of color has been with me ever since.

One can understand that I was in a state of denial about my diagnosis, so in April of 1999, I was able to get a second opinion from one of the most esteemed MS specialists in the country. Initially, he had some doubts about my diagnosis, so he sent me to a rheumatologist for extensive testing. All tests for rheumatoid disease came back negative, so the neurologist ordered an MRI of my spinal cord. Lo and behold, three small lesions showed up. He no longer had any doubt about a diagnosis of multiple sclerosis, and he started me on weekly intramuscular injections of Avonex. The side effects from this drug were so brutal that medication was necessary to counter the side effects.

The big self-administered intramuscular injection of Avonex was done before bedtime, and two ibuprofen tablets were taken along with it. The next day began with two more ibuprofen tablets, and for the remainder that day, I always had a case of the flu so badly that my hair hurt. The headaches were excruciating, along with the temporary inflammation of my optic nerves. I stopped taking it after four and a half years, and I was glad to get off the drug. To this day, I wonder how a drug that made me so sick could have possibly helped my body heal. During the next few months, I was on a mission to prove to myself that I had been misdiagnosed.

In July of 1999, I was doing thirty-mile bike rides in the mountains of upstate New York during an intense heat wave. This was a questionable activity for someone in perfect health, but for someone diagnosed with MS, it was downright idiotic. As a result of this strenuous activity, I began experiencing optic neuritis in my right eye, which was particularly scary because the peripheral vision and color loss in my left eye had never returned. I immediately headed home to South Jersey and began my second three-day treatment of 1,000 mg per day of intravenous methylprednisolone. This dose is the equivalent of 62.5 twenty mg prednisone tablets daily. This course of steroids stabilized things for about one week, then I came down with what I thought was a stomach virus. I began vomiting and was unable to keep down any food or water. This continued for the better part of one week. Against my own wishes, I was luckily taken to the hospital for severe dehydration. I remained in the hospital and on intravenous fluids for four days, until I was given anti-motion sickness medication which stabilized my situation. The neurologist at the hospital recommended I eat something, and I will never forget the first food they brought in after ten days of not eating. It was a greasy cheeseburger and french fries! Needless to say, I passed, and a visitor brought me some organic tofu with brown rice and steamed vegetables.

After being discharged from the hospital, I saw my fifth neurologist, this time at the University of Pennsylvania Hospital. Up to this point, I had been neurologist-hopping, desperately seeking an elusive misdiagnosis. Now, there was no question about a definitive diagnosis of MS. I was barely able to move my hands as the ability to play the cello had been completely taken away. The optic neuritis in both eyes was so bad that I could not read and only saw silhouettes of people. As if that was not enough, I was incontinent and had no physical strength. My body felt like it was receiving a constant dose of electrical current, and my hearing was affected as I was constantly hearing helicopters chopping the air. I was extremely weak and lacking stamina, as walking half a block was as exhausting as running a marathon. I had been in good shape prior to all of this. But now, I was unable to even bench press a forty-five-pound Olympic weight bar with no weights attached.

My latest neurologist at the University of Pennsylvania saw just how dire my situation was, and he ordered a complete set of brain and spinal MRIs with the contrast gadolinium. The results of these MRIs were absolutely shocking. My brain had over fifty active lesions spread out at every level, and my spinal cord had one lesion that measured three and a half cm in length. It encompassed the entire width of the spinal cord. This explained the impaired use of my hands and loss of physical body strength. I did not see the 1999 MRI results until 2013 when I was writing my book. I went back to UPenn after the fourteen-year hiatus, and luckily, they still had them on record. In 1999, my neurologist only explained the severity of the lesions to me and discussed the radiologist's report, but actually seeing the frightening images for myself after so much time had passed was shocking. Here is a slideshow of some of those images: https://www.youtube.com/watch?v=ATjBXvaR7Vo

My neurologist proceeded to put me on ten days of 1,000 mg of intravenous methylprednisolone per day. This was followed by six weeks of tapered oral prednisone, starting with 100 mg per day, gradually reducing to 10 mg per day. This may seem like a radical dose of steroids, but I have to give my neurologist credit for making the right call. To this day, I believe his decision was the right one which stopped the attack in its tracks.

At this point, I went back to my neuro-ophthalmologist at Wills Eye Hospital, who had been monitoring my lack of progress for the previous six months. He proceeded to give me a basic vision test, and I was unable to see even the largest letters on the vision chart. He then administered a visual field test where I was given a thumb clicker to indicate each time a flash was seen in the periphery. During the test, I sat motionless without one thumb click as nothing could be seen in the periphery with either eye. He then halted the test, saying he would write me a note for permanent disability. That was the moment that changed everything for me. I suddenly went into survival mode, and I flatly refused to give up my life. There was a way out of this, and I was determined to find it and regain my life. From that moment, I gained a new mindset, and I would now devote all my time and energy to finding answers that medicine and neurology had overlooked.

Researching multiple sclerosis in 1999 with dial-up internet was a slow and arduous process. My vision was seriously impaired from the optic neuritis, and it was hard to read even with enlarged fonts on a twenty-one-inch computer screen. At that time, helpful books on the subject were few and far between. Dr. Terry Wahls would be diagnosed with MS one year later (in 2000), and her book *The Wahls Protocol* wasn't published until 2014. The one helpful book I found was *The MS Diet Book* by Dr. Roy Swank. I followed some of his dietary recommendations but with modifications.

With my computer screen set to a giant font, I embarked on extensive research to find out everything I could about MS. Until now, I had been passive, unquestionably following the advice of neurologists. The internet did prove to be invaluable, and the first helpful thing I found was Water Cure (*www.thewatercure.com*). It was written by an Iranian doctor who performed an uncontrolled study on Iranian prisoners, which was having them drink half their body weight in pounds multiplied by ounces of water daily. (Example: I weigh 160 pounds, and the recommended intake is 80 ounces daily.) After I started drinking so much water, I was not getting hit with the dreaded fourth MS attack, but I actually noticed my first signs of gradual improvement as my strength was slowly returning.

The next part of my research entailed rates of multiple sclerosis worldwide, which I was able to access on the internet, along with published clinical trials on drugs for the disease. It was interesting to see that the very poorest nations had rates of MS that were about one-third of wealthy industrialized nations. Japan caught my eye because of their extremely low rates of MS, despite high levels of pollution and severe overcrowding. I focused on their diet, which is very different from the Standard American Diet (SAD). The typical Japanese diet consists of far smaller quantities, much less processed food, and a far lower intake of sugar, fat, and salt. While looking into this further, I stumbled upon the Okinawa Centenarian Study. This study entailed an extensive analysis of the diets of more than nine hundred people in Okinawa who were over the age of one hundred, and in perfect health. It is interesting to note that the women in the study had never been screened for breast, ovarian, or cervical cancers. Diseases that are commonplace in the West were almost unknown in this study. I saw this as my winning lottery ticket, and I adopted their lifestyle by telling the waiter, "I'll have what they're having!" It should be noted that they live on a low-calorie, organic, plant-based diet. If they do eat meat (chicken or fish), it's the size of a deck of cards and no more. On average, 67% of their diet is organic Japanese sweet potatoes, and most importantly, they stop eating when they are 80% full. This is quite different from our "all you can eat" lifestyle in America. I modeled my diet after the OCS about two months after my prognosis of permanent disability (about nine months after my first diagnosis). In retrospect, I wish I had made dietary changes sooner, but prior to this, I was busily immersed in a state of denial. I stopped consuming anything that did not belong in my body. This included alcohol, junk food, processed foods, GMO foods, and anything with preservatives or food coloring. I was so serious about this that I did not eat out in a restaurant for close to two years. Even when traveling, I prepared all of my own food to ensure I knew what I was eating.

The next step was devoted to regaining the full function of my body and hands. Determined to rebuild my body, I got serious about practicing yoga, and I followed *The Complete Book of Yoga* by Swami Vishundevenanda. My son was recruited to pitch in Little League Baseball, so to help him I found *Nolan Ryan's Pitcher's Bible*. I was somewhat familiar with Nolan Ryan, the famous fastballer who delayed the aging process of his body for twenty-five years. Having changed my diet to the Okinawa Centenarian Study diet, it was now time to change my exercise regimen to that of Nolan Ryan. With his book as a guide, I added weight training to my daily yoga regimen. After a short time, I was able to bench press a forty-five-pound Olympic bar, and as my strength returned, I incrementally added five pounds at a time.

After discovering I was still able to balance on two wheels of a bicycle, I began extensive cycling outdoors to regain my sense of balance, as well as stamina. Although it seemed like a painfully slow process, there was gradual improvement. After several months, even my vision was improving, along with the use of my hands. I had to relearn how to play the cello from ground zero. To push myself, I even started taking principal cello auditions at other major orchestras around the country. I was practicing several hours a day and gradually regaining my lost ability to play the cello.

While rebuilding my body, I was singularly focused on the mission of getting my life back in its entirety. It was a fight for my survival, and I was not going to lose. Nando Parrado was one of my guides during this fight, as was Lance Armstrong (what we knew of him back in 1999). There were several other people who achieved impossible results, despite the overwhelming odds against them: Roger Bannister, who was the first person to run a sub-4-minute mile; Bobby Fischer, who beat the Soviet Union for the chess world championship; and Jascha Heifetz, who played the violin at an untouchable level for sixty years! To Fischer, chess was a game of life or death—the same way I viewed my health. Two more invaluable books I used as guides were: *A Practical Approach to Strength Training* by Matt Brzycki; *My 60 Memorable Games* by Bobby Fischer.

After the better part of one year on Avonex, I happened to read the package insert, detailing the clinical trial results of the drug. After two years, the success rates of the drug group and the placebo group were nearly identical. This shocking discovery spurred me to research the placebo effect and learn it as a skill. I was given a copy of *You the Healer: The World Famous Silva Method on How to Heal Yourself and Others* by Jose Silva and Robert B. Stone. This book was incredibly helpful as it pointed me in the right direction to train my brain to make physical changes to my body. I designed my own meditation method, specifically tailored to beating MS. It was a fairly simple approach. I started this practice by sitting quietly for five-minute increments while repeating healing commands over and over daily.

Examples of the healing commands are:
My optic nerves are regenerating.
My brain is finding new pathways to the muscles in my hands.
The use of my hands is returning completely.
MS is going into remission and leaving my body.

These five-minute sessions gradually increased to two thirty-minute sessions each day. The cells of the body are constantly dying and being replaced with new and healthy cells; in seven years, all cells in the human body are replaced with new ones (the bones being the slowest to regenerate). My theory was that by training my brain, I would have a say in how those cells are replaced by healthy cells. It took about three and a half years to rebuild my body to the point where it was prior to multiple sclerosis. Not only had I succeeded, but at the age of forty-three, I was in better physical condition than I was at the age of twenty. It should be mentioned that during this extended rebuilding period, I did not go to a doctor for eleven years. Even though I was strong and in excellent shape, a bit of denial existed. I was still telling people I had been misdiagnosed.

Things changed in 2013 when I met Nando Parrado, the remarkable individual who survived the 1972 winter plane crash high in the Andes mountains of South America for seventy-two days. Nando should have never survived the ordeal and most people would have perished. When the plane crashed, he was thrown from row-nine into the bulkhead, and his skull was fractured in four places. Thinking he was dead, the survivors placed his body in the cold with those who had perished. Three days later, Nando awoke from his coma. Seventy-two days after the crash, he showed up in the foothills of the mountains to find help. This man had never seen snow, he had no survival training, no equipment, and no food. He traveled 37.5 miles on foot in one of the most difficult mountain ranges in the world during winter. Nando proved to be an inspirational guide when I was faced with the end of my life. I highly recommend reading two books about Nando's profoundly inspiring story: *Alive: The Story of the Andes Survivors* by Piers Paul Read, and *Miracle in the Andes* by Nando Parrado and Vince Rause.

After meeting him, I went back to my neurologist at the University of Pennsylvania after an eleven-year hiatus. Once again, he ordered a complete set of MRIs of my brain and spinal cord. Miraculously, there were no lesions to be seen. Aside from some permanent nerve damage, there were no traces of the disease. Here is a slide show of those images fourteen years later: https://www.youtube.com/shorts/eSIIiuUAkX0

After self-publishing my book in 2015, *When the Music Stopped: My Battle and Victory against MS*, I was invited to present at a book signing. The featured speaker at this event was the esteemed neuro-ophthalmologist, Dr. Robert Sergott, the Director of Neuro-Ophthalmology at Wills Eye Hospital in Philadelphia. Dr. Sergott is the one who gave me the prognosis of permanent disability. At his speech, he said he had never seen anyone come back from such an advanced case of MS. His speech was fascinating because he spoke of how I had changed my immune system.

Firstly, Dr. Sergott mentioned how switching to an organic, plant-based diet changed the microbiome in my gut. The more I thought about it, the more it made sense. The Standard American Diet (SAD) contains foods and chemicals that are destructive to the microbiome. Consider how alcohol reacts with the microbiome. Within the human gastrointestinal microbiota, exists a complex ecosystem of approximately 300 to 500 bacterial species, comprising nearly two million genes (the microbiome).

Secondly, he addressed my extensive outdoor cycling. I cycled everywhere possible with the sole purpose of rebuilding my body and stamina. When one is cycling, the brain and body are multitasking. The cardiovascular system and muscles are getting a great workout, while the reflexes are hard at work, avoiding everything from potholes to inattentive drivers. Dr. Sergott looked one step further and said I was getting high levels of vitamin D from the sun. He continued by discussing the link between low levels of vitamin D and high levels of MS. He said this was the second way I had changed my immune system. After the book signing, I reflected on what he said. I began to realize there were two other ways I'd changed my immune system.

The third way has to do with exposing my body to cold temperatures. Heat is widely considered an enemy to those with multiple sclerosis as it can trigger an attack. My three previous MS attacks grew in intensity, and I was deathly afraid of a fourth one. As a precaution, I began taking cold showers everyday—even during the winter. I also cycled outdoors in cold weather with minimal protective clothing. My theory was I could still exercise my cardiovascular system without overheating my body. At the time I was unaware, but this was one more way I changed my immune system. The human body was designed to adapt to different climates and temperatures, yet our modern lifestyle has everything at one comfortable temperature. I believe our current state of complacency puts our immune systems to sleep. I am convinced that exposure to cold works to reawaken it.

The fourth way I changed my immune system was by intermittent fasting. When one eats food, the body produces insulin, which changes the glucose to energy, so the body can use it for fuel. What is not used is stored in the fat cells to be used later. The human body was designed to acclimate to different temperatures, but it was also designed to go without food for days at a time. This is where the stored energy is utilized. The problem with today's lifestyle of abundance and comfort is we no longer eat when we are hungry, but we eat because it is time to eat. Not only do we eat because of a schedule, but we consume more calories than our bodies are able to use. When this happens, free radicals (or unstable molecules) are released into the body. In addition, over-consumption of calories combined with the Standard American Diet, leads to high levels of fat, salt, and sugar, creating a seedbed for chronic illness.

When I discovered the Water Cure and noticed my first signs of improvement, I began drinking two quarts of water every morning before doing anything else. As a result, there was no room in my stomach for food. I was unknowingly intermittently fasting for about sixteen hours each day. When the body reaches sixteen hours without food, ketosis is achieved. Ketosis is a metabolic state that occurs when the body burns fat for energy instead of glucose. The keto diet has many benefits. These include potential weight loss, increased energy, and aiding in treating chronic illness. Ketosis also gives the cells of the body an opportunity to heal and rebuild.

The only supplement (or medication) I take is 5,000 I.U. of vitamin D3 daily, which I have been taking for the past three years. I do so because my wife Teresa is a clinical researcher, and she previously worked for Novo Nordisk (the stock you should have bought!) After her position was outsourced to India, she took a position with the Chung Institute of Integrative Medicine. Teresa ran an extensive and detailed vitamin D3 study for Cooper Hospital workers in South Jersey as protection against COVID-19 and other respiratory infections. The study showed a 75% rate of protection against hospitalization for the virus. I piggybacked the study because of what Dr. Robert Sergott once said about low levels of vitamin D and high levels of MS. I got COVID-19 in January of 2022, but I was completely recovered within three and a half days.

Even though I have been completely asymptomatic for twenty-four years, I still live a disciplined lifestyle. My daily routine begins with at least one liter of filtered water. Our house is equipped with a three-stage Granular Activated Charcoal whole house water filter, plus a five-stage Reverse Osmosis filter in the kitchen. While drinking my first liter of water, I begin my daily exercise regimen which can be viewed on YouTube: https://youtu.be/lTofLP9MN0A

My idea of eating out is usually sushi. I'm okay with this because Japan has such low rates of MS. I normally eat organic foods, but only after fasting for sixteen hours each day. My recipes are easy: if you have to read a label of ingredients, move on to something where you don't. Organic Japanese Sweet potatoes are one of the best superfoods, the easiest to make, and they comprise about half of my diet. I get them from my local organic farmer. He custom plants several hundred pounds for me every year. I bake them at 350 degrees until they soften, and after cooling, they are vacuum-sealed and frozen for the winter. Keep in mind they averaged 67% of the diet in the Okinawa Centenarian Study.

My typical diet consists of organic raw nuts and seeds, fresh fruits, and vegetables. Instead of pasta (which I love), I choose zucchini spirals. They are much healthier. I prefer quinoa instead of grains because it is a seed, and it has protein.

My wife Teresa makes a killer quinoa salad. It is one of my favorites:

Quinoa Salad
1 green squash - finely chopped
1 red pepper - finely chopped
4 scallions - chopped
1-2 carrots - I use food processor
1-2 stalks celery - finely chopped
3/4 cup parsley - chopped
(all veggies organic)
3/4 cup organic raisins - depends on how sweet you want it.
3/4 cup organic pine nuts (toasted on stove top)
3/4 cup organic balsamic vinegar
3/4 organic olive oil
2-3 cups organic quinoa - 1 part quinoa to 1.25 parts water. Any more water makes it too mushy. Allow it to cool.

Chop all ingredients. Toast pine nuts on the stove (in a frying pan is fine —no oil needed) until they are a nice golden brown (or darker) color. Constantly stir or wrist-flip the pine nuts while toasting. Mix all ingredients with the quinoa except for the balsamic vinegar, olive oil, pine nuts and raisins.

Whisk the olive oil and vinegar together, so it is homogeneous. You may need to adjust amounts to your liking. Drizzle over mix and stir immediately to evenly cover ingredients.
Stir in raisins and pine nuts.

All of the above ingredients are estimates. I eyeball the quantities. I used to use the food processor for most ingredients but found it was too mushy. Hand-chopped results produce a crispy crunch of flavor.

Lemon Dressing
1 ½ teaspoons white wine vinegar
2 tablespoons lemon juice

5 tablespoons extra virgin olive oil
½ tsp finely grated zest
1 garlic clove
salt/pepper
Mix all but garlic. Smash garlic, and place in mix for about ten minutes. Remove garlic.
You can make this with or without garlic, or you can replace the garlic with finely chopped shallots. Sometimes, if the dressing is too tart, I tone it down with a little agave syrup to taste.

I haven't actively connected with the multiple sclerosis community other than with individuals who have reached out to me, along with the people I've gotten to know from presenting twice at the Wahls Protocol Seminar in Cedar Rapids, Iowa. I must admit to having shied away from organizations that are funded by the pharmaceutical industry.

I have been totally asymptomatic since 1999, and yes, it is tempting to go back to an unhealthy diet. Vietnam veterans have a saying: "When I die, I'm going to Heaven, because I've already been to Hell." I've never served our country, but in some ways, I feel I've been to Hell, and I'm not going back. Out of fear, I continue a diet completely void of meat, chicken, junk food, processed food, alcohol, and anything else that does not belong in the body. I still practice yoga every morning, and lift weights with Nolan Ryan as my personal trainer! There is no one-size-fits-all answer to health issues. But one thing is for certain, a healthy lifestyle will benefit everyone, regardless of their physical state. We live in a society where many people blindly accept a toxic lifestyle. Canceling one's membership to this toxic lifestyle is a move that represents the holy grail of good health.

8

Story by

NASSIRA

Diagnosed in 2018
Currently 48 years old
Lives in Canada
Instagram: @my_natural_ms_lifestyle

My journey began in 2018. I was forty years old, and from what I thought, in good health. While we were on vacation, I started feeling a tingle on my lips, a symptom I had never felt before. A few days later, I noticed that the left side of my face was going numb. This was also something I had never experienced. When I returned from vacation, I decided to go to the emergency room (ER) to make sure everything was okay. At the hospital, they completed blood work, checking to see if I'd had a stroke. I hadn't. The ER doctor submitted a requisition for magnetic resonance imaging (MRI), so they could get a better understanding of what was going on.

I was anxious while awaiting my MRI appointment. My face was still numb, and it wasn't improving. Several weeks later, I had the MRI, and my results were sent to my family doctor. I remember going to the appointment by myself, thinking the conversation was going to be easy. There would be a simple explanation. I was wrong. My family doctor advised that based on the MRI results, I more than likely had multiple sclerosis (MS). He needed to refer me to a neurologist to be sure.

I was in disbelief when he spoke those words. Dazed and confused, I went home to share the news with my husband. It was a big shock to both of us. I knew nothing about MS and didn't know anyone that had it. I didn't really believe the news and held onto hope that it wasn't true. We decided we would take it one day at a time, not jumping to any definite conclusions until meeting with a neurologist.

My doctor advised that the wait for a neurologist in our smaller city outside of Toronto was very long. I was told if I could find a neurologist who would see me sooner, my family doctor would send a referral. Luckily, I found a one who could see me within three weeks. It's important to be proactive and ask what options you have. This is a great example of where being proactive allowed me to see a neurologist much sooner than if I had waited on the system instead of taking action myself.

My first appointment with the neurologist consisted of more tests and another MRI, this time including my spine. I was anxious to go back to see him for the results. Unfortunately, it was the news we didn't want to hear. There was a small lesion on the top of my spine, accompanied by several lesions in my brain. It was official—I was diagnosed with multiple sclerosis. He wanted to refer me to the MS clinic in Toronto. You never think you are going to be diagnosed with a chronic illness. When it happens, it takes some time to sink in. When I was first diagnosed, I shared the news with my immediate family. It wasn't something I was ready to share with everyone. I didn't want people to look at me as a sick person because I didn't view myself as being sick. I immediately went into a warrior-like mindset—MS was not going to get the best of me! I would do everything in my power to support my physical and mental health. What drives me to continue with my positive mindset? My family. They are my world, and I refuse to let MS take my future away.

While waiting to see my neurologist at the MS clinic, I began researching MS and the different ways people managed their symptoms. This included disease-modifying therapies (DMT) and the natural approach by managing through food and lifestyle. The first thing I found was the Swank diet, a diet proposed by Roy Swank that is low in saturated fats. I could feel hope returning. This wasn't going to be the end of my story; this was going to be a new beginning where I chose a DMT or a different path.

I had to wait some time before being assigned a neurologist at the MS clinic. While waiting for my appointment, I had another flare. The right side of my body was going numb. I didn't lose any bodily movement; it was just numb to the touch. My concern grew as I anxiously waited for my appointment at the MS clinic. My first visit consisted of a lengthy conversation regarding my symptoms, the unknown aspects of the disease, and the diagnosis that I have Relapse-Remitting Multiple Sclerosis (RRMS). The recommendation was clear. I should go on DMT as soon as possible to lower my risk of a future relapse, especially since I'd experienced two flares back-to-back. This was a lot of information to digest. While I was scared, I knew I wasn't ready to make any decisions. I shared with the neurologist that I'd researched managing MS via food and lifestyle. He wasn't upset with this information. Rather, he suggested that there weren't enough studies to confirm that this approach worked. He did not share any further information on the topic. I left the hospital confused but knowing I had to continue my research into the disease and how others managed it with a natural approach. I will premise that I have always been open to a holistic approach when it comes to my health. I knew this route was something I wanted to consider if it was a viable option. The neurologist respected that I'd received a lot of information. He told me to consider everything we discussed, and to contact the nurse if I decided to take medication. I was happy he didn't tell me he would stop seeing me if I chose the natural approach. However, he did stress that he highly recommended going on a DMT.

After being diagnosed, it's very important to let the news sink in and process all the options that have been presented to you. You will more than likely find that your neurologist may not suggest the approach of managing your MS by lifestyle, but it is a choice—one that should be considered along with the DMT options.

The symptoms on the right side of my body began to fade as I dedicated time to my research. This is where I found Dr. Terry Wahls (author of *The Wahls Protocol*) and Mathew Embry (creator of *MSHope.com*). Mathew Embry also created the documentary *Living Proof*. This was a game-changer for me. While the documentary carried many hard truths, it validated that managing MS in alternative ways was possible. I found hope in the idea that alternative options to DMT would work for me, too. Please remember that there are excellent MS medications that have helped improve people's lives. I am not against them, but I knew I wanted to try alternative self-care before I said yes to a DMT. My decision to try the natural route first felt right for me.

Listen to your gut. If you know that you want to try the natural route, believe in your decision. There is plenty of research showing that managing your MS through lifestyle changes reduces symptoms and can help prevent relapses.

It was a big decision, but I knew that I had no choice except to go all in. If I was choosing the natural route, it wasn't something I could go in and out of. I had to consider it my form of medication. I also needed my family's support. I shared with my husband and girls the reasons why I decided to try the holistic approach first. My family understood the reasons behind my choice and fully supported my decision. I did stress to them that if at any point we felt it would be a better decision for me to try a DMT, then I would. This helped ease their concern. I started sharing the news with close family friends, but I have never felt the need to tell everyone I know. Now, I choose when and with whom I share it with.

One of the ways I decided to hold myself accountable to my new lifestyle was by creating an Instagram page dedicated to multiple sclerosis. The page holds me accountable to my lifestyle change while allowing me to follow other MS warriors who live a similar lifestyle to mine. This was the best decision I ever made. Having a support system filled with like-minded people helps me immensely.

My Instagram account is *@my_natural_ms_lifestyle*. This account has allowed me to share my healthy food ideas while serving as a platform for sharing positivity regarding the natural MS lifestyle. It is so important to surround yourself with other like-minded people who will empower you in the choices you make.

I began changing my lifestyle, which included going gluten and dairy free, while increasing my daily vegetable intake. I have always practiced living with a positive mindset. I knew a positive mindset would be vital in managing my health. Along with food, your mindset is one of the most important remedies you can give yourself. The mind is capable of remarkable things. Like fueling your body with the right food, it's just as important to fuel your mind with the right thoughts. Never doubt the power of your mind. It will support your health while giving you strength you never knew you had.

Since changing my diet five years ago, I feel great (most of the time). Over the past several years, there have been very few moments where I doubted my decision to choose the natural MS lifestyle. I've made a choice that not only supports my multiple sclerosis, but supports my overall health, as well. What better gift can you give to yourself?

The next step in my lifestyle change was addressing what supplements my body was lacking. Most MS patients have a vitamin D deficiency. In fact, many people do. Vitamin D is crucial for optimal health. When I was first diagnosed, my vitamin D level was extremely low. I went to see a naturopath to discuss this, as well as the other supplements I should be taking. The doctor made recommendations on supplements that would help with inflammation and optimize my health. Some of the multivitamins I take include:

- Vitamin D - 5,000 IU (this can be increased to 10,000 IU in the winter)
- Vitamin K
- Zinc
- B-100
- Fish oil
- Lion's Maine
- Turmeric (something I have taken off and on)

I do my best to take my vitamins daily. There are some days it doesn't happen, but I take them 95% of the time. It's not about being perfect, but it is imperative to follow your best practices at least 90-95% of the time. There is very little wiggle room when dealing with your health. It's also important to conduct research on the brand of supplements you take and the source. One of my favorite brands is Plant Vital. I do my best to stay away from generic brands. I also recommend taking individual supplements rather than a multivitamin, claiming to have everything you need all-in-one. When fighting a chronic illness, it's crucial that your body receives the nutrients it needs from each individual supplement. Five years later, my vitamin D level is finally at a satisfactory level. When my other blood work was evaluated, the doctor was happy with all my levels.

If you can, try seeing a naturopath, even if only for one appointment. Through different modalities, a naturopath can advise what supplements you should be taking. The ones I have shared are very common supplements that people with MS take. If it isn't within your budget to visit a naturopath, the internet is a great resource where you can find tons of useful information.

Over the past five years, I have taken the time to get to know my body. One thing I try not to do is attach everything to multiple sclerosis. One example are the headaches I suffer from. I've always experienced them, and I believe that they are connected to my hormones—not MS. I'm proactive in managing my headaches with different natural approaches before jumping to medication. I purchased an ice cap that helps relieve my headaches. I've found a peppermint roller helps, too.

Trying natural remedies first helps me not to attach every ailment with MS.

Instead of thinking MS is the route to all our bodily issues, try looking at it as a separate entity. This also ensures that we aren't empowering our MS with negative thoughts. Instead, we are considering that we are human, and everyone experiences non-serious medical issues.

I am extremely fortunate that within the five years of managing my MS naturally, I've had only one flare-up. I believe this was triggered by stress, bringing me to another very important piece of the puzzle. I know the damage stress can have on the body. As soon as I was diagnosed, I knew I had to be proactive in reducing my stress levels. I made the decision to share the news with my work. At the time, I was commuting five days a week, driving nearly three hours a day. I knew I had to eliminate this unnecessary stress. I requested that my company let me work from home three days a week. They agreed, and my life became a little easier. For me, telling my company what was going on was the right decision. They were, and still are, very supportive. If you work for an organization that believes in supporting your well-being, you might consider sharing this news.

Some other ways I manage my stress include exercise and red-light therapy. I like to start my day with ten minutes of red-light therapy. During this time, l listen to podcasts often related to health. It's a time for me to set my intentions for the day, which is so important. The red light provides many medical benefits, including reducing inflammation and improved mood, especially during the winter months. I concentrate the red light on both my face and spine.

Exercise varies for me daily, depending on my mood. On busier days where I have less energy, I will go for a walk. On the days that I need mediation and calm movement, I practice yoga. On the days I want to expend a little more energy, I do a high intensity interval training (HIIT) exercise program on YouTube. There are so many great options, allowing you to switch it up whenever needed. My advice is to move however feels right for you. Do your best! If you can, try to move for at least twenty minutes a day. I recommend following Gretchen Hawley (*@doctor.gretchen*) on Instagram for helpful exercise tips for people with MS.

I want to end by reinforcing the importance of food. It is imperative to eat your way to good health. Start exploring new vegetables you haven't eaten before and try different ways of cooking them. An example of this is the way I make my veggie fries. I cut up turnip, sweet potato, beets, and carrots into wedges. Then, I either use coconut or olive oil on top. I season with sea salt, pepper, and herbs, but you can season with any of your favorite spices. I cook them in the oven for about twenty-five to thirty minutes. They are delicious! In this dish, I've demonstrated how to incorporate several veggies into one side dish. It's important not to stop at one vegetable. Instead, add as many as you can wherever you can. Try incorporating vegetables into every meal. I've cut out dairy, gluten, and legumes. Was it easy? No. Is it still easy? No. Is it important? YES! The commitment to reducing food that causes inflammation is key. Have I occasionally cheated? Yes. Has it been worth it? No. I've learned that once you commit to this lifestyle, it's vital to stick to it. After all, it is your medicine.

The alternative approach isn't suitable for everyone. Each one of us is on our unique journey with multiple sclerosis. The one piece of advice I will give anyone just starting their MS journey or looking to try an alternative approach to their health, is to spend time researching the topic. Don't feel pressure to make any decisions or be in fear of changing a choice you have made. You are strong! You have the power to make the right choice for you. I am very fortunate to have been relapse-free over the past five years. I believe the choices I've made have helped me stay this way. Believe in your choices! Be an MS warrior, but also a health warrior. Everything you are doing now is helping to safeguard your future. Not only from multiple sclerosis, but from other possible health issues. Along with everything you practice for good health, a positive mindset is your number one daily dose of medication.

9

Story by
BILJANA

Diagnosed in 2013
Currently 46 years old
Lives in Australia (from Serbia)

It was January of 2013. I awoke in the morning, stood up from bed, and fell to the floor. I had no idea what was happening to me. All feeling had left my leg. It was a living nightmare. I was terrified. At the time of the "incident", I was a single mother, managing two teenage boys. I was overrun with stress, working long hours to ensure the boys had everything they needed (school supplies, soccer gear, food, clothes). Not to mention, allotting plenty of time to talk with them about life since they were growing up. Puberty with two boys is hard.

Somehow, I managed to stand up and get myself to the hospital, where they kept me for an entire month. It was easily the worst month of my life.

At the time, we lived in Serbia. When I was eighteen, we came to Serbia during the war in the Balkans to escape Croatia, giving me dual citizenship in both Serbia and Croatia. I had children from my first marriage. Due to many problems and stress, the marriage ended after fifteen years. The following seven years, the children and I lived alone.

The healthcare system in Serbia is free, making the wait to see a specialist (in my case, a neurologist) very long. The one exception being a trip to the hospital due to a relapse. Then, you will be admitted immediately to receive the appropriate therapy with corticosteroids. This was my case. I'm not sure how it is in other countries, but in Serbia, the official diagnosis of MS comes only with the second relapse. After two lumbar punctures, three MRIs, too many corticosteroids to count, and medications–the doctors STILL didn't have a clear answer. When I was discharged from the hospital, they left me with the diagnosis of "possible multiple sclerosis (MS)".

I felt helpless. Later, I learned what I suffered from that January morning was my first relapse. My family came to visit me everyday in the hospital, but I was angry –angry about life, my body, everything. I could not accept the fact there was nothing I could do to fix my situation. Before the nightmare in January, I was happy, smiling, and full of life. I enjoyed everything, and everything made me happy. Suddenly, life STOPPED.

After my incident, I spent two weeks in a medical spa (similar to rehab for multiple sclerosis patients). It's a sulfur spa. They lifted me up onto my feet where I could feel my legs again, and I began walking normally.

In April of the same year, I experienced problems with my shoulder, giving me the final diagnosis of multiple sclerosis. During this month, I was accepted to be part of a study for a new MS drug. Bad decision. Nineteen months I just want to forget. Every second day, I gave myself an injection. Once a week, I went to the hospital for an infusion. I felt like I was on an emotional rollercoaster or stuck in a bad movie. Pain, depression, and anger continued to pile on. Without the love and support from my family and kids, I don't know if I would have survived.

During the case study for this experimental medicine, I had access to the Clinical Center of Serbia. When I finished the study, they offered me the medication Rebif, which I refused on my own accord. I take full responsibility for that decision. I just couldn't do it anymore. As you may already know, these medications were used to treat multiple sclerosis when the disease was newly discovered. In underdeveloped countries, they are already outdated, and a new generation of medication is dispersed. In my opinion, they are all the same.

Around that time, I married my current husband who is from the same area as me in Croatia. We've known each other since childhood. He lived and worked in Australia. He was divorced, just like me. We started our life together in Serbia. Of course he knew everything about me and my condition, which he didn't mind at all. He always supports me in everything–a wind at my back.

We decided to go to Australia, applying for a partner visa to get Australian citizenship. A lot of paperwork and examinations were involved, including a medical examination. It never occurred to me not to disclose my MS. It is part of who I am. Announcing it led to a three-year struggle for citizenship. In the end, they deported me with the reasoning that I would be a big financial loss to their healthcare system. They estimated I would cost them around $700,000 to treat my multiple sclerosis for the duration of my life, even though I was not taking medication.

We complained to all parties, last being the tribunal. The lawyer informed us we could appeal the decision, but a positive outcome would not be guaranteed. The Australian government is ruthless when incurable diseases are in question. I was disappointed. Not because of multiple sclerosis, but as a human being. I did not choose to have MS– it's part of me now. I can't change that. But the way they treat people with this disease is very dehumanizing. I couldn't stand anymore disappointment. We were forced to pack up and return to Serbia. The right to apply for a tourist visa was taken away from me for three years. Then came corona. After three years, I reapplied and was finally granted a tourist visa. During that time, I was pretty healthy. No major problems, no medication, no relapse.

The last MRI I received was in 2016, during the health examinations related to the visa. I still don't know what the findings were. I have not seen a neurologist in seven years, and I hope to keep it that way.

I think I had multiple sclerosis long before the diagnosis, possibly five years prior. I constantly experienced headaches and fatigue, but justified that it was from being overworked, along with other problems. The first relapse that stole my lower body from me was just the result of wear and tear from the previous years.

Because of everything I'd been through, it took me two years to fully accept that I have multiple sclerosis. Since then, she and I have become BEST friends!

I decided to change everything. It took time and patience, but it was worth it. I rejected every medication offered because I had had enough of everything. I felt a lack of energy, life, and general motivation. I knew I needed to stop and start over. That was my decision–the first good decision on my MS journey!

Afterwards, everything became easier. I started doing yoga, which has become an integral part of my life. It helps me a lot. I've always been mentally strong, but yoga helped me to be even stronger, peaceful, and more stable. I worked on myself constantly.

I read many articles related to MS, listened to countless conversations from different people (including doctors) about how ingredients in food can cause inflammation in the body. Little by little, I changed my lifestyle and diet. My way of thinking, along with my behavior, also evolved. I started eating healthy: no dairy, no red meat, no sugar, sometimes chicken and fish, lots of fruits and vegetables. Of course, sometimes I eat cake on my birthday or at special events, but that's okay. Everything in moderation.

The second decision I made was to remove all people from my life who were negative, boring, and full of unnecessary conversation and empty stories. I have become better for my kids and my family–everyone I love and who loves me.

I started getting massages once a week, which feels amazing. I've learned how to let go of things I have no control over. This helps me manage my anxiety, releasing the major stressors in my life. My daily or weekly routine is very different. I love to dance, and do it whenever I can. I enjoy socializing, going out with friends, and wearing heels! I wear them, even though my legs hurt for two days after. I wear them because they bring me joy. I also like being at home, watching movies, reading books, and just relaxing.

Every morning upon awakening, I drink coffee or cocoa, followed by a trip to the gym or a yoga practice at home. I drink smoothies full of fruit, chia seeds, maca powder, soy or almond milk. I cook healthy meals based around vegetables, chicken, or fish. I don't eat red meat or processed foods. I try to sleep enough. Of course insomnia hinders that occasionally, but it will pass.

I walk a lot, sometimes 10 km a day. I can't run. It makes me very tired and feeling broken the rest of the day. A word of advice: spread your energy throughout the day to make sure you can enjoy every part.

Some days when I struggle with MS and am feeling tired, I've realized I just need a little time alone. Everyone around me understands that and respects my time. Now, I'm forty-six years old, and I feel good. My boys are adults. They both live and work in Austria, and I'm *so* proud of them. My biggest support in life is my husband. He does everything for us to keep me happy and healthy.

I'm grateful for every day I'm granted. I'm grateful to my father who also had MS. While he was alive, he helped me every step of the way. He gave me the best advice about everything. When I was sad and in pain, he always reassured me by saying, "It will all pass and better will come." I have lived with multiple sclerosis (my best friend) for ten years, and I'm good! I'm going to live another ten, slowly and cleverly.

In my country, more than ten thousand people suffer from multiple sclerosis. In my environment, I know about ten people who are fighting this disease. Most of them have major problems relating to their mental health. Poor mental health immediately influences the course of the disease. Many of their family members contact me, asking me to talk with them in an attempt to inspire motivation. I say yes all the time. I do my best to help them by being an example. Sometimes, I succeed; sometimes, it's simply not enough because you have to want it. Some people just aren't willing. It's easier for them to do nothing. It makes me sad to see how hard life is for them. I never tell them what they should do because I know the disease is different for everyone–the struggle is real! All I can do is share my routine. The most important lesson I've learned is to be mentally strong.

What motivates me most is being good to myself, my children, and my husband. Helping my mother not to worry and my sister not to be afraid also makes me happy. I don't burden the children with my condition. It saddens me to see worry painted on their faces. The best times I have with them are when we go out, and they say to me, "Mom, you are a dragon!"

I simply love life because we never know what tomorrow brings. I try to enjoy every present moment. I'm laughing, and it's nice. When there are hard days, I accept them. I don't stay in that mood. Instead, I go on beautifully...

10

Story by

MOHAMMED

Diagnosed in 2018
Currently 30 years old
Lives in Qatar

I am a Yemeni national, born and raised in Qatar. In 2012, I decided to travel to India for my studies. It was there that I first enrolled in an English learning academy and later pursued a bachelor's degree in pharmacy in the fall of 2013. I led an active lifestyle through my younger years, participating in various sports. During school, I was part of a sprinting team, and in college, I played soccer. I regularly worked out and lived a typical, "active" lifestyle, until my diagnosis.

It all started in February 2018. My initial symptom was blurry vision in my left eye. I went to a hospital for a check-up. After a few appointments, they suggested I undergo magnetic resonance imaging (MRI). During that time, I was juggling being a college student and managing hospital visits, which made getting my MRI done challenging. Initially, I shrugged it off as just some vision related problem that would probably require me to use glasses. However, it got progressively worse. It was during the month of Ramadan, while observing my fast, that I began experiencing vision problems in my other eye. By this time, I also started to feel numbness in my extremities. Occasionally, a sudden shock, like an electrical current, would surge through me, causing excruciating pain. During my vacations when I returned to Qatar, I finally had the opportunity to get my MRIs done. Within a week or so, I received the results.

I had never been familiar with multiple sclerosis (MS), until the diagnosis. While we may have briefly studied it during our lectures, I never truly grasped the profound impact it has on people's lives. After the diagnosis, there was little time to process the overwhelming emotions; it felt as if someone had started a timer on my life. I found myself navigating a whirlwind of back-to-back appointments, receiving prescriptions, and being introduced to potential symptoms I would eventually face, alongside the shocking list of side effects that came with the medication. It was chaotic. Taking my time, I made the risky decision to delay starting the medication. Instead, I turned to traditional remedies, researching the healing properties of food and herbs. Adjusting my eating habits proved challenging, as I had to educate myself on food reactions that contradicted what I had known growing up.

It took me a while to identify what triggered my symptoms. Even something as simple as a warm shower would cause me pain if I wasn't careful about the water temperature. Eating processed cheese when I was out with friends would immediately trigger an attack. The weather also affects my MS, so I have to avoid harsh conditions. Before my diagnosis, I could run for miles at a moderate-to-high speed, but as the disease progressed, running became difficult. I started to experience more frequent electrical shocks. Now, I stick to long walks instead of running. My diet helps manage my MS, allowing me to do high-intensity workouts.

Eventually, around 2020, I came across an Instagram page called *Multiple Sclerosis Awareness*, run by Surjeet Kaur. I attended an online meeting, arranged by the page admin, and for the first time, I got a chance to connect with others like me. Not taking the medication for a disease like MS seemed like a big risk to my family and friends and made me anxious, as well. But through this newly found support group, I was able to meet others who had also opted out of taking medications and had been surviving with MS for longer than I had.

As much as it is a physiological disease, MS also affects a person's mental state. That's why it's important to have supportive people who give us strength and courage by our side. Ayona, a friend I met in college, has been a significant source of support throughout my journey with MS. When I was first diagnosed, she took the time to sit me down and explain what MS meant. We would discuss different medications and alternatives, and she would help me research food sources and supplements that could potentially aid in my condition. Ayona even attended the online meeting I mentioned earlier, where she assisted me in connecting with others. Being someone who struggles with meeting new people, her presence provided me with a much-needed boost. I distinctly remember a day during the early stages of my diagnosis when I was on the verge of breaking down, feeling overwhelmed, and struggling to come to terms with having MS. That's when Ayona said something that resonated deeply with me: "You don't have to be known as Mohammad, who has MS. You can just be known as Mohammad, too. Your whole life doesn't have to revolve solely around MS." In hindsight, it may seem like an obvious statement to some, but for me, who was facing the possibility of life in a wheelchair much sooner than expected, those words brought comfort and motivation. They reminded me to strive for more and to be defined by more than just my disease.

At first, I didn't prioritize the role of food in maintaining good health, and looking back, it's something I regret. After the initial diagnosis, I was bombarded with information and encouraged to start taking medication to slow down the progression of the disease. If I had researched the impact of food earlier, I could have potentially avoided the initial years of attacks. I had been on a diet that consisted of organic fruits and vegetables, but it wasn't a well-planned one. However, around May 2020, I decided to take my diet seriously and became more strict with what I should avoid. For instance, I cut out processed sugar, focused on incorporating good fats, and maintained an overall balanced diet. My advice to those newly diagnosed with MS would be to relearn what you know about food and have faith that you can find a way to improve your condition. Despite our bodies having a tendency to attack themselves, it's important to remember that the human body is amazing. With a little support from us in terms of what we allow to enter our bodies, we can effectively fight most diseases.

Life with MS has been challenging. Part of my journey that is very relevant is the impact of my religion. You may or may not choose to believe in God, but I do, and it is the single most constant factor that has helped me endure this predicament. There is a text in our religious scriptures, which translates as, "God does not burden a soul with that which it cannot deal with." These are the words I reiterate to myself during difficult times, when I find myself searching for answers to the questions, "Why me?" and "Why did I have to have this disease?" I do not dwell on such thoughts anymore; I believe accepting reality and focusing on healing is half of the treatment.

Since my diagnosis, I have become more disciplined than ever with my sleep and wake cycle. I've found that the walks I take after my sunrise prayers have been very beneficial. You may not have a personal religious motivation like I do, but I would still advise people to wake up and get moving, refusing to give up on an active lifestyle despite MS. Remember the old saying, "Early to bed and early to rise may not make you wealthy, but it will make you healthy." In addition to long walks, swimming is also an amazing way to strengthen the body, which I highly recommend.

I rely heavily on the knowledge from prophethood medicine, as it has worked the best for me. Some of the superfoods based on the prophethood medicine system are olive oil, black seeds, black seed oil, and Qast-al-hindi (Indian costus powder), which I usually consume by adding a teaspoon to a glass of water. I stick to eating two meals a day and avoid snacking in between. Although my diet consists of protein, vitamins, and fiber, I also consume carbohydrates in the form of dates. A variety of dates called the Ajwa dates, hailed in prophetic medicine as one of the "fruits of heaven", is my favorite. I also take vitamins in the form of supplements. It is important that fat-soluble vitamins are taken with food that helps with their absorption. Therefore, I would advise researching such factors and consulting a doctor before making them part of your routine. Do keep in mind that "supplements" should not become "substitutes" within your diet; you must aim at obtaining as many nutrients and micronutrients as possible from food.

Mathew Embry has been a significant influence on how I've managed my disease thus far. His documentary *Living Proof* is something I highly recommend to those who are newly diagnosed or have family members facing the disease. I also stay informed about the works of Dr. Terry Wahls, another MS survivor, who has remarkably dealt with serious symptoms through dietary measures. It's important to stay updated on the latest MS research and read peer-reviewed articles. Additionally, I want to mention Angie (who is sharing her story in the book, as well), whom I met through the *Multiple Sclerosis Awareness* page. She's an incredibly strong and resilient woman—the epitome of perseverance.

Here is the recipe for the supplement I have been taking. I would like to add that I am not a medical professional or qualified to advise people on such matters. However, an herbalist from Yemen suggested this concoction for me, and it has been working well. Please consult your doctor or be aware of any allergy that may arise if you use it:

- Burdock root 10 g
- Black seeds 40 g
- Fenugreek 30 g

- Cinnamon 20 g
- Licorice 20 g
- Ginger 10 g
- Clove 5 g
- Turmeric 50 g
- Common hop 30 g
- Solenostemma argel 10 g

Living with multiple sclerosis has been a challenging journey, but I have found strength through the support of others and the knowledge gained from inspiring figures. By prioritizing a balanced diet, staying informed about the latest research, and maintaining an active lifestyle, I strive to manage my disease while living life to the fullest. I am determined to make the most of each day, embracing the fullness of life with strength, knowledge, and an unwavering spirit.

11

Story by
KATHRYN

Diagnosed in 2018
Currently 34 years old
Lives in Iowa, United States

My story begins about three years prior to me being diagnosed. My initial symptoms were tingling sensations on the left side of my abdomen, which started after attending an intense hot yoga class. I was seen by several family care physicians during the three years leading up to my diagnosis. Each time I brought up multiple sclerosis (MS), I was told, "You're healthy, you're young, and I'm sure it's nothing." I eventually felt the tingling sensations on the left side of my face. It was then I knew something was wrong. I found a primary care physician who listened to me, and she referred me to a neurologist. I was diagnosed in June of 2018. My life changed from that point forward.

A lot happened in a very short period. The day I was diagnosed, my husband brought home *The Wahls Protocol* by Dr. Terry Wahls, and we began changing our diets immediately. I also saw a functional medicine practitioner shortly after I was diagnosed, who ran labs for me, which gave me a ton of information about my nutritional deficiencies and what heavy metals were in my body. Having this information was key in figuring out what supplements I should take.

My body went through an intense detox for about a month. I was very sick but still maintained all my responsibilities, such as work, volunteer commitments, etc. It took around a year before I started feeling the effects of the changes I was making. During this time, neurologists tried to convince me to get on a drug modifying therapy (DMT). I am not anti-western medicine, but I knew there was another way that didn't require me to completely deplete my immune system and put me in thousands of dollars of medical debt. I was determined to explore holistic healing methods and forge my own path—and I never looked back.

I have no plans of getting on a DMT and generally feel pretty good in my body. I do not fear this disease, nor do I receive regular magnetic resonance imaging (MRIs) any longer, as the neurologists who I was seeing cannot help me.

People hear the words "multiple sclerosis", and they immediately think of the worst possible outcome. I have shared my health status with some but not everyone. Personally, I have never entirely identified with this disease, and I do not plan to hang onto it. This illness and what it has required of me is more than eating healthily and exercising; it has required me to cleanse myself in a way that is profoundly intimate, personal, and at times, very raw. It's not that I'm ashamed of having a chronic illness; I'm not willing to expose myself in a way that would then require me to discuss all of the reasons my body fell weak to this disease. There's too much to share and too much trauma to unpack. There have been no mistakes along this journey because with every setback, I learn more and feel deeper. This disease has allowed me to understand my body in a way that feels affirming. I have always said that my body continues to talk, and it's up to me to listen. My advice to anyone newly diagnosed is to listen and know that nobody knows your body like you do.

In terms of healing practices, I've done it all, and it's changed and taken on new shapes with the different phases of life. Currently, I continue to eat a fairly strict paleo diet. I do not mess with processed foods. I eat a very clean, whole food, organic diet; I know what a privilege this is in this country. I take supplements, and I work out when I can. I love all forms of body work and receive massages and chiropractic care on a regular basis. When it comes to what I expose my body to, I avoid using chemical-based products, and I don't subject myself to anything I cannot unsee. Reading the news is scary enough these days. I am very conscientious about who I spend my time with and what I give energy to, which is another reason I choose not to share my disease with everyone. I don't want to answer people's questions, as I do not have time or energy for that.

My willingness to share my story is not to try to encourage folks to holistically heal themselves but embolden them to make whatever decision is best for them while knowing there are alternative methods. This is a delicate dance. As you know, holistic healing encompasses a wide range of approaches, and there's no "one size fits all" solution, especially with a disease that is systemic.

MS changed my life in countless ways. I'm not going to sugar coat it—it's incredibly hard. But I remind myself that most good things in life are just that—hard. What a blessing to have something that has given me so much in return, taught me so much, and made me realize the flaws in my upbringing and previous path. It wasn't right. The past five years were earth-shattering when I realized my individual strength. I diagnosed myself, I removed the toxins that were poisoning my body and life, and now, I get to heal myself. What a gift!

I will leave you with some soft words of encouragement—listen to your intuition. There is so much information out there about how you should do things, but your body is the best teacher.

12

Story by

CLAUDIE

Diagnosed in 1996
Currently 57 years old
Lives in Hamburg, Germany
Instagram: @claudie_schu

A few days after my last State Examination for Human Medicine in May 1994, I visited the outdoor swimming pool with a friend. Finally, a break and relaxation! The first symptoms occurred while I was walking to the pool. It was vertigo. It started with dizziness in my head. I felt like I was walking on clouds.

A few weeks later, everything was forgotten, and I planned my one year stay abroad in Melbourne with my boyfriend at the time. While in Melbourne, I experienced optic neuritis towards the end of the stay, which was treated with high doses of cortisone.

After undergoing initial diagnostics, a suspected diagnosis of multiple sclerosis (MS) was made. Upon returning home to Hamburg, Germany, I embarked on extensive research, conducting thorough investigations at the university library. Those books were substantial, encompassing the entire collection of publications from the respective journal. I had to make copies of the specific publications that interested me. In 1996, the internet did not really exist yet, so I had to utilize the resources available to me at the time.

I began altering my diet by consistently avoiding gluten and saturated fat. I also included linseed oil for omega-3 (although I now know that isn't enough), cut out dairy, and started drinking aloe vera juice daily. Every day, I had salad with plenty of olive oil and rice cakes topped with banana slices and lemon juice. I ordered soy cheese from England. I was fine with it! I also had my amalgam fillings removed.

Then, unfortunately (from today's perspective), I happened to run into my neurology professor from the University Hospital in Hamburg while shopping, who advised me to visit his outpatient clinic. There were two trials starting at that time, one with Copaxone and one with Interferon Beta. I chose Copaxone, which requires subcutaneous injections. I experienced brief pain, swelling, and a burning sensation at the injection site, but it disappeared quickly within a day.

Within a few months, all the foci in the cerebrum disappeared, and I was doing great. A year later, in 1997, I met my husband. I remember how he was amused by my eating habits. After that, everything happened at once: property purchase, pregnancy, house building, and wedding! I was doing well, even when I stopped Copaxone because of the pregnancy. The pregnancy was not planned, but I was happy to have a break from the injections as a result.

I can't remember exactly when I started eating a "normal" diet again, but at that time, I was free from worries, no longer burdened with night shifts at the hospital where I previously worked. And I was symptom-free! The excitement of our first child and new home filled me with joy.

After the delivery, I made the decision not to resume Copaxone as I wanted to exclusively breastfeed my child. However, about six months later, I experienced my first episode in a long time: optic neuritis. Overnight, I had to wean my child (nowadays, I would continue pumping until the medication had cleared my system) and receive high doses of cortisone. It was at that point that I started the injections again.

For the first two years, I stayed home with my child, transitioning to working one day a week until I became pregnant again. I also stopped taking Copaxone again. At the age of thirty-six, I welcomed my second child. This time, shortly after giving birth, I promptly resumed taking the medication. To ensure a sufficient time gap before the next meal, I always injected after the baby's last evening feeding. Fortunately, Copaxone seemed to be working well for me, with magnetic resonance imaging (MRI) scans indicating no new lesions.

Over the years, my diet reverted to its previous pattern of being vegetarian with fish. I aimed for a supposedly healthy approach, incorporating whole grains, yogurt, or cheese. I also maintained an active lifestyle, regularly engaging in sports, such as inline skating, squash, tennis, jogging, and fitness.

In 2006, I began experiencing foot drop, which made running difficult. Unfortunately, it never crossed my mind to reintroduce the diet I had initially researched. Maybe I lacked the mental strength to pursue it with my responsibilities of work, two children, and managing the household. Eventually, I started looking for alternative options, specifically after learning about studies or experimental individual treatments that seemed relatively safe. For six months, I received immunoglobulins, but they didn't have a noticeable effect. Sometime later, I underwent a procedure where mesenchymal stem cells (MSC) were extracted, multiplied, and then administered intravenously. Though it did result in the unexpected disappearance of my hay fever, it was not what I had hoped for. Around 2010, I participated in a study called "Establish Tolerance in MS" that involved autologous modified lymphocytes. Unfortunately, the desired outcome of stopping the progression of MS was not achieved. More about this study: https://www.ncbi.nlm.nih.gov/pmc/articles/PMC3973034/

I experimented with various treatment options in my search for relief. For six months, I tried minocycline, which unfortunately only resulted in blackened teeth (thank you, professional teeth cleaning!) In another attempt, I tried consuming pork tapeworm eggs in hopes of triggering an immune system response, but it was ineffective. In addition to my ongoing use of Copaxone, I also took encapsulated dimethyl fumarate (half a dose). However, as my white blood cell count plummeted, I had to stop taking it. Over time, my foot drop weakness worsened, accompanied by knee instability and a weak hamstring. My entire right leg was affected by these symptoms. Thankfully, I was fitted for myoelectric orthosis (Bioness) which improved my running considerably, and I still wear it today.

Although my right leg had limitations, my left leg was unaffected, so I bought an adult scooter. It was in the trunk of my car, so I had a reasonably large radius. I put my lame right leg on the running board, and off I went. In the car, I had a left throttle pedal installed, and after three hours of driving lessons, it was no problem.

At the end of 2013, there was a "Visite" health program on TV, covering the topic "Nutrition in MS". It discussed the benefits of a ketogenic diet. Since I had no other options, I signed up for a nutrition consultation at Medicum Hamburg. It was a very high-fat, low-carbohydrate diet (butter, curd, eggs, etc.), which I then implemented. In June 2014, I heard a lecture by Dr. M. Bock from Berlin, who in a conversation afterwards strongly recommended a gluten-free diet. Apparently, someone else had to tell me before I believed it.

At the end of 2014, after a span of eighteen years since my diagnosis, I finally discovered Dr. Terry Wahls. Her book had just been published in German, which I then bought. I was on fire and turned my entire refrigerator upside down. To be honest, at first, I didn't know what to eat anymore and lost a few kilos until I had settled into this new way of eating. After a short time, I achieved a reduction in my fatigue. That was really sensational! I stuck with this diet, snacked on giant salads daily, and was a fan of the "Wahls Buttertoffees".

Recipe: Wahls Buttertoffees
1 cup of coconut oil
1 cup of raisins
1 cup of walnuts (soak beforehand)
1 avocado
1/2 cup of dried coconut
1-2 teaspoons cinnamon
1 teaspoon of cocoa powder
Mix all ingredients in a food processor until smooth. Press the mixture into a glass mold (20 x 20 cm) and place in the refrigerator.

During 2017, I had heard about the Coimbra Protocol for the first time (coimbraprotocol.com). I looked deeply into vitamin D itself and was sure that there really must be a causal link here. I had my first appointment with the protocol doctor in December 2017 and started with 60,000 IU of vitamin D per day!

In retrospect, vitamin D deficiency was most definitely the core cause of the onset of my disease. It's very likely that I experienced a severe deficiency in my mother's womb. As an infant, I did not receive vitamin D or cod liver oil. At one point, I just collapsed, revealing clear signs of a serious deficiency. I did not have my first vitamin D supplementation until after the birth of my first child in 1999. My neurologist never prescribed it to me before then. Rather, I happily asked myself at the time why the child was getting vitamin D and I was not. It is also interesting that I, as a medical doctor, did not learn anything about this in my studies! I was appalled by the revelation, especially considering my background in "Hemapheresis", Department of Transfusion Medicine at the University Hospital Hamburg Eppendorf. It is a very important hormone in the body, on par with the thyroid hormone, which can be deduced from the fact that every cell in the body has vitamin D receptors.

Fortunately, during my first pregnancy, I had plenty of exposure to the summer sun, so I assumed that my child didn't experience any vitamin D deficiency. Even my gynecologist failed to suggest vitamin D supplementation. So, in 1999 I started taking one thousand units per day, which is quite insufficient given the vitamin D receptor defect found in autoimmune patients (as discussed by Carsten Carlberg in Finland). Thus, the required level is not even remotely reached in the cell, leading to severe consequences.

As a child, I naturally received all recommended vaccinations. Today, I know that harmful substances such as mercury and aluminum are in them. It is true that vaccination side effects were not even discussed in medical school. Truly unbelievable. Vaccinations can trigger and increase autoimmune diseases, especially with a poorly developed immune system due to vitamin D deficiency. I really regret having vaccinated my children in their early childhood.

The numerous MRIs performed throughout the course of the disease have their drawbacks, particularly due to the frequent use of contrast agents. The agents contain gadolinium, which can accumulate in the brain. This accumulation, in combination with heavy metals from vaccinations and dental fillings, and glyphosate from our food, creates a chain of events. It is evident that we are being poisoned!

With the start of the Coimbra Protocol in parallel with Wahls Protocol, I got better in the sense that I became much clearer in my head. The number of falls I had noticeably reduced, and that was after only a short time. It must have taken me a year to find my individual dose of vitamin D. Over time, I was able to gradually reduce it (35,000 IU currently) and realized that this reduction signifies a restoration of the vitamin D receptors.

In 2018, for approximately a year, I also tried Low Dose Naltrexone (LDN), but I could only take it for a short time. The taste was bitter and nasty. Unfortunately, my motor function restrictions did not improve at all. On the contrary, by the end of 2020, my second hamstring was weakening. I contribute that to COVID and the stress that it brought to us. The stress from my work also caused me to feel sick. Because of this, I no longer work.

I now have time to myself. The kids are grown and going their separate ways. Last year, I conducted a lot of research, and I'm going in new directions. Initially, my focus was on detox. I have been using special drops (Clean Slate Root) since March 2022 as part of my routine. During the year, I also realized the importance of hexagonal water.

Hexagonal water is characterized by the fact that the H2O water molecules combine in hexagonal ring structures. It is crystalline-like and, therefore, stable. Hexagonal water represents the living, energy-rich structure found in natural, very healthy glacier water. In contrast, common drinking water consists of larger water molecule compounds compared to hexagonal water. In normal water, due to its dipolarity, around twenty to twenty-five water molecules combine to form a macro cluster, which is too large to enter cells through the small aquaporins (cell openings). As a result, the body experiences dehydration, and a lack of fluid. On the other hand, hexagonal water has a smaller structure and easily splits, allowing it to enter all cells. It possesses optimal cell permeability and availability, making it the most important means of transporting nutrients, oxygen, and waste products within the body. Hexagonal water has the potential to aid in the following: Improved hydration, optimal nutrient absorption, improved cell availability, optimal flow rate of all body fluids, effective detoxification, more efficient metabolism, increased cell communication, energy production, increased protection of the cells, and DNA deacidification/ optimal pH value.Source: BRIEF INFORMATION NO. 3, CELLTUNER

I use a special water carafe for energizing, and I have been filtering the tap water for some time. In September 2022, I bought a frequency generator called Diamond Shield Professional from Alternativ Gesund (alternativgesund.de). I was fortunate to find frequencies for myelin sheath repair, which prompted me to buy the device. I dedicated up to two hours a day for "zapping" with these frequencies, hoping that the discoverer got it right with these thirteen frequencies. Diamond Shield aims to liberate the meridians. It is also possible to create custom programs using the provided frequency primer. Furthermore, I regularly run a detox program, along with another program, targeting various bacteria and parasites. These programs involve cleansing organs, such as the liver, kidney, and gallbladder.

Recently, an acquaintance from a support group recommended the book *Comeback* by Dr. Stefan Hainzl. He started the Coimbra Protocol ten years after his MS diagnosis and initially began with the Wahls Diet ™. Later, he switched to a vegan, gluten-free diet. He is back in complete remission after hard training, which he also attributes to his daily meditations, according to Dr. Joe Dispenza. Inspired by this, I bought Dr. Joe's book *You Are the Placebo: Making Your Mind Matter* and worked through it. I have never had access to real meditation and have been trying it now since mid-February. As you can guess, I need new myelin sheaths! My lesions are stupidly all in the spinal cord, and the nerve impulses don't reach there without myelin sheaths.

I sometimes wonder why there is not already a transmission device of electrical impulses from above the lesions in the spinal cord to below the last lesions. You can do so many things wirelessly. You can measure the currents, why can't you reroute them or transmit them differently? That would be a good topic for a PhD thesis!

The more you read and research, the more you get confused and often question your own way. This will always be a challenge. One should remain true to oneself and one's findings, that is what I have learned. I had to create this experience when I heard about Overcoming MS (OMS) in early 2020–vegan (but with fish) and gluten-free, according to Prof. Dr. George Jelinek. That went well for a while, but my gut rebelled against the legumes and seeds. Not everything applies to everyone. Through trial and error, I now have a long list of supplements that work for me.

In addition, I put collagen powder in my breakfast: coconut chips with wild blueberries, mulberries, psyllium husks, cinnamon, and cashew or almond milk. More recently, I have also started adding barley grass powder to smoothies.

For me, it was never the case that I equated the diagnosis with ending up in a wheelchair. It was always clear to me that there had to be another solution. When the doctor told me I had MS, I didn't feel fear. I reacted very soberly and started researching right away. I never let it influence my dreams. There have been slight deviations from the course. For example, I didn't become a cardiologist, but a transfusion physician. But I have two great children and was able to play sports for a very long time. It wasn't until my left (supporting) leg was also affected, just over two years ago, that I first felt I was no longer in control. Suddenly, I was increasingly dependent on help! Negative thoughts and fears came up, as well. It was awful, especially after I had quit my job. I was suddenly confronted with a lot of free time to go in depth with my thoughts undisturbed. I was disappointed that the Coimbra Protocol had not improved my motor functions. This was the case with so many, but I simply learned about it too late.

In retrospect, if someone were to ask me what I would have done differently to avoid my loss of mobility, I would have maintained my diet with more discipline. Instead, I was given medication and relinquished my responsibility. I also would have started with the Coimbra Protocol, but I didn't know about it then. If this had not led to remission, then an autologous stem cell transplant would have been an option for me (a reset for the immune system, especially in the case of lesions in the spinal cord). This is followed by the implementation of the Coimbra Protocol (remedy vitamin D deficiency), as a stem cell transplant does not cure the vitamin D receptor!

I would like to elaborate on my daily "rituals". They have evolved over time, and I have continued to develop them. First thing in the morning, I get on my Powerplate for ten minutes to prevent osteoporosis. After that, I do some stretching exercises on the exercise ball. Unfortunately, I can't do anything on my yoga mat because I wouldn't be able to stand up by myself. I also start my day with a big cup of warm water with freshly squeezed lemon juice. Then, I have breakfast (listed above).

I bought gymnastic bands, which I use to perform arm exercises throughout the day based on my mood. Between four to five in the evenings, I usually make myself a salad, and I take long breaks between meals. In the evening, I have a big vegetable dish: once a week with chicken breast, once a week with fish, and once a week with two eggs. I like to eat koniac noodles and soups with which I use bone broth. I ferment cabbage, which I eat daily as a side dish. My go-to snacks are nuts and cashews. As soon as the house is quiet, I do a meditation by Dr. Joe with headphones on the couch. However, I can't wait to meditate outside in the woods, alone in nature. Hopefully, it will warm up soon!

During the day, I zap as it fits, and in the evening, my near-infrared therapy mat is waiting on the sofa to put on my back (for the spinal cord) for thirty to sixty minutes. Once a week, I go swimming and do water aerobics. My brain cells also need exercise, so I am learning two new languages. I would still like to try hyperbaric oxygen therapy and explore the potential benefits of a drug called Clemastin, which is believed to promote myelin formation.

Basically, I only buy organic food and hygiene products. I have banned plastic from my household. I use fluoride-free toothpaste and rinse my mouth with Finnish birch sugar (xylitol) and coconut oil. When possible, I work with LAN to reduce radiation, but it's not optimal yet. When it is nice outside, I go to the garden and tend to my raised garden beds. I grow wild herbs, which allows me to keep a small medicine chest. I often try to mix wild herbs into my salad or smoothie.

My myelin sheaths must have already been completely damaged because I experience a range of limitations from head to toe. Starting with mild facial paresis, I also have hearing loss on the right side and mild vision loss on the left. In terms of mobility, my right hand and arm function are limited, and I have scapula alata on the right side, causing my shoulder blade to protrude. Additionally, my right leg is completely non-functional, except for the use of fashion accessories. I've also noticed a weakening in my left hamstring flexor. I walk outside with walkers and have a myo-electric orthosis on the right to stimulate the right foot elevator muscle. For walks, I use the Alinker (adult running bike with three wheels). When I don't want to take the car, I have an electric trike that can do twenty-five km/h and has a range of fifty km. To be in nature and exercise my legs, I ride a recumbent bike (Hase Bike). However, I need calf braces for both legs to keep them from wobbling back and forth. It's a lot of work keeping everything tightened.

Fortunately, Dr. Joe came into play, and now I have the feeling that everything is possible again! Also, frequency therapy gives me confidence. Furthermore, we are planning to relocate to the Canary Islands, where we will experience different climate zones and hopefully find a new home. I am aware that my recovery will not be as rapid in northern Germany as it would be in the subtropical climate there, so we are taking this big step.

Living with this disease takes a lot of strength, optimism, consistency, and determination. Fortunately, I am a fighter, supported by dear ones who provide me with assistance. I hope to give back valuable information from my research to prevent such diseases like MS. By educating the next generation about the importance of vitamin D, omega-3, proper nutrition, and connecting with nature, we can help protect them.

13

Story by

LAILA

Diagnosed in 2010
Currently 30 years old
Lives in Connecticut, United States

I was a senior in high school in Connecticut. I'd spent my time, like most teenagers during these years, active in sports, hanging out with friends, and eating junk food. One day during drama class, I noticed what felt and looked like a piece of fuzz in my eye that wouldn't rub away. A few days later, I told my parents. Photos of my optic nerve were taken, showing current inflammation. Turns out, it was optic neuritis. My first magnetic resonance imaging (MRI) showed eight inactive brain lesions. I was diagnosed with multiple sclerosis (MS) on the spot.

My parents were both devastated and confused. They thought the best and only course of action to take was medication, especially my dad with whom I lived at the time. My two older brothers did not have much of a reaction because we were all relatively young. Solu-Medrol (a prescription glucocorticoid) eventually restored the blurry spot in my vision. I'd like to add as a disclaimer that Sulo-Medrol is not a multiple sclerosis medication.

Naturally, I googled multiple sclerosis because I knew nothing about it. The search results were terrifying. My research told me I'd soon be disabled. I freaked out like any 17-year-old would. I started medication quickly after being advised to do so. Being so young, I also thought it was the best decision. I do not feel comfortable naming the three medications I took from 2010-2014. Every case of multiple sclerosis is different, causing medication to be the best course of action for some.

Later in 2014, I decided to get off medication because I was still experiencing problems with my vision. Letting go of the medication was the start of my natural healing journey, ongoing still to this day. I gave up red meat, desserts, and tap water. This eventually led me to build a more routine diet, which is very similar to the paleo diet. In addition to dietary changes, I began regulating my sleep schedule and slowly eliminating stress. Learning to manage life stressors became extremely important. Deep breathing helped. I try to do some form of stretching and exercise daily.

I scheduled MRIs for every six months. My first MRI was the most emotional. I have now undergone so many that I've become used to the loud noises and enclosed space. Sometimes the noises even lull me to sleep. I'm usually not nervous about results because I can sense what they will be based off how my diet and symptoms (or lack thereof) have been progressing. I'm pretty in tune with my body and can feel when something is off, unless there is an asymptomatic lesion. Some have appeared but not a lot. Unfortunately, my neurologist, whom I'd seen for thirteen years, passed away. As of 2022, I'm seeing a new neurologist at the same clinic.

I married in 2021 to a man I met previously and decided to reconnect with. I was upfront about having MS from the beginning. I was open and honest because it is part of who I am and how I live. Anybody who fears that cannot be on my team. Which goes without saying, if you meet someone who can't accept ALL of you, then you are better off without them.

This brings me to my next milestone with multiple sclerosis: pregnancy and having a baby. Pregnancy itself was a breeze. The neuroprotective hormones did their job, while all dieting went out the window for nine months. My husband imports pink salt for work. I relied on stone massagers and salt foot soaks for relief from non-MS related aches and swelling. The delivery was all natural, no epidural, and I pushed for only an hour! I drank red raspberry leaf and ate dates during the third trimester. Right after delivery, I had to take a five-day course of three antibiotics to treat sepsis and Group B Streptococcus (GBS). Goodbye, microbiome!

Two weeks later, I returned to the hospital for malnourishment due to a lack of nutrients while nursing. A full MRI of my spine and brain was conducted to determine if the weakness was MS related. There were no lesions. One month had gone by without any regrowth of beneficial gut bacteria, accompanied by a cute, crying, sleepless newborn. It's only natural that a lesion came next. It was the most impactful and noticeable lesion I've had since being medicated. Fortunately, IV steroids restored a lot of the walking and visual impairments, coupled with the strictest paleo diet I had ever followed. I noticed if I drank a latte or ate something sugary, my vision got blurry. There was no room for cheating on the diet.

My multiple sclerosis diagnosis ultimately changed my life for the better. I eat organic foods, exercise, and sleep regularly. You may have gotten the takeaway above but keeping good gut bacteria on your side will only serve to benefit. A healthy microbiome plays a vital role in your overall wellbeing. I've recently found all sorts of articles published on this topic. There is no way I would be taking these steps to improve my lifestyle without MS.

Before my diagnosis, I lived a very erratic lifestyle. The bottom of my food pyramid was littered with Slim Jim's and chocolate. I barely slept. Multiple sclerosis was the catalyst that turned it all around after about a decade of slow and steady changes. (Diet/lifestyle changes mentioned above.) My daily routine is to be as routine as possible. That can be tough with a newborn. Before pregnancy my routine was cookie cutter— I'd wake up and go to bed at the same time every day, while nourishing myself with healthy paleo meals.

One piece of advice I would give to someone looking to explore more natural approaches to MS is to not get discouraged—take it day by day. Initially, the diagnosis can be overwhelming. But, if it manifests earlier in life, you can slowly shift your routines and habits around for the better to see what works for you (diet-wise, supplement-wise, and lifestyle-wise). Everyone is different, so get to know your body. Through trial and error, test what works/doesn't work for you. Doctors are great, but they do not know YOUR body better than you.

I learned about the power of black seed through the Prophet Muhammad (peace and blessings be upon him). He narrated it has the ability to cure every disease except death. Post medication, I had nothing to lose. I tried it, and my MRI activity took a turn for the better. I have taken it every day since (minus pregnancy). It is taken orally through the forms of seed, oil, or pill. I heard about the power of olives as they are mentioned in the Quran. After reading about how their leaves protect the tree and their properties, I decided to take the extract.

If you are reading this and taking an MS medication that works for you, that's great, also. Do not take any of this as instruction, rather just a shared experience from me. There is no intention to treat or diagnose by sharing my story.

The Wahls Diet ™ served me for some time. These days, I listen to the podcast "The Autoimmune Doc", hosted by Dr. Taylor Krick. I also like to read white papers on multiple sclerosis and its effects on the nervous system. I dream one day of receiving mesenchymal stem cell therapy (MSC), but it's not offered at my clinic.

Because of the baby, I'm getting pressure now more than ever to start medication in order to control my symptoms, although I'm very apprehensive. I am in the process of weighing my options, leaning towards taking it one MRI at a time. Meaning, if I can get things to stabilize, then I will not start medication again.

I would like to have more children, but I am first prioritizing my health by weighing all my current life factors. If the MS did not exist, I would have ten kids—they are so cute! But I know my body needs to be strong and stable to raise them. If my journey has taught me anything it is to listen to my body. So, I will take the steps I have in place and revisit this topic later down the road. Until then, I remain hopeful. The human body is an amazing machine! It is always trying to heal itself, despite the immune system attacking the myelin sheath.

Clean eating overall has helped me and is something I will continue to implement. Ironically, fasting from food and drink has helped me detox my body, as well. I feel better after a traditional fast (no food or drink from sunrise to sunset.) Agota, the creator of the Instagram page "@beatingmyms" is an inspirational figure to follow. She has a great support system and attitude about multiple sclerosis. This is vital for moms with MS!

14

Story by

ADRIA HUSETH RDN, LD, NASM-CPT

Diagnosed in 2020
Currently 41 years old
Lives in Urbandale, Iowa, United States
Instagram: @livingproof.nutrition
Email: livingproofnutritionllc@gmail.com

Fate whispers to the warrior, "You cannot withstand the storm." And the warrior whispers back, "I am the storm."

When I contemplate the first forty-one years of my life, the best analogy I can come up with is a house. Thinking about what I have been through thus far is like that of building a home. You must have a solid foundation. Once that foundation is cured, you can start framing out the walls. You enclose those walls and make that house your home. You decorate and make it homey. Over the years, your taste may change, and you "redecorate". You feel safe within those walls. However, your walls aren't immune to toxic environmental factors. A tornado could take out your roof, or a house fire could damage that frame. But when damage happens to your house, you don't just turn and walk away. You grieve that damage; you thank God (or whatever higher being you prefer) that you're still alive, and you rebuild those walls—maybe even better the next time around. You get back up and fight to reestablish your home.

The Foundation

I grew up on a farm in rural America (Iowa) as an extremely active and healthy child. I was exposed to a lot as a child, being the daughter of a veterinarian and chiropractor. I had the happiest childhood anyone could ask for, filled with adventures, a large organic garden, animals, two brothers, loving parents, extended family, and cousins nearby where our imaginations could run wild. I wasn't abnormally sick. I was breastfed as a baby, no chronic use of antibiotics, I had mono (EBV) in high school, and never broke any bones. (Trust me, I should have broken plenty with trampoline shenanigans and with as many trees as we climbed while exploring the open land.) I point this out because there was no childhood trauma. We were surrounded by nothing but love, positivity, encouragement to follow our dreams, and ample support. I think my passion for sports and a competitive nature evolved early on. With two brothers and many older cousins, I either kept up or got left behind. That drive led me to success in many competitive sports throughout my younger years. I competed in anything that involved "winning!" Throughout junior high and high school years, I found myself craving that competition. It wasn't uncommon for me to finish one sport and merge into another. In the fall, there was volleyball, leading to basketball in the winter, track in the spring, and softball in the summer. I managed to play varsity sports as an incoming freshman. I was an athlete and that defined me for half my life. Being competitive involves giving nothing less than 110% effort every day, being a leader, never giving up, and practicing until I succeeded—then practicing more! If something didn't go my way, I tried harder, never taking no for an answer. And if I didn't want to do something, then I wouldn't. What I didn't know at the time was that this training, mindset, and discipline I put myself through would not only one day save my life, but it would also set me up for success in more than one battle of a lifetime in 2020. I look back at the first twenty years of my life and am beyond grateful to those who influenced me so deeply: aunts, uncles, coaches, teachers, friends, classmates, siblings, parents, and God. If it wasn't for that solid foundation of what made me who I am, I'm not sure I'd be sitting here, sharing my success story with you.

"You, me, or nobody is gonna hit as hard as life. But it ain't about how hard ya hit. It's about how hard you can get hit and keep moving forward. How much you can take and keep moving forward. That's how winning is done." - Rocky Balboa

In college, I took an active interest in health, specifically nutrition. I eventually made a career out of it and became a registered, licensed dietitian and certified personal trainer after earning a bachelor's degree in marketing. Together, these unique skill sets allowed my career to evolve through educating others on the impact of nutrition and health. I also delved into human nutrition research. Dietetics is an evidenced-based profession, and I found an interest in how food can profoundly impact disease and health. In 2018, I furthered my training and explored functional nutrition. Functional nutrition considers every aspect of health, diet, and overall lifestyle when giving nutrition recommendations. It aligns with the ideologies of functional medicine. Hindsight is 20/20, but I know God, once again, was guiding me down a path that would set me up for success for the second half of my life by using my education.

The First Build

In 2015, I married the perfect man for me. We had a lot of similar interests and hobbies. We were what you could call the perfect match. Marriage is hard under normal circumstances. Little did we know just how far we would be put to the test in the unforeseeable future. At the end of 2015, we welcomed our beautiful son Jack, and in late 2018, our precious daughter, Charlotte (Charlie). Both pregnancies were hard on my body, and the deliveries even more so. After twelve hours of labor, they determined Jack was breeched, and we had to have an emergency C-section. That experience was traumatizing. There were complications, but at the end of it all, we both came home and were doing well. The recovery from the C-section wasn't a picnic. It took me a lot longer than I would ever imagine getting back to "normal." Charlie wasn't breeched, but I wasn't dilating as fast as the doctors wanted. I ended up having another C-section, even though I was adamant about a VBAC. This time around, I didn't recover well. After twelve weeks, my incision split open, and my body began expelling the staples that should have been dissolved by my body. I was having tremendous pain during this time and headaches that would take me out. I saw a pain specialist and my OBGYN. It took the better part of a year before the pain and headaches subsided. I used over-the-counter pain medication to help alleviate the headaches and pain. If I had to pinpoint the start of my health demise, I would say it was the trauma to my body from my second child, the over-the-counter pain medication that, more than likely, was causing gut permeability, and low vitamin D3 status. For autoimmune (AI) diseases to occur, we must be born with the genes.

You can do genetic testing to determine what genes could make you susceptible to AI diseases, but there is no DNA test available specific for multiple sclerosis (MS). Changes in 200 genes are linked to the disease, but not everyone with MS has them, and most people with these changes don't have MS. The changes are polymorphisms, not faulty genes. MS has a genetic component but isn't hereditary. This could definitely change in the future with the advancement of technology and testing. Source: https://pathology.jhu.edu/autoimmune/development

I've spoken with my pediatrician about potentially testing my children for AI disease susceptibility. I haven't done so yet but will consider it in the future. I plan to educate them on food choices when older and monitor their vit D3 levels to help prevent any disease activity as best I can. Having a balanced diet, exercise, not smoking and keeping their Vit D3 levels at optimal ranges is the best preventative measure I can take for them as of right now.
Source: https://www.genosalut.com/en/genetic-testing-and-counselling/autoimmune-diseases/

There's only about a 1.5% chance of a child developing MS when their mother or father has it (meaning around one in sixty-seven get it). Source: Adrienne Dellwo. "Is Multiple Sclerosis Genetic Testing Available?" https://www.verywellhealth.com/multiple-sclerosis-genetic-testing-5201481 - 27 September 2021.
We can go our whole lives without the genes becoming activated. We can experience trauma or be exposed to lifestyle and environmental factors that, after so long, activate those AI genes.

The House Fire
September of 2019 was a poignant time in my career. Reorganization of my past employer had been occurring off and on for the last year. It was becoming clear the organization was taking a different path of business operations, and my role in that was not clear. I felt there was no transparency, a lack of communication from upper management, and gaslighting throughout the whole process. This took a toll on my mental and emotional health, and eventually, my physical health. The chronic stress began and continued over the course of the next year. I dedicated ten years of my life to building programs and a solid nutrition foundation for an organization. Feeling that my work was undervalued and unappreciated had a profound effect on me—in a negative way. I feel I held those that needed to be held liable accountable with the help of a kind, smart lawyer who believed in me. I did what I did because I felt I needed to stand up for those before me who couldn't or wouldn't. I pioneered as a leader to help those who will come after me, at the expense of my mental and physical health. I hope my small stance changes the future for my children.

"She was powerful, not because she wasn't scared, but because she went on so strongly despite her fear." - Author unknown.

In the height of my stress at work in the fall of 2019, I was beginning to experience anxiety, panic attacks, and sad moods. I wasn't sleeping well —two small children and a stressful job will do that. I was so hyper focused on work and trying to survive that I couldn't focus on anything else. The damage stress can cause to our bodies is often overlooked. It's no secret that stress can wreck your emotional well-being, but chronic stress works quietly behind the scenes to wreak havoc on your physical health, too. They call it the silent killer for a reason. I specifically remember my first and only MS attack. It was just before Halloween in 2019. I was getting ready for bed and walked out of my bathroom. I reached to turn the light off. As I stepped out of the room, it felt as if the light switch went off in my body. A bolt of electricity went down my left side. There was a numbing, buzzing sensation from head to toe on the left side of my body, and it did not stop. Initially, I thought it was a pinched nerve. In true fashion, I ignored it for several days. It went on for a week or so but lessened over time. When it wasn't improving, I decided to see a doctor at a walk-in clinic. They sent me to the emergency room (ER), which eventually led me to neurology. I remember being in the hospital and getting nervous, thinking to myself, why aren't they being direct with me? Not to mention we were missing trick-or-treating with my kids (who were one and four at the time). I remember looking at my husband with tears in my eyes, asking, "What if it's multiple sclerosis?" He dismissed that idea because I was so healthy —not even possible. The buzzing eventually stopped, and I returned to what I deemed normal after a week. I still saw the neurologist at the request of my mother. In my mind, the buzzing stopped, so why go? Had I not gone, I could have progressed more. This first visit essentially "caught it early". In December of 2019, they diagnosed me with transverse myelitis. I had a lesion on my cervical spine. I had never heard of this diagnosis. The neurologist kept talking to me about MS. I remember being so angry at him. Why did he keep bringing up MS? Why would he allude to the fact that transverse myelitis could lead to MS? Since I had recently completed my functional nutrition training, I had the knowledge to request specific blood values be tested since deficiencies can mimic that of autoimmune diseases, like MS. I requested my vitamin D3 be checked, along with my B12 and inflammation markers, including CRP and homocysteine. I wouldn't be notified until months later of the results. According to functional medicine ranges, my D3 was deficient, and my inflammatory markers were high (this told me my body was in a chronic state of inflammation). According to western medicine, they were within "normal" limits.

In true Adria fashion, I began researching all things transverse myelitis and did not like what I was learning. I agreed to do a follow-up MRI in six months to monitor my progress. January 2020, I was progressively having more anxiety, panic attacks on the way to work, in my office, and at home, accompanied by sleepless nights. I was still experiencing extreme fatigue, plus joint pain like nothing I had experienced before. Every joint hurt. I couldn't run because my ankles and knees hurt so bad. I couldn't lift my arms above my head because my shoulder joints were so painful. I couldn't sit for extended periods of time because my hips ached. I experienced what I call heavy legs—it was as if I had sandbags strapped to my legs, and I had to concentrate on moving my legs to walk. I had a baby the year prior, and I couldn't lose my baby weight. I was barely eating and working out harder than ever to combat the stress, but I was only getting worse. I was deteriorating. I was experiencing Lhermitte's (when you look down, an electrical sensation runs down the back and into the toes). It sounded like tissue paper in my neck every time I moved it from side to side. I was riddled with anxiety attacks, depression, and hopelessness. When you're so far in, you don't realize how dark your world has become. You have adapted and lost pieces of yourself. You stop laughing, smiling—trying to survive one day at a time. You chalk it up to a new baby, breastfeeding, lack of sleep, a toddler, everything that comes with working full time, running a home, and producing meals. Relationships become strained. One day you look in the mirror and don't recognize the person looking back. Who and what have I become? What's wrong with me?

No one on the planet could predict what the whole world would endure over the course of the next two years. COVID. I was traveling abroad for work and was in Budapest when COVID broke. Initially, like the rest of the world, I shrugged it off as just another virus. As the months progressed and things were locked down, my health deteriorated. In February of 2020, I lost my job. Less than three weeks later, the world was in lockdown. To say my stress was heightened was an understatement. I had a one-year-old and a four-year-old, loss of significant income, and now my health—my whole family's health—was at risk. The world shut down, and it was the perfect storm of my world falling apart. Never in the history of humankind had we experienced anything like this. Like the rest of the world, we adapted. We stayed home, we took walks on the trails, we made rainbow hearts on our windows, we cooked, we drank, we binge watched all the shows, we facetimed, and we kept our family safe.

In June of 2020, I went for my follow-up MRI. I was given the diagnosis of multiple sclerosis on July 9, 2020. It was the worst day of my life. I remember the doctor delivering the news as nonchalantly as a weather report. What I remember is him showing me the MRI image with the lesion on the right side of my brain and saying, "You'll take a pill the rest of your life and most likely won't end up in a wheelchair. We don't really see that anymore." I remember sort of blacking out. I will NEVER forget the look on my mother's face. I know that look. As a mother, you never want to have your child diagnosed with an incurable, debilitating disease. She instantly went into "mom" mode, and I am grateful to her for asking the questions I couldn't, having the strength to stay strong and levelheaded. Not once breaking—not one damn time. I admire her strength and courage because right then and there, I was shattered into a million pieces. Who would pick up my pieces? I remember my mother and the doctor speaking, but I couldn't tell you what they said. My whole world stopped. I couldn't see or hear anything around me. My life flashed before my eyes.

I remember thinking my life is over. I'll be in a wheelchair by the time my daughter is in kindergarten. I'll be dead before they are married. This isn't the life my husband signed up for. It's bizarre how the most irrational thoughts instantly enter your psyche after receiving devastating news, and it's even scarier how quickly this disease will make that mental space dark.

I remember leaving the doctor's office in a daze, and my mother saying, "We need to make a plan—we'll beat this," as matter of fact as she could. I think a small part of me wanted to believe her. I had to break the news to my husband, my dad, brothers, aunt, and my four closest friends since grade school. I remember most of them teared up and were speechless. No one expected this. I just floated through the next couple of days. At one point, I remember lying in bed one night, convincing myself I was a complete burden to my family. My husband didn't sign up for this. He shouldn't have to take care of a disabled wife.

How would this affect my children? Would I embarrass them? Would they get sick of having to answer that question of, "What's wrong with your mom?" In my darkest moment, I decided they would be better off without me. The kids were young enough that they wouldn't remember me, so there'd be no emotional pain to deal with. Let's face it, my kids are adorable—who wouldn't want to take them on? My husband was young and vibrant. He would easily find someone to love again without the burden of an incurable disease dampening his "happily ever after". That night, I made the decision for them. When I got bad enough, I would end it (thinking this would be sooner than later at the rate I was feeling).

I slept well that night. Early the next morning, I woke up to Jack, my son, telling me I needed to get up and make him breakfast. He was hungry. I looked at the baby monitor, and Charlotte (Charlie) was bopping up and down in her crib, and the dog was barking to go outside. I got out of bed and started the process of "mothering". I got the dog out, the kids set up for breakfast, and started making a cup of coffee. An overwhelming feeling came over me. I didn't want the kids to see me crying, so I turned away from them. I wiped away my tears and swallowed the lump in my throat. When I turned back around, they were all at my feet, staring up at me silently. Jack asked me if momma was crying. Daisy, the dog, was dancing on her hind legs as if asking to be picked up, and Charlie was just smiling at me like she was seeing me for the first time. If this were a movie, *Eye of the Tiger* would start playing, and Mickey would shout at me, "Get up, you son of a b*tch cause Mickey loves ya!" (Rocky V 1990). If you can't tell, I'm a diehard Rocky Balboa fan.

But this is real life. At that moment, I knew I was the ONLY person for them. I would fight like hell to stay here and be healthy FOR THEM. If that meant some days, I was only operating at 10%, then my 10% would be better than zero. But let's be real, I trained my whole life thus far for this moment, and I would give nothing less than 110% to being the best damn mother on earth. That meant starting then and there with finding a cure. And for me, I eventually found it. My babies can't read right now, and they will never fully understand the profound impact they had on me at the darkest time in my life, but they truly saved me that day. They are my heartbeat, a literal extension of my aorta, and my reason WHY I fight so hard every day to be here. I hope one day, they know just how much they saved me. I love them more than words can describe, so I won't try.

I have never shared these details with anyone. I hesitated to even write it down. What would people think? In the end, I decided to include this overwhelming moment because it shines a light on how dark, lonely, and dire this disease can take a once profoundly positive, outgoing, life of the party kind of person. It changes everything about you—physically and mentally.

Growing up, and even into adulthood, I never experienced anxiety, depression, or dark thoughts. People used to tease me that glitter ran through my veins because I was extremely happy and outgoing. The darkness was all new for me, and I was not equipped to handle it. Healing my mental health would prove to be my biggest challenge as it was the hardest hurdle for me to clear. I attribute my best friend for bringing to my attention how depressed she thought I was and encouraging me to seek professional help. She made me look inward when I didn't even want to leave the house. She designed a journal personally for me when I didn't even know what to say, so I wrote. I am deeply thankful for her support in my mental health journey.

Taking care of your mental health is such an important part of healing this silent disease. I share my experience because I know I am not alone on this journey. There are others out there. If reading my story can help save another MS warrior or make them feel less alone, then that is my duty to fulfill.

I cried nonstop for weeks, months even. I still choke up thinking about those first few weeks and what my inner circle and I went through; how impersonal and cold that doctor was. After a couple of days, it sank in. I was terrified to even speak the words multiple sclerosis. It felt like a dirty secret to me. I was feeling shame and guilt around it. I was a health professional! How could I let myself get to this point? Why did I take pain medication knowing the damage it could potentially have? Why didn't I push back more when having my second child and insist on a VBAC? Why did I fight for a job where they didn't want me? Why did I keep pushing myself to the edge of exhaustion?

I decided to not accept this diagnosis, and the first neurologist had gotten it wrong. I said no to the drug reps who were stalking me every day, calling me multiple times a day to start their MS drug. There is money to be made, and I'm a walking dollar sign to them. The problem was, I just didn't feel it in my gut that meds were the answer. Something was telling me there had to be another way. The side effects of the drugs sounded worse than the disease, and with my luck, I'd be the one who ended up with the rare brain cancer they can cause. I asked the pharma rep to please stop calling, and I would reach out when I felt the time was right to start.

As I was overanalyzing what to do with my unknown future and health, I started to research natural approaches to treat the disease. I came across Dr. Embry and his son Mathew's work on treating MS naturally. Unintentionally, I ran across Mathew's documentary, Living Proof, and for the first time in a month, I had a glimmer of hope. I thought that maybe things would be okay. I won't sugar coat it; it was hard to watch. It's triggering to see MS warriors and their declining health. It's hard not to ask yourself, is that how it will be for me? Mathew's documentary led me to his site MSHope.com. Mathew's story and his father's research and development of the Best Bet Diet is truly inspiring. I continue to follow Mathew and his father's work. I am grateful for their trailblazing path while sharing evidence-based research, and their commitment to disseminating the information for anyone who will listen.

Within the Living Proof documentary, Dr. Terry Wahls is featured. Dr. Wahls was dependent on a tilt-recline wheelchair for four years (because of progressive MS), until she reclaimed her health using a diet and lifestyle program that she designed specifically to restore her cellular health. She now pedals her bike to work each day. Dr. Wahls is a clinical professor of medicine at the University of Iowa Carver College of Medicine in Iowa City, Iowa, U.S.A., where she teaches internal medicine residents in their primary care clinics. She also does clinical research and has published over sixty peer-reviewed scientific abstracts, posters, and papers. I live seventy miles from the University of Iowa (my alma mater). It is as if fate was stepping in again. I inquired to see if she was taking on patients and set up a discovery call to see if we'd be a good fit to work together. Until then, I researched and purchased her book, *The Wahls Protocol*, and dove in.

In the meantime, I managed to get into the Mayo Clinic in Rochester, MN. I got a second opinion from the head of neurology in mid-July of 2020. For weeks I had full panels of blood work drawn, more MRIs, and met with various doctors that weren't convinced it was MS initially. The lesion in my cervical spine had healed, and there was only one lesion on my right parietal lobe that seemed to be getting smaller. Eventually, they encouraged me to get a spinal tap. Initially, I was completely against it. After the trouble I had with my C-sections, I didn't want anything in my spine ever again. I did eventually agree after many tests came back normal. The spinal tap would be a determinant of what course of treatment to take. Just my luck, I had a spinal fluid leak after the procedure and was bedridden for almost a week with severe pain and headaches until my body could heal itself. The results of the spinal tap showed that what they were seeing in the cerebrospinal fluid (CSF) was consistent with what they would see in a typical MS patient. I was disheartened, but nothing like the first time the news was delivered. At this point, I had a plan.

The Rebuild
I decided then, with the support of my neurologist at Mayo, I would attempt to treat this naturally, monitoring the disease with MRIs every six months. I have done so since July of 2020. When I asked her about diet and lifestyle changes, she stated that diet had no impact on the course of the disease, but it didn't hurt to eat healthfully and not smoke. She stated her biggest concerns were her patient's mental health. Depression is one of the most prevalent psychiatric conditions in MS

patients. Today, lifetime prevalence of major depression in MS patients is estimated to be around approximately 25–50%, a number two-to-five times greater than in the general population.

Source: Feinstein A, Magalhães S, Richard JF, Audet B, Moore C. The link between multiple sclerosis and depression. Nat Rev Neurol. 2014;10:507–517.

On the way home from Mayo that day, I was mentally exhausted and unsure of the future. The little research I had done on treating MS naturally didn't seem too idealistic. If we don't have hope, then what do we have? As we exited off the interstate, I closed my eyes and asked God to show me a deer if I was making the right choice. I took a deep breath and opened my eyes. In the ditch, a large buck seemed to jump out of nowhere, looked at me, and bounded off. Other than the birth of my children, it was probably one of the most miraculous experiences I've had. I don't know why at that moment I asked God to show me a deer. It just popped into my head, and He answered. It wouldn't be the last time God winked at me. Nearly one year later, as I was preparing for another MRI, I was feeling anxious that week. A sense of doubt was creeping in, and I asked God for another sign as I was driving home. I kid you not, in the exact same spot as last time, He showed me another deer. I had to look twice to make sure I wasn't imagining things.

Last spring, the kids and I were planting flowers, and I found myself wondering, would I always be able to do this? Would I always be mobile and active? Just then, three butterflies landed on the flowers I was planting. They rested for a minute, fluttered their wings, and eventually flew off. The significance of the butterfly refers to the normal appearance of the choroid plexuses on the axial imaging of the brain in an MRI. Butterflies are symbols to me and MS patients worldwide. I felt a sense of calm, and I still carry those winks with me each time I spiral with negative thoughts. I know He's got me. Whatever your belief, look for the signs; find comfort in those moments to help ease the uncertainty that comes with this disease.

I connected with Dr. Wahls at the University of Iowa in fall of 2020. I was going to work with her individually as a patient; however, she was recruiting for a clinical trial for those with Relapsing-Remitting MS (RRMS) and had not started on any disease modifying treatments to treat MS. I instead opted to be a subject in her RRMS research study for the next year. Throughout fall of 2020 and all of 2021, I followed a very strict, modified paleo diet, targeted supplements, mental health and breath work, and exercise to complete the study as a compliant subject.

Surveys and phone interviews were conducted. Journaling and support calls were encouraged with other subjects in the trial.

That first year connecting with Dr. Wahls, her team, and the other subjects in the study was truly a gift from God. I can say with 100% certainty I would not be doing as well as I am today if it was not for that experience and the specific education provided. It saved my quality of life, my health, and provided me support through those who were "walking in my shoes". My family and friends provide me with the support and love needed to keep going each day, but the small group, whom I still stay in contact with today, lifts me up and can relate to life with MS. They, too, are working towards good health daily. Our group motto is, "If Dr. Wahls can get out of a wheelchair, then we can keep ourselves from getting into one." And we live by that. If there is an opportunity to be a part of Dr. Wahls's team and her clinical trials, I highly encourage it. She is my hero and an angel on earth who wants to change the way healthcare treats incurable diseases like MS, and give us hope that we can thrive in life after diagnosis. I will never be able to repay her for giving me my quality of life back, but I will honor her legacy each day by staying true to the cause and paying it forward to those who are diagnosed after me.

One of the hardest parts for me was not personally knowing anyone who was diagnosed with MS and thriving. My only experience with the disease was a family friend who had passed away from complications, along with others who were quite limited in mobility. I was terrified. I thought that was how life would be. Throughout my journey, I have met so many wonderful souls who are thriving after diagnosis, and we all treat the disease differently. It is important to find support in your community for those living with MS. In Iowa, I was lucky to connect with a non-profit, MS Moments, just this past winter. Their mission is to provide financial assistance in the form of grants to Iowan's and their immediate families. It is so much more than that. It is unique in the way it brings MS warriors and their families together in positive, fun ways to keep the community engaged, active, and supportive of a cause that affects more than just those living with the disease. Another group I have ran across is First Descents. First Descents provides life-changing outdoor adventures for young adults impacted by cancer and other serious health conditions like MS. I encourage you to seek out their information. Research similar organizations in your state or country to find support throughout your healing journey.

MS affects everyone differently. I think that is why it is so difficult to diagnose and treat. We are all individuals, and we must choose the healing path we feel is right for us and what we can stay consistent with as life evolves. There is no right or wrong way to treat this disease. For me, I am one giant walking experiment. Over the course of the last three years, I have tried many holistic approaches and feel confident I have found what works best for me.

To treat MS the way I do takes discipline, and you must want it enough to be consistent and dedicated each day. It is not for everyone. If medication is your chosen route to treat the disease, I still believe a paleo diet and supplements should be implemented. The disease modifying drugs (DMDs) are not treating the root cause of your disease. It is essential to work with a functional doctor, or a doctor who supports your treatment course. Look inward at your lifestyle to help you determine what the root cause is. Most people with an autoimmune disease like MS are vitamin D3 deficient, according to functional medicine ranges. There more than likely was some chronic stress, trauma, or exposure to environmental factors that occurred before diagnosis. Consuming a Standard American Diet (SAD) can cause chronic inflammation, as well as stress with work and family responsibilities. Pinpointing the where and why of the disease can prevent you from repeating the habits that are contributing to the progression of the disease. Treating the root cause and stopping the inflammation is key in managing this disease. DMDs address inflammation, but they also suppress your immune system. I was diagnosed during COVID, and the thought of tampering with my immune system during the pandemic didn't feel like the answer. There is a reason the drugs stop working overtime, and you may have to try multiple drugs over the course of your life. DMD's might be needed in certain cases, and many choose this route. This is completely acceptable. I am not against medication. I do feel strongly, however, that finding the root cause of your disease is just as important as treating it.

The way I treat my disease is through a very strict, modified paleo diet. Initially after diagnosis and throughout the clinical trial I was involved in, I eliminated all gluten, dairy, soy, corn, nightshades, legumes, alcohol, grains, eggs, sugar, processed foods, and oils. If you do nothing else, give up dairy and gluten. Scientific data shows the proteins in gluten contribute to increased gut permeability and food proteins can leak through the intestines, firing up the immune system. With MS, the body attacks the myelin sheath. Avoiding gluten can help keep those gut junctures tight. Science shows that dairy proteins closely resemble the proteins in myelin. When the immune system encounters dairy through consumption, it gets sensitized to the myelin and attacks the myelin sheath. This is what we are trying to avoid with MS.

After the food elimination phase, I slowly reintroduced certain nightshades and grains to see if I had any reactions to them. This is a strategic process, and if interested, I encourage you to work with a functional medicine or nutrition expert to help educate and guide you on how particular foods can affect you. Since the research trial has ended, I still maintain the paleo diet for the most part. I have reintroduced organic, pasture-raised eggs with no issues but only eat them one to two times a month. I do eat more nightshades than I have in the past. I know which ones I do well on and in certain amounts. I have incorporated rice into my diet at a minimal amount—this girl loves sushi! I may have rice a couple of times a month, and I'm satisfied with that. I also love popcorn, so I pop my own at home a couple of times a month (organic non-GMO), drizzled with olive oil, salt, and nutritional yeast.

In addition to a varied plant-based diet with quality protein, fiber, and healthy fats, fermented foods are another important aspect for a healthy gut. Most fermented foods contribute bacteria that have a potential probiotic effect. This means that these bacteria may help restore the balance of bacteria in your gut, support digestive health, and alleviate any digestive issues. A healthy gut makes for a strong gut-brain axis and is essential in managing MS. The gut-brain axis is a bidirectional communication network that links the enteric and central nervous systems. This network is not only anatomical, but it extends to include endocrine, humoral, metabolic, and immune routes of communication, as well.

Throughout this process, I have become so in-tune with my body that I now know what foods I need to incorporate each day to feel my best. If I slack on that routine, I feel it. I try to buy in season produce and organic when available, as well as grass-fed beef, organic meats and wild seafood. Green smoothies are almost a daily staple. I call it a salad in a cup. This is one way for me to knock out six cups of leafy greens, with a serving of brightly colored frozen fruit (i.e., dark cherries, wild blueberries, aronia berries, or raspberries, etc.), a chunk of organic fresh ginger, cold flax oil, a tbsp of nut butter, a scoop or two of Paleovalley dried bone broth protein, matcha powder or cacao powder, camu and acerola cherry powder, all incorporated into one large smoothie. Not only does this provide a nutrient dense meal, but it is anti-inflammatory, as well.

Investing in a commercial grade blender will provide a huge advantage. I use my Vitamix blender daily, and it pulverizes the smoothies. I make sure to have a quality protein at every meal, in addition to a sulfur-rich food (arugula, brussel sprouts, asparagus, bok choy, cruciferous veggies like broccoli or cauliflower, cabbage, onions, garlic, etc.) or brightly colored fruits or veggies. There is a science to eating this strategically and why it is important to incorporate particular foods and food groups daily to maintain health. This education is already widely available and would take another thirty chapters for me to go through. I encourage you to seek out Dr. Wahls's Protocol or the Best Bet Diet for more information.

I won't pretend eating this strictly was easy initially. I am a dietitian and still had to drastically change the way I looked at food and how I fed my body to heal. I cried in the grocery store on more than one occasion and was completely overwhelmed. Reading food labels and ingredient lists will be key. Your once go-to comfort meals and family staples will need an overhaul. You'll grow sick of cooking some days and just want to eat whatever you can get your hands on. For a couple weeks when I initially overhauled my diet, I felt unwell, like I had the flu and wanted to give up (my body was detoxing). I assumed it wasn't working for me. But one morning after sticking to it for a couple weeks, I woke up and felt better than I had in years—and I never looked back. I think I felt sick because I quit all foods cold turkey. Had I eased into it, I would have had an easier time.

The biggest tips I can provide are to find your food staples and stick to them. Reading food labels is helpful as they must call out common allergens at the end of the ingredients list. For me, especially when I travel, meat sticks like Chomps or Nicks are my go-to. Paleovalley superfood bars (my favorite flavors are chocolate and apple) have been a lifesaver as far as convenience and travel items. Many paleo brands like Siete, Simple Mills, Hu, Jovial grain-free pastas, and Primal Food products offer compliant substitutes for your pantry. There is a plethora of paleo food products out there. Some are great to help calm that craving or a great substitute for products you miss.

Food prep will become so important. I always have a compliant soup, a meat prepared like organic rotisserie chicken or ground beef, and chopped veggies to assemble meals quickly. Not being prepared is setting yourself up for failure. Find ways that work for your schedule to always have compliant foods ready to go after a long day. Because of COVID, we did not eat out for close to one and half years. As awful as COVID was for so many, it did force me to deal with my mental health and familiarize myself with cooking dishes at home that didn't leave me feeling deprived.

Don't limit your meals to what society deems meal appropriate. Breakfast foods were the hardest for me. Now it is not uncommon for me to eat leftovers for breakfast, make a green smoothie, have a sausage scramble with some kind of veggie, or have soup using bone broth for added nutrition and protein. Sipping on bone broth after some water first thing in the morning can be very nutrient dense and healing to the gut. One cup offers nine grams of quality protein and contains the amino acid L-glutamine that is extremely healing to the gut if you're dealing with "leaky gut" or gut permeability.

In addition, I do a natural fast since we typically eat an early dinner with kids around 5:30 pm, and I tend to not eat before 8 am the following morning. Fasting is tricky. If it works for you and you feel great doing it, then continue to do so. If you feel you struggle with it or feel unwell, shorten your hours of fasting. Fasting can be hard on women, specifically when trying to balance and manage hormones. I also encourage you to not drink coffee on an empty stomach. Fasting, plus caffeine on an empty stomach, is setting yourself up for an imbalance of hormones and cortisol spikes, which can lead to insulin resistance.

Over the course of the years, I have found staple dishes I never grow tired of. They leave me full and satisfied. Examples of my go-to dishes are tacos or taco salads with organic grass-fed beef, spaghetti squash lasagna bowls, dairy-free clam chowder, salmon patties, pork lettuce cups, and cauliflower rice. My family loves shrimp fried cauliflower rice or buffalo chicken bowls with cilantro lime cauli rice. We also enjoy smoked trout and roasted potatoes and veggies, various soups and stews, as well as stir-fries and scrambles.

I try new things—sometimes they work, and sometimes they flop. Look for paleo recipes online, knowing you'll have to modify ingredients to be compliant for what works for you. Over the years, I have found online food bloggers like paleorunningmomma.com, cookprimalgourmet.com, 40aprons.com, againstallgrain.com, and Dr Wahls have plentiful recipe options for inspiration.

Lean on family to help, try new dishes, get the kids involved, and/or get your family to eat like you! It will only set them up for success in the future. As my kids have grown older and understand mommy can't have gluten or dairy and I must eat healthy for my brain, it makes them interested in how food provides nutrients to their little bodies. We have not discussed the words multiple sclerosis with them. I feel they are too young to understand at this point, but we do spend a lot of time discussing health and how what we do today affects our bodies as we age.

I allow my family to still eat gluten, dairy, and have treats in moderation. I know my children are more at risk of developing an AI disease. When they are old enough to understand, I will educate them on the importance of limiting some of their food intake. But most importantly, making sure their vitamin D3 levels are in optimal ranges is the most preventative measure I can take for them right now.

Having food around that I cannot consume doesn't bother me anymore. When someone offers me something, I politely say no, thank you. When we go out to eat, I tell the server I have a gluten and dairy allergy, and I've never been met with any disputes. Early on, I would bring my own salad dressing in a small container or cassava chips for a side. I review the menu before going to a restaurant. If attending a social gathering, I bring a dish I know is compliant.

I often get asked if I cheat, and the answer is no. There really isn't anything I truly miss that I haven't found a substitute for. The only thing I do still think about is a good slice of pizza, and that's because of the ooey gooey cheese. I desperately miss cheese. There is no dairy-free substitute that truly embodies a good, aged cheese. I was the queen of dairy prior to my diagnosis. I had it at every meal. But no food is worth being in a wheelchair. Dramatic, I know, but that is how I think of it.

In addition to a strict diet, I incorporated acupuncture, chiropractic care, psychotherapy, and massage therapy monthly. These have made a huge impact on me regaining my mental and physical health. I'm lucky to have a mother and brother who are chiropractors and a father and brother who are veterinarians. We come from science-backed training. My family has been instrumental in not only supporting me, but also talking through the physiology of the disease. There were many days or nights I'd call any one of them sobbing about one of my symptoms, and they would listen, discuss the mechanisms with me, and calm me with the reassurance that I was not progressing or that my lesion wasn't active. Early on, that is where my thoughts immediately jumped with any twinge, tingle, or twitch. Now I know that sometimes things pop up, and it is not always MS related. It can be due to aging, injury, sickness, or just life in general. Over the years, I have learned what affects my body negatively. For example, alcohol doesn't work well with my gut health. Consecutive nights of poor sleep negatively affect me. Oats make me tingle.

Stress brings on fatigue or tinnitus. We will never escape stress, but having resources to manage stress is imperative to controlling disease activity. Viruses like COVID or the flu linger on for me longer than "normal" people and can cause symptoms related to MS to flare-up. I had COVID at the end of 2021 and was in rough shape for about a month. I had to receive fluids daily at the walk-in clinic, and the nausea kept me from being able to eat or drink much for weeks. I lost about fifteen pounds in one month and was so fatigued and weak, I could barely function. I lost 60% of my hair, had gut inflammation for eight months afterward, and continuously lost weight. I could barely eat anything without GI distress and had to heal my gut all over again.

In December of 2022, I had the flu virus like I had never experienced before. I quickly recovered in general, but the lingering effects of fatigue, low blood pressure, and dizziness remained. Had this happened a couple years ago, I would have been riddled with anxiety and panic attacks thinking something was wrong, but I now know this is just life with an autoimmune disease, and I am armed with education and resources on what to do to alleviate the occurrences. It took years to get to this point. When I start to feel off, I ask myself, what did I eat the day before or even days ago? Did I get my rest? Did I do my breathwork? Do I need to slow down? Was I recently sick? Asking yourself these questions is a way to check yourself on where you might be slacking and where things might need to be tightened up. In the beginning, keep a journal to track your habits and symptoms. Life is going to throw us curve balls—be prepared to swing.

I have discussed the importance of mental health work throughout my journey. Psychotherapy was influential for me when I realized I couldn't fix what I was going through on my own. I had no experience with poor mental health. It is important to find the right therapist for your needs. I am not one that likes to "talk" about my issues. I prefer to just forge on. I wanted to be armed with tools and resources to revert to when issues arose. Eye movement desensitization and reprocessing (EMDR), accelerated resolution therapy (ART), acceptance and commitment therapy, brain spotting, manifesting, and guided self-hypnosis were influential tactics used to help me work through my problems. I started a gratitude journal and still do this each morning. Even if it is five minutes of writing down what I'm grateful for—even if it hasn't happened yet. I visualize stable and clear MRI's. I envision a Pacman in my brain chomping down on all my lesions to produce a clear and healthy brain. This is particularly helpful when lying in the dreadful MRI machines.

Another imperative aspect of my mental health is meditating, prayer, and breathwork. Any of these you can find on YouTube or phone apps. I particularly use the *Headspace* app for guided meditations each morning or when feeling particularly anxious or stressed. Breathwork can be as simple as breathing in to the count of four, holding your breath to the count of seven, and releasing the breath to the count of eight (4-7-8 technique). There is also the box method, along with countless types of breathwork methods, and other ways to stimulate the vagus nerve to calm the nervous system.

Exercise is also imperative in managing any disease and stress. If you rest, you rust. For me, learning how to exercise and not overdo it was a challenge at first. As an athlete and someone who relished challenges (i.e., mud runs, marathons, triathlons, intensive hikes, waters sports, snowboarding, etc.), it wasn't a workout unless I was left dripping in sweat or spent two hours at the gym. There is such a thing as working out too much. It stresses the body and can contribute to inflammation. Slowing down and working out less intensely has helped me improve over the years. What does this look like? I do something every day. It could be a walk, run, weight training, yoga, biking, stretching, swimming, or chasing my kids at the park. The key is it doesn't have to be a high intensity workout every day. Just moving your body, getting steps in, and raising the heart rate for a short period of time will be beneficial. Doing more weight resistance training and building solid muscle mass as I age will be a key factor in managing my disease for years to come. I don't go to any fancy gyms or classes anymore. I have a treadmill and free weights in my basement. I tune into apps, Youtube or Netflix for yoga or short HIIT sessions, and I modify according to my needs. You don't have to push yourself to the point of exhaustion—you just need to move your body daily and consistently.

Over the years, I have watched or listened to what feels like every podcast, movie, or book written on autoimmune disease and functional medicine. I devour anything related to Dr. Wahls's work. Her movie *Defying All Odds* was a beautiful inspiration. I receive her e-newsletters and follow her on social platforms. I read her research publications and keep a finger on the pulse of any upcoming work she has in the pipeline.

Other podcasts I have tuned into are: *The Doctor's Farmacy* with Dr. Mark Hyman, *The Genius Life* with Matt Lugavere, *Wholistic Matters*, and countless others. MSHope and Dr. Embry and Mat Embry's work, including their question-and-answer segment Tuesdays on Facebook live, is educational. There are numerous functional medicine doctors I follow on Instagram and many MS books that allude to different ways not only to look at the disease but how to manage it spiritually and physically. As I said, I am my own science experiment. I keep learning and incorporating new health techniques to see if I feel any benefit. I am an ever-evolving human living with MS.

I have a Durasage sauna I sit in three-to-four times a week, and immediately take a cold plunge or shower after. I do cryotherapy every couple of months, and I exercise daily. We have installed a reverse osmosis water filtering system in our home for our drinking water. Most city waters aren't as clean as I would like. The reverse osmosis system is wonderful at removing all the contaminants you would not want in your drinking water; however, it also removes the trace minerals you do want in your drinking water. This means you'll have to add back trace minerals to your drinking water. This is important so your body is not depleted of the trace minerals needed for proper biological functioning.

We use an AirDoctor air purifier in our bedroom. We have had our home tested for mold. I have incorporated more plants throughout the home. I have a year-round herb garden in my kitchen on the wall, so I have access to fresh herbs even in the winter, and we plant a garden every spring. I swapped all food storage containers to glass. We no longer use plastic in our home when storing food or water bottles. We incorporated new cookware like cast iron or ceramic. I no longer use any pans with PFAS, also known as the forever chemical. You typically see PFAS in nonstick coatings. I upgraded our mattress to one that is organic with no "off-gassing" and use organic, cotton bedding. I gradually switched all my skin and beauty products over to safer ingredients. This was a process. I changed what makeup I used, skin care, toothpaste, soap, lotion, deodorant, and hair care. Thankfully, there are so many cleaner options out there. Find what works best for you and your family. It took me some trial and error.

A great tool I use to look up clean products is the *EWG Healthy Living* app. Not all products are on there, but it is continuously being updated. You can look up products by category, and it shows the ingredients with their rating according to the Environmental Working Group. I have switched over to safer cleaning products, hand soap, and laundry detergent, using Branch Basics.

I stick to my sleep schedule, even on the weekends, and make sure I'm getting my eight-to-nine hours of sleep each night in a cool, dark room. If you struggle with sleep, as many MS warriors do, there are many sleep habits you can incorporate into your daily routine to improve your quality of sleep. Sleep is so important because it is your body's time for cellular repair. Getting natural sunlight first thing in the morning can help regulate your circadian rhythms. Circadian rhythms are physical, mental, and behavioral changes that follow a twenty-four-hour cycle. These natural processes respond primarily to light and dark and affect most living things. Being out in nature and limiting light exposure at night can help regulate this natural process.

My supplement list feels extensive and ever evolving, but what I have found that works for me over the years is as follows. I take vitamin D3 + K2. Vitamin D3 is not only a vital fat-soluble vitamin, but it's also a hormone that is essential for initiating several important biological processes. Vitamin K2 is essential for their completion and expression. When diagnosed, I requested my vitamin D3 levels be checked. They were at 25 ng/mL. I was told that was normal. With my functional nutrition training, I knew better. Anything below 70 ng/ml will affect how I'm feeling. It is essential to have your vitamin D3 levels checked one-to-two times a year and know your numbers. Don't rely on western medicine ranges to make that decision for you. Listen to your body. My sweet spot is in the 80's. This winter I had my D3 checked, and it had dropped to the low 60's. That, coupled with the flu virus, had me feeling off. I upped my D3+K2 intake and have been feeling better. Now, this recommendation isn't for everyone. It is best to know your body, numbers, and what works for you. More is not always better either. You ideally want that D3 sweet spot of 70-100 ng/mL when dealing with autoimmunity. Talk with your doctor to see what works for you.

In addition to D3+K2 each morning, I take Nordic Naturals omega 3 fatty acids, magnesium threonate, NAC, phosphatidylcholine, and a methylated B12, B6, and folate. The methylated forms are important because they are already activated and more readily absorbed and bioavailable for the body to use. In the afternoon, I take an activated B-100 complex, organ meat supplements (because I just can't tolerate eating organ meats), curcumin, and every other day, chlorella. In the evening, I take magnesium glycinate, zinc, selenium, a spore-based probiotic, and mushroom adaptogens. It is important to have testing done to tailor the right supplement regimen for your body. The supplements I take have specific and targeted purposes. For example, there are seven different forms of magnesium. They can serve different purposes. Knowing the forms of the supplements you take, and their purpose, is imperative. It is a highly unregulated industry, so choosing reputable companies is crucial. Many of the supplements in my regiment are antioxidants with anti-inflammatory properties. Others are targeted for mitochondrial health. The classic role of mitochondria is oxidative phosphorylation, which generates ATP by utilizing the energy released during the oxidation of the food we eat. ATP is used in turn as the primary energy source for most biochemical and physiological processes, such as growth, movement, and homeostasis. Dysfunction of the mitochondria and a resulting depleted energy supply is thought to contribute to the damage of nerves and subsequent disability. That is why minding your mitochondria is so important in managing MS and its symptoms, particularly fatigue.

I take CBD oil some nights or arnica for when I have menstrual cramps, or any pain that needs alleviating. I no longer take NSAIDS. I had a stool analysis done to check for parasitic infections. I have dabbled in parasite cleansing using specific herbs, but this is something I only recently began educating myself on. It is important to understand herbs can interact with specific medications and are dangerous at copious levels, so I would only advise this under a health professional's guidance.

I had a hair tissue mineral analysis done (HTMA), and it showed I was under A LOT of stress! YA THINK? And that my body was depleted of a lot of trace minerals. It also showed the heavy metals aluminum and mercury in my system at low levels. I have two mercury fillings (hello, I'm an 80's baby) that I am considering having removed.

Aluminum exposure is from aluminum filled deodorants, which I have stopped using, and food/beverage packaging. Because of this testing, I know I have a fast metabolism. I run through my minerals, for example, copper and magnesium, quickly—especially when stressed. Because of my fast metabolism, I need to use a B-100 complex. Not everyone will have the same results. You can order this testing from a functional or holistic practitioner, per your request. I know @nutritionbyrobyn on Instagram is a functional RD, and she runs HTMA testing bundles where she sends you the kit.

I also had a food sensitivity test done (ELISA). Now, food sensitivity testing is controversial. I think if done properly and with the right testing, it can be a helpful tool to help you navigate your healing journey. When I tested myself for food sensitivities, the company I used was US BioTek. It uses three main immunoglobulins in their testing: IgG (1,2,3), IgA, and IgG4. They test these antibodies separately to establish a clear picture of what food triggers may be the root cause of patients' symptoms. I used BioTek because as a practitioner, I could order my own testing. It is important to understand if your body is under chronic inflammation, this test might yield a different result than if your body is at a calmer state. When I took this test, I had not eaten dairy, gluten, soy, corn, sugar, eggs, etc. for a year. All those items showed up as "safe" foods because I had not been exposed to them. That doesn't mean I am not reactive to them.

It means my body had not been exposed to those foods, so there was no intolerance at that point in time. It did show intolerances to bananas, Brazil nuts (two Brazil nuts a day meets your daily selenium needs which is important for thyroid health), some cruciferous veggies, vanilla, and some other foods. I have never noticed any issues with bananas, nuts, or vanilla, but I'm conscious of my consumption of them. Because of my food elimination diet and reintroduction phase the year prior, I was aware of the effects some veggies had on me, particularly some of the high sulfur ones. I know I can't eat a lot of veggies raw, or indigestion, gas, and bloating occur. Same thing happens with some nightshade veggies. Food sensitivity testing is expensive and can lead to inaccurate results. The best way to truly understand your food sensitivities is through an elimination diet, followed by a reintroduction phase. A nutrition expert can help assist you with this.

I'm happy to report that since 2020, my MRI's have always been stable, no new or active lesions (I've had four MRIs since 2020), no inflammation, and no disease activity. The lesion margins appear to be shrinking. This has shocked my doctors at Mayo. They tell me to keep doing what I'm doing, and they'll see me next year, unless any issues arise.

As you may know, regardless of how one chooses to treat this unpredictable disease, it comes at an extreme cost. Not only financially, but mentally to the individual and family. I did not incorporate all these changes overnight. It takes time and money. These are all things I have managed to slowly incorporate over the last three years. I think it is important to note that early on, you will be consumed with learning, devouring anything you can get your hands on related to the disease. It's natural to want to educate yourself and compare other people's stories; however, I think it is beneficial to not let it consume your every thought. It is important to take a step back and still enjoy life, finding happiness in the interests and hobbies that make you "you".

You define your life. Don't let this disease, or one doctor's opinion, write your life's script. I will continue to explore and dedicate my time and energy to health and happiness, not only for myself, but for my family. As of today, I am living proof that nutrition and lifestyle can be one possibility used to control and manage this incurable and unpredictable disease.

I can say that I'm 100% healthier now than I ever have been. It is not just ONE thing that has changed my health. It is the synergistic effect of ALL THE THINGS. I can't eat healthy and not exercise or address stress. That is like bringing a spray bottle to a house fire. It doesn't help! You must get the body back in balance while staying positive and consistent, knowing when to pivot when something is out of whack and having the tools and resources to know how to accomplish such an undertaking.

My family teases me that I'll outlive them all. I have almost gotten back to my "old self", but I am forever changed. I think with this disease, it is important to grieve your old life and find passion in almost a rebirth of yourself. Cry over that food you miss, cry over the inconvenience this disease can have on our daily lives, be angry, scream, shout, get it out of your body! It is important to release those feelings. There is no timeline for healing. It is what feels right for you.

It took me a year before I could speak the words "multiple sclerosis" out loud. It was even longer before I could talk about it and not cry. Early on, the support of my husband and his unwavering positivity and compassion of allowing me to choose the path that was right for me was essential. I went against what all the medical professionals were telling me, and he never questioned my choices. He is the most selfless human and works so hard to provide for our family. I know the last three years have not been easy. There were moments where I wouldn't have blamed him if he wanted to walk away—but he never did. He was strong when I couldn't be. He was a positive light when I had been dark for so long. I have fallen in love with him all over again because in marriage, it's the hard times that truly test your strength, love, and compassion for one another. I'm grateful my husband stands with me.

"The ultimate measure of a man is not where he stands in moments of comfort and convenience, but where he stands at times of challenge and controversy." – Martin Luther King, Jr.

The support from my parents from day one has been profound. Not only the emotional support through some excruciatingly painful moments, but the physical support, too. Both my parents also incorporated the dietary changes that I made into their own lives. They both have improved their overall health and have come off several medications. I know when they look at me, they hate that I go through all this. But they have faith in me because they raised me to be strong, stubborn, and determined to defy the odds of what most doctors have told me. As a chiropractor, my mother has been key in my treatment with her unique training in sacral occipital technique (SOT), activator methods, trigger point, myofascial release and unwinding, and bioenergy synchronization technique (BEST). I'm so grateful for the parents who raised me. They are the true definition of what parents should be.

Good parenting involves parents living their lives as role models. I've been blessed with the best, and this includes my father-in-law. Both of my brothers, their spouses, my extended family, my in-laws, and my best friends will never fully understand the impact they have had on me through my healing journey. Never once has anyone in my inner circle questioned or made me doubt my choice on how I'm treating my disease. I know this support is rare after speaking with others. I encourage you to surround yourself with those who support and lift you up. It is not the quantity of people around you, it's the quality of those you allow into your safe space. Choose the ones that will improve your happiness, lessen your misery by doubling your joy, and who will divide your grief. To this day, I haven't announced or told many people about my diagnosis.

Treating MS in any way is hard! What is going to motivate you to stick with it? You must find your reason "why". What motivates you to want to get better? For me, that "why" is my children. I can honestly say if it wasn't for them, I'm not sure I'd still be here. Looking in their little faces each day, knowing they need me keeps me going. They are the reason I get out of bed each day. They need me as much as I need them. I want to be there for them when I'm old! I want to chase after my grandbabies and be a part of their life as my parents are for my children. I'm in it for the long haul.

"The secret of change is to focus all your energy, not on fighting the old, but on building the new." – Socrates.

Redecorate
Plan A for me was treating my disease naturally, and I have done so through trial and error for the last three years. I'll continue to do so, as long as it keeps working. I know what I'm doing now is something I can sustain for a lifetime, God willing. I will always be evolving and modifying to fit my life, but I have a benchmark of non-negotiables. I do monitor the disease through annual MRIs. I cannot say for certain this is something I will continue every year. The anxiety, stress, and anticipation of the results is far more stressful and dreadful than it's worth.

One of the most memorable pieces of advice I received during the Wahls clinical trial was from the physical therapist. She always reminded us that an MRI is just a snapshot in time—a picture. It does not define the overall representation of our journey. It is more important to focus on how we are feeling in general. If we are feeling stronger and symptoms are subsiding, that is more telling of our health than an MRI image. Don't put too much stock in that "snapshot".

If for some reason my health declines, my plan B is a hematopoietic stem cell transplantation (HSCT). HSCT is an intense chemotherapy treatment for MS. It aims to reset the immune system by wiping it out and then regrowing it, using your stem cells. It comes with huge risks, side effects, and financial costs. Having a plan gives me peace and comfort. I think the most jarring thing when I was newly diagnosed was not having a plan, hope, or answers. It took me years to find them, and looking back —it was a hard, dark journey. I don't wish those dark moments of hopelessness on anyone. Over the course of the years, I have found myself asking "why me?" Why do bad things happen to good people?

The answer I have found is looking at this disease as a gift. I had to find a silver lining in the darkness. I have concluded that God is showing me my purpose for the next chapter of my life. He had to break me to show me why he created me. There are some people who will be content just "being", but some of us have been chosen by God to be "broken". I had to suffer with this disease. But when the breaking was done, I was able to see the reason for which He created me—for me to live a healthier life for my family and educate others to do the same.

As a dietitian with a focus in functional nutrition, I have slowly started a private practice and want to have a more online social presence to educate others about additional ways to treat MS. Ideally, when my kids are in school full time, I'll be able to focus on helping other newly diagnosed MS patients find hope and light through the darkness of those first few months after a life changing diagnosis.

I wish I had someone when I was first diagnosed to guide me on my options. Thankfully, I had the support, education, and awareness to ask questions, do the research, and make my own plan on how to treat my disease. I know my treatment is rather unconventional and will not work for everyone, but I think people should have options, regardless of their decision on how to treat the disease. I want to be the person that holds the new MS warrior's hand and tells them it will be okay. We can live healthy, meaningful lives. We are here to support one another—to be the light at the end of a dark tunnel. Whatever you are going through, the sun will come out. Never. Lose. Hope.

"Above all, be the heroine of your life, not the victim." – Nora Ephron

15

Story by

MARA REZO-MEDEIROS

Diagnosed in 2004

Currently 41 years old

Lives in Hamilton, Ontario, Canada

Instagram: @madame_mara9

I experienced my first flare in the year 2000 while in my first year of university. It happened during first semester exams. I noticed that I had a numb feeling on my left side from the bottom of my breast to the bottom of my feet. I went to my family doctor, and he said it was just a pinched nerve, and it would go away. The numbness lasted about a month. Thinking it was a pinched nerve, I continued with life, not giving it much thought. It came back four months later during exams. This continued happening to me for four years—always around exam time.

It was not until June 2004, when my best friend, Evelin, said, "Enough is enough. We are going to go to the emergency room to get some real answers." This is when my multiple sclerosis (MS) journey began to take shape. In the emergency room, they asked me questions about my symptoms and told me that they were going to refer me to a neurologist for further testing. Within two weeks, I saw the neurologist, and a month later, I had brain and spinal magnetic resonance imaging (MRI). On

August 24, 2004, my neurologist, Dr. Michael Francis Mazurek, diagnosed me with multiple sclerosis. When he diagnosed me, he said, "You have multiple sclerosis. You will not die from this. This is not cancer. I want you to go home and read the good and the bad about MS, and I want you to come back in two weeks and let me know how you want to proceed."

So, I did just that. I read the good, the bad, and the ugly. When I finally returned to his office, I told him that I would be the girl who cures herself. He had a big smile on his face and said he would want his own child to say the same. This incredible doctor sat down with me that day, encouraging me to take my own approach to this disease. He helped me learn that my mind is my biggest ally. We also spoke about how I would be starting Teacher's College in Australia with my best friend in a few months. He said I could not have picked a better career for someone with multiple sclerosis.

After I got diagnosed, my mom obviously called my grandmother who lived in Munich, Germany. My grandmother recommended that she bring me to Germany and then to Croatia to meet her priest who was also a naturopath healer. So, my mom took me to Germany and Croatia for a month. My best friend and my boyfriend at the time also came to support me. We first arrived in Munich in September of 2004. We were there during Oktoberfest. We stayed for nearly two weeks. We did a lot of sightseeing and partying in the beer houses and clubs before heading to Croatia.

When we got to Croatia, we stayed for a week in a house by the Adriatic Sea in the region of Istria. There, we met with the Priest and brought a copy of my MRI scan, which he had requested. He looked at the results, and although I do not recall what he said about the scans, I do remember him saying that we could treat this. Each day, he performed reiki on me and had me take different herbs and supplements that he had compounded into capsules. Unfortunately, after all these years, we have lost touch, and I cannot remember exactly what was in them.

We came back to Canada, and I lived my life normally and left for Australia in January 2005. My parents told me to enjoy my adventure and just live my life as if I did not have MS. I did just that and did not have any more flare-ups because I had figured out that stress was triggering them. I finished Teacher's College, came back to my hometown, got hired as a French teacher, and have enjoyed a seventeen-year-long career, which I absolutely love.

For most of my time living with multiple sclerosis, I did not really disclose that I had the condition. I continued to do the normal things that women my age did. In 2010, I met my husband. We got married in 2011 and had our son, Niko, in 2015. I chose to have a natural birth with my son because I was told by the anesthesiologist that if I wanted to have an epidural, I had a high chance of exasperating my MS and ending up in a wheelchair, so I chose not to and had my son naturally. I also breastfed him for two years. I felt incredible throughout my pregnancy and after.

In 2018, I gave birth to my daughter. Two months into that pregnancy, I experienced a flare-up; the same flare-up I had had back in my university days. The left side of my body from just below my breast to the bottom of my toes felt numb. It did not affect me in any other way; it just felt strange having a different sensation when touching my left side compared to my right side. I was not nervous or scared at that point because I knew exactly what it was, and I also knew that since I did not have any with my son, the chances were that I was having a girl. This flare-up, like the previous ones, lasted a month.

I gave birth naturally the second time, and because I knew what to expect, I felt much more confident. I would talk to Mia while rubbing my belly every day, telling her that labor was going to be two hours and two pushes. It was a beautiful pregnancy, much like the one I had with my son. About a week before Mia was born, I had my hypnobirthing coach come to my house to give me a quick refresher. She told me that the hospital where I was giving birth had a transcutaneous electrical nerve stimulation (TENS) machine, and it would be beneficial for me to use it throughout my labor. She was right. My labor was beautiful and smooth. Mia came out in exactly two hours and two pushes with the most beautiful smile.

I believe breastfeeding my daughter for over two years kept my MS at bay. In fact, I exclusively breastfed both of my children for a combined duration of four years and eight months, taking only a four-month break when my son did not want my milk anymore.

When it comes to how I manage my multiple sclerosis, I have decided not to get any more MRIs, and my neurologist agrees with this choice. The thought process behind this is, if they discover more lesions, how will it affect my state of mind? Personally, I do not think I need to know that I have more or that nothing has changed. I think I just need to move forward and continue managing through the struggles I have. It will not make a difference to my journey.

I have never taken any multiple sclerosis medication. I have chosen to take vitamins and supplements (like vitamin D, magnesium, Lion's Mane, and multivitamins), based on my own research and informal recommendations from naturopathic doctors I have seen over the years. I pay attention to how my body is feeling when taking them to see what is working and what is not. I usually take between 5,000 to 10,000IU's of vitamin D daily. It just depends on the season. I forget here and there, but in the summertime, I do not take as much. I did not have my vitamin D levels checked when I was diagnosed because I chose to live my life as if I did not have the disease. I do not know if this was a good thing; it was just how my twenty-three-year-old mind wanted to handle the situation. I have been going to physio, doing Pilates, and following Instagram accounts, like The MS Gym and Dr. Gretchen Hawley, who specialize in physical therapy for multiple sclerosis.

If I can, I buy organic vegetables and fruits. I have also found that dairy, gluten, and sugar affect my body in a negative way. I try to avoid them the best I can. I have not always been strict on my diet. I go through phases: from being really into what I am eating, sticking to no gluten, dairy, or sugar to going into phases where that is all I want to eat. Doing this is probably worse for me as I get older. I always feel better when I cut them out of my diet, but I think that sometimes everyday life, along with any inconvenience, makes me forget, and I cheat. When I am going through these stages, my body feels horrible, and I try to get out of it as fast as I can.

Marijuana is my choice of medicine. I smoke every night once my kids are in bed to relax and help my body rest. It has been my go-to option since I was diagnosed. It works for me, although there can be some negatives. It does give me the "munchies" and depending on the amount I smoke or the THC potency, it can make me a little anxious. After all these years, I have finally figured out that I do best with sativa strains containing lower THC. I also must mention that I am obsessed with healing crystals, particularly rose quartz and amethyst. There is something about them that makes me feel stronger in coping with this disease.

I will say that for most of the time since I have been diagnosed, I have completely ignored this disease. I did not want to read much on it or participate in anything to do with it, like the MS walks and charities. I suppose I never wanted to admit it to myself. However, about three and half years ago, that changed. It happened when I was at my husband's cousin's house, and his wife introduced me to one of her friends. The lady was a former French teacher at the school I currently teach at, and she also happened to have multiple sclerosis. She asked me if I wanted to join a local group of people with MS who went out for dinner every few months and talked about their experiences. I accepted and went to a few dinners up until COVID ruined everything. Sadly, I lost touch with them all.

Last year, I met a young lady who told me about how she had been diagnosed with MS. I listened to her story, and I believed God had sent her to me, so I could show her that everything was going to be okay. I explained to her that she would also have a great career, get married, and start a family. I wanted her to look at me and know that her diagnosis was not a death sentence—that she would be able to live all her dreams. We have kept in touch since and are always in each other's corners.

Nearly twenty-three years after experiencing my first flare-up and nineteen years since my official diagnosis, I have no regrets in choosing not to take any multiple sclerosis medications. Although it is visible that I have something that is affecting me through a limp when I walk and the weakness I get from walking too long, I think about how blessed I am. I have now lived longer with MS than I have without it. Multiple sclerosis has not stopped me from living a beautiful life: traveling the world, getting married, having children, having amazingly supportive family and friends, pursuing a fulfilling career, and receiving guidance from a wonderful neurologist I have had for the past nineteen years. I want newly diagnosed people to know that they can and will get to live their dreams! It might not be the easiest of paths, but the journey is yours. Trust yourself. You are amazing. XOXO

16

Story by
KELLY KIDD

Diagnosed in 2015
Currently 44 years old
Lives in Gainesville, Florida, United States
Instagram: @Lazybiohacker

Before multiple sclerosis (MS), I was an active, healthy, fitness-obsessed mom of two kiddos. I was married to my now ex-husband, who was a professional basketball player. We met when I was a junior in college. Within three months, I was living in Europe with him where he played in the Italian and Spanish professional leagues. Within two years, my son was born. By our fourth year together, he retired, and we settled down in Birmingham, Alabama. We married after thirteen years together, and my daughter was born a year later.

My undergraduate degree was in International Business, but my passion was always fitness. I was a soccer player when I was younger and always found confidence in being strong and fit. I started weightlifting in college, got certified as a personal trainer, and ended up working most of my adult professional life in fitness, with brief excursions into private investigation and teaching.

It was during my excursion into teaching that my journey with MS began. I was three weeks away from beginning the school year as a first-year kindergarten teacher. As a mid-career change and not the grade I planned to teach, I was running around like a maniac, trying to get materials ready, writing lesson plans, and trying to get the classroom organized and decorated. This was following two years of working full-time while pursuing my master's in education. I had been running a marathon at a sprint pace for years. I also wasn't sleeping very much, often less than a couple hours a night…sometimes not sleeping at all. I was exhausted, mentally and physically.

Looking back, there was one moment that defined how I felt at that time. I remember lying on my office floor at home, surrounded by laminated materials for the classroom I was cutting out, and thinking to myself that I was so exhausted that my brain actually hurt. Not like a headache, but more like a weird, deep aching I had never felt before. I told myself I needed to stop and just go take a nap. Then I thought, I probably won't be able to fall asleep anyway. What's the worst that could happen if I just kept working? That thought, "What's the worst that can happen", has haunted me ever since that day.

I started noticing a gradual haziness in my left eye, similar to when you get lotion or soap in your eye. Everything was becoming progressively blurry. I made an appointment to see an optometrist, thinking it was just a vision issue or a mild infection. After an exam, he suggested a stronger prescription, saying it was just age-related vision deterioration. He ordered new glasses that would take a few weeks to arrive.

A few more days passed, and the haziness was getting worse. During this time, I developed an aching feeling when I looked up or to the side. I realized it was more than a vision issue. Worried, I made an appointment with my uncle, who happened to be a prestigious ophthalmologist, for a second opinion. After examining my eye, he didn't see anything suspicious but referred me to a neurologist colleague for further evaluation. This was about three o'clock on a Friday afternoon. By four that same day, I was in a magnetic resonance imaging (MRI) tube, getting a brain scan.

The MRI determined that my symptoms were caused by optic neuritis (ON). Optic neuritis occurs when swelling (inflammation) damages the optic nerve—a bundle of nerve fibers that transmit visual information from your eye to your brain. Common symptoms of optic neuritis include pain with eye movement and temporary vision loss in one eye. Findings also included three brain lesions, which were later explained to be evidence of previous demyelinating activity. The neurologist explained the results of the scan that evening. "Kelly, this combination of findings leads me to believe you may have multiple sclerosis (MS)." He recommended a high dose of Solu-Medrol (a glucocorticoid) to shorten the duration of the optic neuritis. He also referred me to a neurologist who specializes in multiple sclerosis, Dr. Emily Riser, for further testing.

I began treatment that night. Over the course of a week, my vision slowly improved. Unfortunately, the doctor neglected to order a proper tapering protocol for the steroids, and I had a terrible reaction that was much worse than the optic neuritis. One day after I finished the steroids, I had to call the nurse to request a tapering dose just to get off the couch.

When I met with Dr. Riser a week later, she took a thorough medical history and ordered a variety of tests, including extensive blood work and a spinal tap to rule out other potential causes, like lupus and Lyme disease. The history uncovered a variety of symptoms I was experiencing periodically but never considered serious. Those included tingling in the legs, sensations of hot water spilling on my thighs, chronic insomnia, chronic hives, sun sensitivity, and numbness. Watching her nod as I described the weird symptoms made me even more nervous than the waiting room filled with disabled people when I arrived for the appointment. Once the history was taken and all the exclusionary tests were complete, the diagnosis was confirmed as multiple sclerosis.

When explaining the results, Dr. Riser said we could consider it as clinically isolated syndrome (CIS) and delay treatment. The statistics were scary though, with more than 70% of CISs progressing to full-blown MS within five years. She said that with the combination of optic neuritis and multiple brain lesions, I met the criteria for diagnosis. She recommended starting treatment, which included medication for the rest of my life. She explained that her diagnosis was Relapsing-Remitting Multiple Sclerosis (RRMS), meaning that I might have future relapses, but I would likely resume normal function after the relapse resolved. She also explained that most people with RRMS go on to develop Primary-Progressive Multiple Sclerosis (PPMS) when the loss of function occurring as a "relapse" is permanent.

After explaining the statistics, Dr. Riser asked me if I needed more time to consider my options. In shock and deathly afraid of becoming handicapped, I asked her, "What do the other 30% of people do that keeps them from developing full-blown MS?"

She replied, "The research is mixed. We're not really sure…" I cut her off mid-sentence with tears in my eyes, grabbed her hands, and asked her, "Off the record, please. I have two young kids, I'm thirty-six years old—please tell me. Your waiting room is full of people every day. You know what people who do well with this diagnosis are doing differently. Please tell me what to do."

After a few moments, she replied, "Listen, if you were my daughter, I would start medication now. Copaxone is a safe drug, and it has very few side effects. Some people experience no side effects. It's not worth the risk to wait. You're young and healthy. Start treatment, and then reduce stress drastically, workout, get good sleep, eat healthy, don't join a support group (they're full of depressed people), and go on with your life. Take vitamin D every day until we get your levels up. Don't think about MS all the time." I thanked her, took out a pen, and wrote down exactly what she said.

She referred me to a sleep specialist to treat the insomnia, which was pervasive by that point. She also set me up for a nurse to come to my house to teach me how to give myself injections three times a week.

Shock and fear were understatements when remembering how I felt leaving her office that day. It all seemed unreal. I worked out three-to-four times a week religiously, ate a low-fat diet, and took pride in being healthy. I was a personal trainer in a past life, and even owned a gym, at one point. I didn't look like any of the people I saw in that waiting room. It felt like I was in a twilight zone.

I had to go home and explain to my husband that I had been diagnosed with MS, and I would have to be on medication the rest of my life. I told him that eventually, I might end up disabled if I didn't follow their advice. He was in more shock than I was. His first reaction was maybe it was a mistake. In tears, I assured him it wasn't a mistake, and I would understand if he left me because I ended-up disabled.

I told my parents, siblings, and a few friends. They were all devastated and shocked. They also questioned the diagnosis, but since my uncle was so well connected with the doctors he referred me to, we trusted their findings.

I told the new school I had just started teaching at that I may have to miss some days early in the year to travel to see the sleep specialist, and for other appointments. They were shocked and a little concerned about it being my first year and having health challenges, but they were 100% supportive.

I told my kids, who were thirteen and eight at the time, that I had an illness, but they had a great medicine for it. Even though I'd have to give myself shots a few times a week, I would be fine. Inside, nothing felt further from the truth.

A nurse, sent by the Copaxone drug company, came to my house and taught me how to give myself injections. Since the first injection, I've given myself three a week for almost eight years. I started out using the auto-inject device they give you. Once I got the hang of it, I transitioned to manual injections. The auto-inject device was more painful and left bruises sometimes.

I used to rotate through the eight sites they recommended to inject into (both thighs, both backs of arms, stomach, and hip flanks). Once I started to see skin denting (tissue breakdown) in my thighs, I stopped injecting there. The same thing eventually happened where I was injecting it in my stomach, so I stopped using that location, as well. The backs of my arms were hard to reach, and I hit a nerve once (very painful), so I stopped using that location, too. Now, I just inject it in my hip flanks. Think of the skin that spills over your jeans in the back if they're too tight, which is the only area I really have any fat. I've always been pretty lean, so finding a good fat pocket has been difficult anywhere else on my body.

Copaxone is a brand name for glatiramer acetate. I now take the generic form. The medication is about five thousand a month, billed to the insurance company. My copay would be around three hundred dollars a month, but both Copaxone and the generic product have medication assistance programs that you can enroll in for a zero copay. There are no financial requirements to qualify. It's just a five-minute phone call. With the medication assistance program, the medicine doesn't cost me anything. I figured this was a way for the drug companies to charge the insurance companies for people like me who probably wouldn't continue treatment otherwise. Either way, I'm grateful for not having to make that decision.

During the first three years, I did MRIs twice a year, as recommended. Then, I went once a year after all the previous scans had shown no evidence of progression. I haven't done an MRI in two years because of the cost and how much I hate doing them. The last one cost me over fifteen hundred dollars, and that's with good insurance. A brain MRI is different than when you get an MRI for something like your knee. Your head is strapped down, there's like forty-five minutes of super loud banging (magnets), and it's a tiny, closed tube. I didn't think I was claustrophobic until I had to slide into that tube. It's a mental challenge every time. I even took medicine for anxiety once out of fear that I was going to have a panic attack if I didn't.

Given the cost, anxiety, and lack of physical progression, my current neurologist and I have agreed that we will do another MRI at the ten-year mark, in 2025, before considering stopping the medication. Apparently, the immune system involvement in MS becomes less prevalent as we age, also reducing its involvement in relapses.

According to the *Cleveland Clinic*, the benefits of disease modifying therapies (DMTs) appear to diminish as inflammation naturally wanes. In the normal, healthy population, the immune system becomes less functional around age sixty. Observation of MS patients indicates that relapses also tend to diminish after that age, and that subsequent disease progression may not be immune-mediated, as it tends not to be associated with MRI-detectable inflammatory activity. While this current study suggests that therapy directed at the immune system may no longer benefit older patients, prior studies involving patients of all ages indicate that outcomes of DMT discontinuation based on disease stability alone tend to be less successful. Source: https://consultqd.clevelandclinic.org/disease-modifying-therapy-for-ms-discontinuing-after-age-60-appears-safe/

At the ten-year mark without progression or relapse, there is an argument that I may be categorized as having benign MS. According to my doctor, only 5-10% of people with MS ever achieve this designation. Upon more recent investigation, I've learned that the research is still evolving on this exact percentage. Some stats are as high as 64%, but most medical and peer-reviewed sources are much closer to what my neurologist told me (5-15% range). The main reason for the confusion is there's not a standard definition for benign MS.

As a single mom, I've chosen to use medication as an insurance of sorts. The ten-year mark also coincides with my daughter's high school graduation. I credit my health and lack of progression to my lifestyle, but I don't want to be so arrogant that I stop medication and end up being wrong. I consider it my responsibility to launch my kids into the world as adults capable of taking care of themselves. Until I feel like I've achieved that, I can't, in good conscience, discontinue medication. Especially since it costs me nothing and I have zero side effects other than the skin issues at the injection sites, which are largely resolved now that I'm injecting into the fat pockets on my flanks.

The first year following my diagnosis was a blur. I was a first-year kindergarten teacher and had two very busy kids who were both involved in athletics. They both struggled in school with learning challenges. It was actually my son's struggle with dyslexia that inspired me to leave fitness to get my master's degree in education. Although I was married, most of the activities, including school support, fell on me. I was working full time, cooking breakfast every morning, dinner every night, and cleaning a massive house by myself. Basically, I was trying to prove to everyone that despite the MS diagnosis, nothing would change for them.

I traveled to see the sleep specialist my neurologist recommended. He reviewed my MRI, confirming that one of the lesions in my brain was in the sleep center. He gave me extremely specific instructions that I followed to the letter. Although he wasn't a fan of medication as a therapy for insomnia, he prescribed me Remeron, which is characterized as an antidepressant but also improves insomnia. It helped me sleep but caused continuous food obsessions. I was literally thinking about food every second of every day and swiftly gained ten pounds.

After implementing the other sleep hygiene advice, I tapered off the medication and, thankfully, lost the extra weight. Aside from the obvious sleep hygiene advice he gave me, the most useful advice was, "You're resting even if you are laying in the bed and not sleeping. Don't worry if you don't sleep. Just rest. The anxiety of worrying about not sleeping makes it infinitely worse."

The sleep hygiene tips are corrective in nature. I don't have to maintain all of these unless I experience a few nights of poor sleep. Then, I revert right back to this list for a few weeks to get things back on track.

- No television or electronics within an hour of bedtime.
- Don't watch television in the bedroom, or engage in any other activities there, other than sex and sleep (especially not arguing or stressful discussions).
- No caffeine after my morning coffee.
- No eating late.
- Keep the bedroom cold and completely dark.
- Get up and leave the bed if I can't sleep after thirty minutes or an hour to teach the brain the bed is for sleep.
- Same bedtime and wake up time every day, even weekends (don't sleep in).
- Exercise every day but avoid evening exercise.

- My own addition: make sure I've eaten enough during the day. I tend to forget to eat sometimes, which can adversely affect my sleep.

By year two, I was sleeping better. I usually slept about seven hours a night, with only one or two sleepless nights a month. That said, I was still exhausted most days from juggling motherhood, an unhappy marriage, and teaching.

After my first year teaching kindergarten, I moved to another school to teach fourth grade. I was starting over again, and to my surprise, in a much worse situation. It was a struggling school with a lot of dysfunctions. There were a lot of kids below grade level in reading and math. There wasn't a real curriculum for math or reading, which was not a coincidence. By midyear, I was exhausted trying to develop the materials the kids desperately needed. That was in addition to teaching the kids the social skills they were missing, coming from dysfunction at home also. It was a real wake-up call into how bad public education can be in some schools.

One day during my break period, I was so tired I actually fell asleep on the break room floor. It was then that I knew something had to change. The way I felt reminded me of the day I laid on the office floor at home with that awful headache, several years prior. I knew that if something didn't change, I would trigger another episode like the optic neuritis. I went back to the list Dr. Riser gave me. I was doing everything on the list, even sleeping better. The only area I was failing in was reducing stress. I decided at that moment I would aggressively tackle stress. I resigned from teaching mid-year, which was one of the hardest decisions of my life. I was very attached to those kids, many of which had very few heroes in life. The way I convinced myself to do it was by realizing that if I continued with that level of stress and had a relapse, I would let my own children down. I accepted a remote fitness sales job, and I scheduled an appointment with my general practitioner for a check-up.

When I met with my general practitioner, she asked me how I was feeling lately. I said fine, but my stress level was higher than I wanted. She asked me how I was coping with the stress, and I said, "Okay, I think."

Her next question was, "How would your husband and family say you're doing?" I teared up. Somehow, I couldn't advocate for my own mental health. But when she asked the question that way, it made me think about how it was impacting people I love.

Through her skillful interview questions, she was able to identify that my stress was manifesting as anxiety. She insisted that anxiety is treatable with medication and prescribed me Zoloft. She also encouraged me to start making the hard decisions necessary to reduce stress.

The Zoloft took the edge off and allowed me to evaluate things more clearly. I hired a housekeeper and scaled back my hectic life. Cutting back and taking better care of myself caused friction in my marriage. When my husband and I met, I was twenty years old, but he was much older, being twenty-nine. I spent most of our early relationship trying to do and be everything—the ultimate homemaker and a full-time career woman. It's not his fault he got used to having the best of both worlds, but it was slowly killing my spirit, wearing me down. From the outside, I looked fine, and my husband couldn't relate to why I needed to scale back. He liked the division of labor with him just worrying about his work, maintaining the yard, and tending to his extended family while I handled everything else.

As I tried to establish a new balance that honored me as a whole person and not just a wife and mother, the friction increased. It became obvious to me that I would have to choose myself and my kids or him. It was becoming impossible to keep everyone happy. I wouldn't say that the MS diagnosis caused our divorce, but it did help me regain a sense of self, which brought a lot to the surface.

Within two years, I moved with my kids from Alabama to Florida. The trigger for the move was a scholarship offer for my son to play basketball at a prep school. Again, doing something I knew was better for my kids was the way I set myself in motion.

My kids and I moved from a huge home in Alabama into a tiny, two-bedroom apartment in Florida. When we moved, my husband cut us off financially. He didn't want us to leave but refused to tell my son he couldn't take the offer. In the end, I had to make the final decision. Without any financial support, we barely had enough money for groceries most weeks. My daughter and I shared a bed for a year. I had to travel for work frequently. When my mother came into town to stay with the kids for me, there would be nights before I left, and when I returned, when my mother, my daughter, and I all slept in the same bed.

The only furniture we had was donated by family or from a thrift store, but we were happier than we'd ever been. We had a peaceful, happy home. Over the course of the next two years, we upgraded apartments, bought furniture, and eventually bought a home as our financial situation improved. One step at a time, I worked to restore our lifestyle as much as I could, while keeping peace as the ultimate priority.

A big part of restoring our lifestyle was taking a much better job with a company I love and still work with today. It took me about two years to disclose to anyone at work that I have MS. One day at a huge event we hosted, where we had dozens of customers attending, I spontaneously told my story on stage.

It happened when I was explaining why our company mission meant so much to me personally. I explained that bringing in strength training and making it accessible to as many people as possible fulfilled a deep desire I have to make people healthier. I explained how the gym, lifting weights, and making my health the ultimate priority had kept me healthy despite the devastating multiple sclerosis diagnosis.

As soon as the words came out of my mouth, a hush went over the room. Anyone who was texting or halfway paying attention looked up. All the sudden, I had a completely captive audience.

After the revelation, I felt like a weight had been lifted. By that point, I had already proven my worth to the company, clearly showing that my diagnosis didn't prevent me from doing everything that was required for the job. It was so much more powerful that way, and a lot less scary.

Their support was overwhelming. Since then, I don't announce it everywhere I go, but I'm not scared to tell people. The one area where I'm still a little reluctant is dating. I've found that guys will act like it's no big deal when you tell them. But after they've googled it, they're a little more reluctant. To be honest, it sucks since I'm super healthy and symptom-free, but there's really nothing I can do to change it. I've had to realize that whatever guy is truly okay with it deserves the amazing life we'll have together. The other guys just aren't for me.

Soon after the move to Florida, I began eating more of a keto diet. I started it to lose a little weight. I knew several people who had used the diet to lose a lot of weight, and from what I read, it seemed really safe. I was still fit and worked out regularly, but I just didn't feel as toned as I used to feel. It's hot in Florida, and I wanted to be comfortable wearing shorts. Not long, weird mom shorts—cute, little shorts. Once I started eating keto, I easily lost about ten pounds in two months. Beyond the weight loss, I was surprised how much my energy improved on the diet.

After about a year on keto, I started intermittent fasting, and eventually ended up mostly carnivore. Currently, my diet is about 80% red meat, 10% carbs (mostly low sugar fruit), and 10% healthy fats, including full-fat, organic dairy. I avoid alcohol almost entirely due to the toxin load it creates.

My kids have gradually moved towards my style of eating on their own. My son, who is a division one basketball player, eats steak almost every day. The only carbs he eats are usually rice, sweet potatoes, or fruit. He's become a great cook! When he can eat at home, his diet is super clean. When they provide food for him, he does the best he can.

My daughter is a talented high school volleyball player, who has suffered from irritable bowel syndrome (IBS) and anxiety. I recently brought her to my physician, who put her on a gluten-free diet. Now, she eats very much like I do. Her symptoms of IBS are almost completely gone, and her anxiety is improving. As a teenage girl, she cheats periodically, but overall, her diet has improved dramatically.

I never forced my kids to eat like me. For a long time, I would cook a protein, vegetable, and carb for them, and I would just skip the carb for myself. Over time, they started loading up on protein also and gradually eating less bread, pasta, and refined carbs. Neither one of them eats sugar or sweets regularly.

I used to say that 80% of the time, I ate very clean, and 20% of the time, I ate whatever was available. Over time, it's really become more like 90/10. If I'm at a special place with a signature meal, like the Italian restaurant I visited in Little Italy in San Diego a month ago, I might eat pasta. In those situations, I enjoy it and get back on track with the very next meal. I'm not legalistic or annoying about it. I just try to eat the way that makes me feel the best most of the time.

I started feeling so amazing that, with the help of my amazing doctor, Stefania Bray, MD, who is board-certified in family medicine and integrative holistic medicine, I was able to taper off the Zoloft. Before beginning the tapering protocol, she recommended a blood test to check for a MTHFR gene mutation. She explained that many people with anxiety have this mutation. Sure enough, the test determined that I am homozygous for the mutation, making the effects very pronounced. According to the *National Library of Medicine*, the MTHFR mutation makes it more difficult to purge toxins from the body, making people who carry this mutation more prone to anxiety. It also has an impact on stroke risk, blood clots, cardiovascular risk, and fertility. Source: https://medlineplus.gov/lab-tests/mthfr-mutation-test/

By reducing toxins (like alcohol), taking supplements, and doing things like visiting the sauna, I was able to reduce my anxiety naturally and taper off the Zoloft completely. It was difficult and took about six months to completely be free of withdrawal symptoms, but it was 100% worth it.

I also removed as many other toxins as I could tolerate from my beauty routine and home environment. All of my personal care items are unscented; I use aluminum-free deodorant and filter all of our drinking water. Additionally, I use Free and Clear laundry detergent and white vinegar as fabric softener. I only use pure soy or beeswax candles in my home, with either essential oils as fragrances, or no scent at all. I never use commercial fragrances. Essentially, I'm very careful about what is in the air and what I put on my skin. With this gene mutation, I can't clear out these chemicals very easily, so I try to avoid them.

Since then, we've done several more tests (some covered by insurance while others are not) to identify underlying risk factors. This approach has allowed me to continuously optimize my health and reduce my dependence on prescription medications. Currently, I take a variety of supplements, all the result of actual blood work and genetic testing. While I'm not disciplined about taking all of these daily, I take them most days. This list will evolve with further blood work and is updated periodically in the "Lifestyle Guide" I share with my followers on Instagram.

The supplements listed below with an asterisk are the priority ones I try to take, even if I don't get to them all. One of the most important ones listed is vitamin D and K2, which is implicated in all MS patients. I take everything daily unless otherwise specified.
- Omega 3 - Nordic Naturals
- Zinc - Jarrow
- *Vitamin D and K2 - MicroIngredients (brand I found)
- Vitamin C - 500mg - Solgar
- *Magnesium Glycinate
- *ONE Multivitamin - Pure Encapsulations
- Curcumin - Pure Encapsulations
- Taurine - Jarrow
- Melatonin - Life Extension, gradual release, as needed at bedtime
- Methyl CPG ortho molecular – three times a week

I used to have chronic hives that would last for weeks, sometimes a month or more. When I changed to the carnivore diet, the hives went away. If I ever have a recurrence, I take the supplement Quecetin, made by Jarrow, and nettle tea. My doctor recommended flaxseed oil and eating one Brazil nut per day for selenium, but I chose not to include them in my regime because they make my skin break out. I also take creatine monohydrate for a variety of benefits, including muscle building and cognitive benefits. I take 5mg a day after workouts in my protein shake. The brand I like is from Bulk Supplements, and it's in a powder form. I never "loaded" creatine and don't believe that loading is necessary. It's one of the safest and most studied supplements on the planet.

One very important point to consider is the quality of any supplement. I only use specific brands, recommended by my general practitioner. Also, combinations of supplements need to be balanced appropriately. For example, vitamin D doesn't function well without K2 and magnesium. There are many other examples of cofactors and imbalances that can occur by improperly prescribing yourself supplements. Having a general practitioner, who is also board certified in integrative holistic medicine, has been invaluable in getting the correct combination and quality of supplements.

There are five basic principles that guide my eating strategy. I eat very little carbs, avoid packaged and prepared foods, prioritize protein, leverage supplements, and use occasional fasting. I usually have my first meal around 12pm-2pm. I don't snack much because I'm not hungry all day, and I want my body to experience low or stable insulin levels for as much of the day as possible.

The books that have guided me the most in developing my current eating philosophy are listed below. In my view, these should be required reading if you have any chronic health concerns. Or even better—before you develop a problem. Most of these are available in paperback and on Audible. These books changed my life and taught me the "why" behind the "how" to live this lifestyle. Without this knowledge, I think most of the lifestyle changes I adopted would have faded over time as I started to feel better. For me, it's always been important to understand why I'm doing something.

Notice anything about the authors? These aren't fly-by-night quacks— they're MDs, with the exception of Jessie Inchauspe, who is also brilliant. If I had to choose one book to read first, it would be *Lies my Doctor Told Me.*

- *Lies My Doctor Told Me* by Dr. Ken Berry
- *Obesity Code* by Dr. Jason Fung

- *Why We Get Sick* by Dr. Benjamin Bikman
- *Carnivore Code* by Dr. Paul Salidino
- *Undoctored* by Dr. William Davis
- *The Salt Fix* by Dr. James DiNicolantonio
- *Glucose Revolution* by Jessie Inchauspe

I consider myself a keto/carnivore because most of my calories come from animal protein and fats. I keep carbs very low (20-50g/day) to stay in ketosis most of the time. This means I don't eat pasta, bread, rice, grains, oats, white potatoes, sugar, or vegetables high in carbs. Many of these contain inflammatory oils and added chemicals, food additives, etc. I eat mostly food without labels, which are natural, whole foods. I cook at home as often as I can. When I eat out, I'm careful about what I order.

I am especially careful to avoid monosodium glutamate (MSG), maltodextrin, and fake sweeteners, like sucralose and aspartame. I cook at home much more than I eat out to control ingredients. The week before my diagnosis, I went to a family reunion where I binged on Diet Coke all weekend. I still think that may have had something to do with the optic neuritis onset. It didn't explain the brain lesions, or I might have blamed that toxic sludge for the entire multiple sclerosis diagnosis. I focus on protein at each meal. I shoot for 1 gram per pound of ideal body weight. I'm around 140 pounds, so I aim for a minimum of 100 grams per day, ideally 140 grams. I only count animal proteins because of the bioavailability of the protein and the complete amino acid profile. Plant proteins are never my preference.

When I first started tracking protein, I used an app called *Protein Pal* and a cheap food scale to learn how much protein was in my food. After tracking for a few weeks, I was able to gauge how much protein I was eating. I prioritize ruminant animals for their unique ability to digest plants and extract their nutrients without being affected by their antinutrients. Ruminant animals include cows, sheep, goats, and deer. I don't eat deer or much goat, but they are both solid proteins.
1. **Beef -** (all cuts) Preferred cuts: ribeye, grass-fed ground beef, all other fatty cuts. Okay cuts: NY strip and other lean cuts.
2. **Eggs -** Pasture-raised when possible.
3. **Lamb -** I usually buy ground lamb.
4. **Chicken -** (dark meat w/skin when possible) Preferred cuts: thighs, wings. Okay cuts: breast and tenderloins.
5. **Pork -** Preferred cuts: bacon, ribs, and other fatty cuts. Okay cuts: loin.

6. **All other seafood** - (shrimp, all small fish). Avoid fish high in mercury, like shark, ray, swordfish, barramundi, gemfish, orange roughy, ling, and southern bluefin tuna.

I drink a protein shake most days to add protein to my diet in a convenient, easy to consume way. On workout days I have it after workouts. On rest days I have it whenever the mood hits. Marigold is my favorite brand, and I like unflavored and chocolate malt.

Other forms of nutrient rich protein I want to add more often include oysters (one-to-two times a month) and beef or chicken liver (one-to-two small servings a week). When money is tight, I focus on ground beef, chicken thighs, and eggs. I purchase most proteins at Sam's Wholesale in bulk and keep the freezer stocked. Hamburgers are a great way to consume beef. I get an eight pack at Sam's and cook four at a time in the oven in a casserole dish, which is less messy.

Currently, I alternate strength training and yoga if I'm not traveling. I usually take one day off a week. I have been strength training for over twenty years, have a background in personal training, and work in fitness technology. I say that to point out that I love fitness and feel very comfortable in the gym environment. I love working out, but also must be time efficient with my hectic schedule. On the weekends, I tend to train a little harder and take my time.

The following is an example of my typical workout routine:
Full body strength training: 2-4 days/week, 40-60 mins. Using a weight that's hard to do more than ten repetitions. 2-4 sets, depending on time. If time is limited, I do the exercises marked with an asterisk only.

- Legs - leg extension, leg curl, single leg leg press, Bulgarian split squats, kickbacks, glute kickbacks
- Chest - push ups, chest press
- Back - lat pulldown, seated row, pull ups
- Shoulders - overhead shoulder press, front & lateral raises
- Biceps - dumbbell bicep curls, cable bicep curls
- Triceps - overhead tricep extensions, tricep push ups or bench dips, dips
- Abs & Stretching

Find my routines and workout videos on YouTube:
https://www.youtube.com/@lazybiohacker4075/videos

I do yoga two-to-three days per week. Yoga lengthens muscles, improves spine and joint mobility, mindfulness, and is a great tool for stress reduction. I prefer to do it at home, using the *Down Dog* app. I used to teach yoga, and I'm particular about the flow and pace. I also don't like a lot of the "fluff" comments from instructors like, "This is your time, focus on connecting with the earth, find your peace"—yada yada. I like more of a minimalist approach. The app and home practice gives me that control. I miss the community aspects of yoga. That might be the one thing that could tempt me back into a class environment.

In the app, you can customize your class. I choose the filters that select "Hatha style" and "flexibility focus". Those filters don't include a lot of balance or strength postures, which is ideal for me since I work my muscles in the weight room. When I travel and can't strength train, I sometimes take off the "flexibility" filter and do a full class, which includes strength postures. I go to the sauna a few times a week and do cold plunges occasionally at my local gym. I've also plunged in some beautiful lakes and rivers when I've traveled North during colder months. Those outdoor experiences were nothing short of magical. I've released a lot of emotional baggage in lakes and rivers.

Cold plunges have been particularly helpful with anxiety during sad times or times of stress. The best way I can describe the effects of cold plunging is that the cold water immediately disrupts negative or sad thoughts. There's also an intense feeling of euphoria afterwards that lasts a few days. Everyone's experience is different, but for me, it's like a natural high. I've used it as an anxiety tool and a mental reset. Cold plunging can also help stimulate brown fat, which improves metabolism.

I started with three minutes and gradually built up to a max of fifteen minutes for most sessions. More is not better with plunging because most benefits happen at three minutes, and all benefits max out between eleven-to-twenty minutes, depending on the temperature of the water. I never cold plunge alone, which can be dangerous, especially in really cold water. There was one time in a lake in Virginia where I almost couldn't get out of the water. The water was very cold (probably below the ideal fifty degrees), and I was in the water for twenty minutes, which was probably about five minutes too long. When I tried to push myself up onto the dock, my arms just gave out. Sometimes muscles don't cooperate when they get really cold. Thankfully, I was able to get back onto the dock, but it took a few attempts. I almost pulled the woman watching me into the water when she offered her hand. Now, I always keep safety in mind.

It's worth noting that both cold plunging and sauna would be contraindicated, according to most MS advice. Extreme temperatures can supposedly trigger relapses for some people. I took the opposite approach, deciding that if extreme temperatures were problematic, then I should build a tolerance and stamina in those environments. I had no intention of hiding from cold or hot weather the rest of my life. The benefits to both therapies were immediate and never triggered any symptoms.

I use box breathing as a tool to control the "fight or flight" response. It's a breathing technique Navy Seals use to calm down during missions. It's easy to find free videos online demonstrating the technique, but it's basically a four second inhale through the nose, four second breath hold, four second breath out through the mouth, then hold breath there for four seconds. I actually use seven seconds for each step now, but I've built up to that point.

I also meditate during times of extreme stress, and I prioritize sleep. Mediation is something I'm still learning. I used to teach guided meditation when I was a yoga instructor many years ago. The easiest way to learn is to sit or lay on your back, place your left hand over your heart, and your right hand on your stomach. Breath deep into your belly and exhale completely. Focus on that process, the rise and fall of your stomach with the breath. Allow the mind to rest. Don't fight intrusive thoughts, just let them pass through, letting the mind rest again. Start slow with a few minutes, gradually building up as your stamina increases. The cue I used to use for students was to imagine you're hitting pause on a movie or show. That's the effect you're looking for in your meditation at first—just a pause. Over time, you can explore free guided meditations online that focus on visualization and manifestation. I find that starting with those methods is difficult for most people, and they never really learn how to quiet or pause the mind, which I consider a fundamental skill.

Using the methods I described, I firmly believe that without MS medication, I would be healthy and relapse-free. That said, as a single mom, I have a profound responsibility to my children. If I come off the medication and I'm wrong, they will pay the price. I've been healthy and relapse-free for eight years. Each of my follow-up MRIs showed no progression. All of the routine manual evaluations they do every visit show zero progression and sometimes even improvement (gait test, balance, reflexes, etc.).

I'm concerned about disrupting that positive momentum. Similar to how Remeron helped me learn to sleep again and Zoloft took the edge off of the anxiety so I had the strength to make the changes, everything has its place. I have zero side effects from the MS medication and zero cost. The risk of being wrong could be steep. That said, I expect to come off the medication in 2025, after a clean MRI.

Much of my journey since 2020 is documented on my Instagram page @Lazybiohacker. I created the page to support other people trying to restore their health and connect with likeminded people. I also created a lifestyle guide that outlines all my current lifestyle choices. You can request it through email or Instagram. I'm a continuous learner, and as such, my diet and lifestyle continue to evolve as I learn. Topics covered include exercise routine, diet, grocery lists, influencers I follow, and books I love. I try to update it every few months with new information.

When I reflect back on my journey with multiple sclerosis, it makes me emotional. Mostly, I'm proud of myself for not leaning into hopelessness. My life could have been so small. There were so many times when I felt defeated, and it would have been easier to lean into depression and self-pity. But each time I felt close to that point, I used what little strength I had to take the next step and then the next step. Each step strengthened me mentally and physically. I now live a life more amazing than I would have ever thought possible. I'm grateful for where I find myself in life and for the journey that brought me here.

17

Story by

MICHELLE

Diagnosed in 1996
Currently 56 years old
Lives in Florida, United States
Instagram: @mysaladbowloflife

In January of 1993, I was twenty-five years old and newly pregnant with our third daughter. My husband was traveling to China for three weeks, while I was preparing to fly across Canada with our two daughters (ages two and four) and the dog to stay with my parents. Two days before I was set to leave, I started noticing one of my eyes was not quite right. I couldn't see clearly. By the day of travel, it was as if a cotton ball was clouding my vision. When I arrived in my hometown, my mom took me to the University hospital where there happened to be a neuro-opthalmologist in residency. After an examination and vision testing, he diagnosed me with optic neuritis (ON).

Because I was pregnant, there was nothing they could do for me. I was sent on my way, told that it should resolve itself. If anything else odd happened to me, I was told to see a doctor. Sure enough, my vision improved, correcting itself over the next couple of months. Our healthy baby girl was born, and I dove into the chaos of being an overly tired mom of three little ones.

For the next two years, nothing out of the ordinary happened, aside from being exhausted. But then again, what new mom isn't? One day, as I was preparing the main course for a "moms' dinner club" night I was hosting, I snuck a mouthful of chocolate chips. I thought to myself, "Wow, this brand of chocolate chips is awful. They taste like wax!" I didn't give it much thought until later, while enjoying dessert and coffee with my friends. I realized I couldn't taste or feel temperature on half of my mouth. A few days later, after confirming the loss of sensation, I went to the doctor, who then recommended me to a neurologist. Because I was living in Canada, it took nearly four months before I was able to get into the specialist.

During my first visit to the neurologist, I shared my health history and received a neurological exam. For some reason, this doctor did not want to tell me about my condition because he didn't want me to live my life differently. The one thing he did say was that the myelin around my nerves was breaking down. I was perplexed, to say the least. I went home, and being the sleuth that I am, immediately grabbed my husband's college biology book to look up "myelin" in the index. When I turned to the assigned page, I found this shocking explanation: "When the myelin breaks down around the nerves, it is most often multiple sclerosis (MS)." Everything I'd heard about multiple sclerosis before this moment was scary and overwhelming. My neighbor had it, and she was struggling to walk.

Two days later, I reached out to the MS society, requesting any informational brochures they had. When they arrived, I read through them and was positive that I did, in fact, have multiple sclerosis. I began reading everything I could about MS. What I found were the worst-case scenarios, over and over. My brother-in-law's father was a neurologist in Canada. One of the first books suggested to me was *Multiple Sclerosis: A Guide for the Newly Diagnosed* by Jock Murray. The fifth edition of the book was published in 2017, so I must have read an earlier edition. It gave me very little hope, confirming my thoughts that I had no choice but to live the rest of my life with this.

My next definite MS attack was trigeminal neuralgia (TN)—an awful stabbing pain in the side of my face. Back to the original doctor I went, for a new referral to a neurologist who was actually interested in confirming a diagnosis. She also prescribed an anti-seizure medication to quiet the TN. It resulted in me being unable to function or take care of our girls. So, I got off it. Again, I had to wait to see the neurologist, followed by another long wait to undergo magnetic resonance imaging (MRI). In Canada, you often wait up to a year to get an MRI. I remember getting a call that someone had cancelled, so I got in after only eight months. A month later, the neurologist confirmed that based on my clinical symptoms and a positive MRI, I indeed had MS. The time span from the presenting case of ON to official diagnosis was over three years.

I told my husband of my diagnosis after he arrived home from an overseas trip. We were both shaken, unsure of my future. This became even more overwhelming when we shared my diagnosis with a couple from our church. He'd been diagnosed years prior. They were both emotionally distraught at my news, causing my husband and I to be even more scared. We didn't have family living near us, so we had to share our news by phone with most of the family. It was a mixture of tears and great concern. I was blessed to have a group of close mom friends who were my support system. As I shared the news with them, they shared in my sadness, promising to be there for me if I needed anything. I was twenty-nine years old and incredibly unsure of what my future held. In Canada at that time, multiple sclerosis medications were not available. Over the next few years, I treated attacks with oral steroids, trying to live my life as normal as possible.

In November of 1997, we moved from Canada to the United States. For the first couple of years, my MS was fairly quiet. I was still dealing with bad fatigue but didn't experience any real attacks. One Florida day, I spent hours in the sun and heat, playing with our girls. The next day, I felt as if I'd been hit by a truck. The MS decided to show itself again with back-to-back attacks. I found a new neurologist and did my best to replay the tape of my MS history for him. Since I had been diagnosed, I dealt with severe vertigo, Lhermitte's Sign (a shock sensation when bending my neck), MS hug (a tight band-like sensation around the chest or torso), loss of feeling in my arm, a collapsing knee, along with other MS symptoms. And, of course, the presenting optic neuritis and trigeminal neuralgia. These attacks would appear then disappear within a month or two.

Looking back, so much of this was a blur. I had three young daughters, a husband who traveled one hundred fifty days a year, and multiple sclerosis. My husband was amazing! When he wasn't working, he took the girls on lots of fun adventures. It took a couple of years after our move to the U.S. to build up a support system of incredible friends.

The first and only neurologist I have seen in the U.S., Dr. Harris, confirmed that these attacks warranted the start of Copaxone (a multiple sclerosis agent). For the next two years, I took Copaxone daily. Despite my fear of needles, I gained some solace by being in control of the injections. My MS continued in an active state during this time. I'd had several attacks, requiring IV Solu-Medrol (a glucocorticoid). I started noticing divots at my injection sites. My gums were also receding. After examining these serious side effects, Dr. Harris determined that continuing with Copaxone would be detrimental to my health. It was time to try something new. Next up was Avonex (another multiple sclerosis agent). It's administered through weekly intramuscular injections, which I continued for a year and a half. During this time, my quality of life plummeted. I administered the injection on Fridays, so my husband would be home with the girls during the most intense post-injection side effects. For the following forty-eight hours afterward, I experienced severe flu-like symptoms. I dragged myself around as best I could the rest of the week, often sleeping sixteen broken hours out of a twenty-four hour day. I was in and out of bed throughout the day as my body would allow, and then back in bed before the girls went to sleep. I'm so grateful my girls were very responsible and able to put themselves to bed most nights. This was a dark time. I found myself slipping into a deep depression. I tried treating it with antidepressants, but they left me with nothing but suicidal thoughts. I gained a great deal of weight. Being active felt almost impossible. After one too many days of this, I decided I could no longer deal with the horrible feelings. I took myself off the Avonex.

In 2008, after six months off all meds, I returned to my neurologist, explaining what I had done. Dr. Harris immediately ordered an MRI with contrast. The results showed a new, large, active lesion. I was told I needed to start Tysabri, a once-a-month IV treatment. I had to stay in the office to fill out the paperwork and arrange a nurse for a home visit to qualify me for the treatment. Upon a bit of research, I found out three women had died during the trial! Not only that, but it also had a black box warning! There was no way I was starting a treatment that came with a possible chance of death. No, thank you!

The next day, I went to Barnes and Noble and found myself wandering over to the health section. I stumbled across a book called *The MS Recovery Diet Book* and bought it. I took it home to discuss with my husband, who agreed to support me in trying the diet. My sister, who was visiting at the time, also encouraged me to give it a try. That day was fifteen years ago, and it was the best decision I have ever made in my life (aside from marrying my husband and having my three amazing girls).

I read the book and immediately started the elimination diet. I removed seven foods: dairy, gluten, legumes, sugar, corn, eggs, and yeast. I found it easiest to precook and freeze individual servings of protein (chicken and salmon) while upping my veggie and fruit intake. The rest of my family continued with their regular diets. When I decide to do something, it is all or nothing. So, I followed the diet strictly. It wasn't easy removing the specified foods as I have always loved all foods. I was raised not to be a picky eater, so the adjustment was hard, especially when eating out or at someone's house. I never wanted to appear picky to others. I was able to set myself up for success by always having safe food available. I would cook for myself with the foods I could eat, and then add to it, making it more interesting (and palatable) for my husband and girls. Being addicted to sugar made it tough to eliminate. But, after two months of giving it up, I could successfully stand in front of a bakery case without craving one item!

I avoided all processed foods and stopped drinking alcohol. At the same time, I started swimming on a local Master's Swim Team. Within two weeks, my husband and our girls started noticing a difference in me. I was thinking more clearly, and my energy level was much higher. I still took my afternoon nap, but I wasn't in bed for most of the day anymore. I found eating at home proved to be the easiest because I could control what I ate. If we ate out, I opted for a piece of protein (no seasoning or sauce) and veggies. As the weeks went on, I was feeling better and better. In the first three years, I let myself slip a couple of times. Within hours, I was in bed, exhausted and not feeling well, often lasting several days. I was so incredibly thrilled when I felt well. It was all the encouragement I needed to stick to the elimination diet.

Three years after making my drastic life change, my husband thought it would be a good idea to get an MRI to make sure the multiple sclerosis wasn't doing anymore damage to my brain. I wasn't experiencing any attacks, but I agreed. When I walked into my neurologist's office, he exclaimed, "Michelle, you look amazing!" I smiled as I was feeling amazing. I explained to him that I chose not to go on Tysabri, but instead, made a huge lifestyle change. He could see I was doing much better than before, but he also wanted to order an MRI. Two weeks later, my husband and I sat across the desk from Dr. Harris. He asked what MS meds I was taking, and I replied that I hadn't taken any in over three years. I told him about my decision to use nutrition and exercise to manage my symptoms, instead. Then, he pulled out the MRI from three years ago, putting it side by side with the most recent. He looked back and forth between the two, as if he was having a hard time deciphering something. He asked me again what medication I was taking. My answer was still none. He immediately rose from his chair and went to get another doctor, along with a resident, to review the MRIs. Confused as to what was happening, my husband and I were holding our breath. Finally turning to me, Dr. Harris said, "I am seeing no new lesions, and the existing ones are shrinking." We were overjoyed! What I was doing was working. He followed it up with, "Whatever you are doing, keep doing it! If you have anything come up, come see me." When I left his office that day, I knew I had to keep taking care of myself. It was my only option. I was healthier than I had been in many years.

It wasn't long after that when I decided to slowly begin adding eliminated foods back into my diet, watching for any odd symptoms. The MS recovery book I spoke of earlier did have a good section on reintroduction. I tried adding back only one food per week. I first added soy sauce to rice. That was a big "no" for me. Within fifteen minutes of consuming, a patch of burning skin would appear, often lasting twenty-four hours. Next, I tried frying an egg. It resulted in intense brain fog. If I eat an item with egg as an ingredient, I don't seem to get as intense of a reaction, i.e., gluten-free pancakes. I tried eating a piece of bread and felt tired afterward. Gluten is the one food I wish I would have fully taken out of my diet from the beginning. I know you can't have just a little gluten because it stays in your system for a long time. Its biggest side effects were a skin rash and fatigue. It wasn't until years later that I connected gluten to the appearance of rheumatoid arthritis attacks. I can't remember what I did to reintroduce diary, but it was probably ice cream. It caused me to get all stuffed-up. You could guarantee there would be snoring that night. This is another food I know should not be in my diet, but I save it for special dessert opportunities. This had happened to me before starting the elimination diet. Back then, I attributed it to being overtired or stressed. My body told me if I ate something it didn't like—I just had to listen! Occasionally, when I slip up and don't take care of myself, the MS gives me a reminder.

I am so grateful for my good health and how it has changed my life in so many ways. I continue to swim a few times a week, travel, and live an incredible life. I stick to a paleo diet and try to source the best quality food possible. I have spent the last 15 years researching nutrition and modalities to keep myself the healthiest I can be. I've found that massage and stretching is a good addition to my regime. About ten years ago, I had all my amalgam fillings removed. I went to my regular dentist and asked her to read an amalgam removal protocol, so she could remove them for me. Back then, holistic or biological dentistry wasn't a well-known thing (at least to me).

About three years ago, I started experiencing muscular pain with no known cause other than possibly MS, thyroid issues, or menopause. I was working with an integrative doctor at the time. I asked if she would prescribe me Low Dose Naltrexone (LDN) 4.5 mg. It's an off-label drug, typically used in treating alcoholism or drug addiction when taken in 50 mg doses. In the eighties, a doctor discovered that it helped his multiple sclerosis patients. I read *The LDN Book* by Linda Elsegood, along with *The Power of Honest Medicine* by Julia Schopick and Don Schwartz, and decided to give it a try. I joined an LDN support group on Facebook where I've met many other members with autoimmune diseases. The medication has made the muscular pain much more bearable until I'm able to complete more functional testing to find the root cause.

I've volunteered at the Multiple Sclerosis Society and spoken to others with MS. I decided it wasn't for me when I was told more than once, "You can't have MS. You look too good." I've offered to share my story and successes with others. Often, I get in return, "Oh, that would be so difficult. I could never do that." It pains me to hear people selling themselves short.

In 2021, I completed my certificate to become an Integrative Nutrition coach after a one-year online course. I received my Integrative Nutrition Health Coach certificate from The Institute for Integrative Nutrition. I may practice when I complete my other certificate. Time will tell. Last month, I started a one-year program to become a Functional Medicine Coach. This is very important to me as I believe in a functional medical view, which is to look for the root cause of a disease or disorder. Ultimately, with the two certificates, I will be able to help others, as well as friends and family.

For me, turning to nutrition and exercise was an absolute game changer in my life. Today, I am thriving as a wife, mother, and nana to five amazing grandchildren.

Back when I was diagnosed, I thought I was destined to be wheelchair bound. Instead, I am living my life actively and plan to keep on doing just that.

My book list is extensive!
These are since 2008:

I have read all of Terry Wahls books
Managing Multiple Sclerosis Naturally by Judy Graham
Thrive: The Vegan Nutrition Guide by Brendan Brazier
The Gold Coast Cure by Andrew Larson
Staying Healthy with Nutrition by Dr. Buck Levin
Eat to Live by Dr. Joel Fuhrman
MS - Living Symptom Free Daryl Bryant
Kitchen Cures by Peggy Kotsopoulos
The Immune System Recovery Plan by Susan Blum
The Body doesn't lie by Vicky Vlachonis
Healing Multiple Sclerosis: Diet, Detox and Nutritional Makeover for Total Recovery by Ann Boroch
The Food Babe Way by Vani Hari
The New Health Rules by Frank Lipman
The Autoimmune Wellness handbook by Mickey Trescott
Eat Fat, Get thin by Mark Hyman
Paleo Principles by Sarah Ballantyne
Food Rules by Michael Pollan
Eat Dirt by Josh Axe
The Paleo Cure by Chris Kesser
The Paleo Approach by Sarah Ballantyne

18

Story by

JOANNE MAKWANA

Diagnosed in 2009
Currently 38 years old
Lives in Ontario, Canada
Instagram/Facebook: Joanne Makwana
Podcast: Tipping Point Nutrition

For nearly five years, I had been dealing with strange, yet seemingly unconnected symptoms. In 2004, I experienced a squeezing sensation throughout my ribs and a "pins and needles" feeling that traveled up and down my leg. At that time, my initial doctor's visits were focused on a potential blood clot or pulled muscle. Eventually, the numbness I was experiencing led my family doctor to refer me to a neurologist. After a round of magnetic resonance imaging (MRIs), it was noted that I had a small spot on my brain. The neurologist stated that although uncommon for someone my age (nineteen), it wasn't enough for him to "hang his hat" on or diagnose me with anything.

While going through testing, I had simultaneously begun seeing a naturopath at the suggestion of my dad because my leg heaviness got really intense. He called around to find a local naturopath that would see me for an emergency Saturday appointment. He had an experience where he was overmedicated at one point in his life and had started making healthier changes for himself. When I told him what was going on, he immediately began printing off information he was seeing online about lifestyle and dietary changes that were helping people with chronic illness. Whether I was diagnosed or not, he didn't want to see me on intense medication at such a young age. He also knew that further testing and MRIs were going to take time. Why not get started on lifestyle changes that could help in the meantime?

After making some changes to my diet, I found that many of the strange symptoms had vanished—amazing! Not only did I not have MS, but my symptoms were gone! That's what I thought. Fast forward to 2009. I switched jobs and was burning the candle at both ends. All the healthy habits I'd begun to incorporate in 2004 started to go out the window. Symptoms returned more intensely than anything I'd experienced before. Extreme fatigue: There were times I had to pull over while driving because it would randomly hit me so hard that I'd feel like I was going to fall asleep at the wheel, even after a full night's sleep. Neuropathy: numbness and tingling, as though both feet were asleep 24/7. Extremely heavy legs: they felt like they were bricks of cement that were impossible to lift. Vertigo: laying down and holding the carpet because the room was flipping. Cognitive decline: extreme brain fog, trouble organizing my thoughts, feeling confused about what I was doing, and forgetting things. Loss of balance: feeling as though people would think I was drunk, based on how I walked. Swelling and edema in feet/lower legs. Headaches/migraines and sinus pressure (especially in the morning). Muscle spasms and twitching. The MS "hug": A tightening sensation that felt like a boa constrictor was squeezing me around the rib cage.

All of this had resulted in a massive loss of confidence and self-esteem. I would arrive early to work, so I could get out of my car without feeling like a colleague might see me struggling to walk. I'd linger behind in meetings, so people wouldn't see me graze the wall or a meeting table for balance. I wrote everything down, so I could remember as much as possible. I worked in public relations and was a company spokesperson. I needed to be able to think clearly to find my words in media interviews.

I went back to see the neurologist and began the process of MRIs, once again. This time there was no question about it, there were lesions on both the brain and the spinal cord.

"You have lesions all over your brain; you definitely have MS."

Tears filled my eyes. After many doctors and late-night magnetic resonance imaging (MRI) appointments, it was the diagnosis that had long been suspected. Even though I knew multiple sclerosis (MS) was a possibility, receiving the label hit me hard (not to mention delivery of the news wasn't how I imagined). I stared blankly at the neurologist and felt as though my mind hovered outside of my body. He seemed surprised that I was affected by the diagnosis.

"Oh...do you need some tissues?" He awkwardly asked before launching into high-level treatment options, where to pick up copies of my MRIs, my need for an occupational therapist, and timing for seeing a specialist. Although I saw his lips moving, I didn't take in a word he said. I left feeling empty and overwhelmed. In July of 2009 (at the age of twenty-four), I was officially diagnosed with multiple sclerosis.

My family was shocked but were most upset about the way I was diagnosed. The first time I had gone for MRIs, I had to call the neurologist's office for the results. Several years later, when I had to follow-up for results a couple of weeks after my MRIs, I figured nothing was flagged, or they would have proactively notified me. I was naive and thought they would encourage me to bring someone if they were delivering bad news. They did not, so I went alone. I wish I'd brought my parents with me.

After being diagnosed, my symptoms immediately got worse. Isn't the power of the mind incredible? I initially felt sorry for myself and spent every spare minute watching videos of people documenting their MS struggles. I'd cry while thinking about the future—the possibility of losing my vision, being wheelchair-bound, or not being able to feed myself. My legs were weak, and I was having so many issues with my balance that being in public was a huge source of anxiety for me. I couldn't imagine things getting worse than they already were and was suddenly forced to think about the possibility. My mind constantly gravitated to worst case scenarios.

In the weeks following my diagnosis, I did a lot of research and came to two realizations. Firstly, I understood that my mindset was going to determine everything moving forward. Anyone I had encountered with MS, who was doing well, had a positive outlook. Secondly, there is power in food and in taking better care of myself. I knew this based on my experience with the naturopath years before receiving a diagnosis. I had once been able to get rid of my symptoms by changing my lifestyle. I could do it again, regardless of a "new" MS label.

After my initial diagnosis, I had to wait for an appointment at the MS Clinic to see a specialist and discuss my treatment options. I was nervous and spent lots of time documenting my symptoms, filling out paperwork around my needs for an occupational therapist, etc. While physical therapy focuses on improving the patient's ability to move their body, occupational therapy focuses on improving the patient's ability to perform daily activities. I had no idea what this was at the time, but the MS Clinic asked me to complete several forms prior to my appointment that would determine my need for this type of support. I also compiled some of the latest research I'd come across on vitamin D and MS.

My appointment could not have been more of a letdown. The neurologist seemed rushed and annoyed by my questions. I knew there were several medication options and was curious to see which one he would recommend and why. He firmly stated there was one medication he wanted me to go on—Rebif. I was looking for some rationale behind the recommendation and stated that I wasn't sure I wanted to go on medication, given I'd had good results with changing my lifestyle. I relayed my hesitations, along with some of the latest research on vitamin D, and was immediately met with hostility: "All vitamins are placebos. They aren't going to do anything for MS." I was surprised by his unwillingness to discuss my findings.

"Well, if you look through some of the studies I've provided, there's some really promising research taking place. The vitamin D connection makes sense to me, given that Canada has one of the highest rates of MS in the world." I could tell there was no interest in what I was saying. I continued: "I have a pretty stressful job…do you think that will have implications for how things progress?"

"Stress has absolutely nothing to do with MS," he quickly retorted.

With that single statement, he lost me. Stress plays a role in EVERYTHING! I wasn't a doctor, but I absolutely recognized this, and it was concerning to me that he did not. As the appointment came to an end, he pushed a paper towards me with a drug identification number for Rebif written on it.

"Check and see if your insurance will cover it. Then, call me when you're ready to start."

It was clear he had zero interest in working with me if I wasn't going to go on the disease modifying therapy (DMT). As I left the office, he handed me an informational packet from the MS Society. I opened it up, and the very first page was all about limiting stress and how much it affects MS! A relationship with a healthcare provider should be a partnership. You have every right to voice concerns, questions, and your own findings.

I left feeling extremely disappointed. He had belittled me and made me feel like I had no say in my own treatment, or what was happening with my body. I didn't know exactly how I was going to move forward but working with the naturopath had left me feeling so much more empowered and hopeful.

I knew several people with MS. The potential side effects of the MS medications weren't particularly pleasant, and it was something I wasn't ready to resort to at the age of twenty-four. If I was able to change my lifestyle and impact my symptoms, it seemed logical to first attempt this. Given that I was dealing with a serious condition, I would have to be very disciplined. This wasn't just about going on a diet; it was about using my food and healthier lifestyle choices as my medicine. I dove in and quickly began to see results. I was amazed at how good I started to feel again, and even noticed improvements to issues not associated with MS. Every day I found things were getting better. I was reducing inflammation, and my digestion started to improve for the first time in my life. The heaviness in my legs subsided, neuropathy in the feet went away, and I no longer had the traveling sensation in my leg or squeezing feeling throughout the ribs.

I wasn't eating gluten or dairy. I had drastically reduced sugar and was trying to avoid processed/packaged foods. I also started to try different foods for specific therapeutic properties (ginger, turmeric, tahini, new vegetables, lots of berries, and greens). I was drinking more water and focusing on organic, overall food quality (avoiding genetically modified ingredients or food laden with pesticides). I also began taking supplements to address nutrient deficiencies and inflammation. I spent my spare time reading and following the latest research on autoimmune/ neurological diseases. I stumbled upon the work of Dr. Terry Wahls, who has Secondary-Progressive MS (SPMS) and was able to restore her health and get rid of her wheelchair, using her education and experience in the areas of research, medicine, and nutrition. Seeing others relieve chronic disease symptoms was incredibly inspiring and helped me to BELIEVE that I, too, could restore my health.

By 2011, most of my major symptoms had gone into remission, and the changes I'd implemented had really made a difference in my overall health. I did have some lingering issues I was hoping to resolve though, such as fatigue, numbness, and headaches. In an attempt to address some of these symptoms, I opted to pursue a new, controversial treatment for Chronic Cerebrospinal Venous Insufficiency (CCSVI), or the "Liberation" Therapy. CCSVI was a term coined by Dr. Paolo Zamboni. It describes the theory in which the head/neck veins are narrowed or blocked and are unable to efficiently remove blood from the Central Nervous System. The pressure caused by the build-up of blood, in turn, causes reflux of blood back into the Central Nervous System through new blood vessels which develop when the others are not working. Dr. Zamboni suggested that because these new blood vessels don't have the same structural integrity as larger veins, they tend to leak blood into the surrounding tissue, depositing iron into the Central Nervous System, triggering an immune response associated with MS. The procedure leverages an angiogram (a balloon that helps open the vein), so blood can flow through.

The first clinic I went to told me I had no issues. Something in my gut said to keep pursuing, so I went to another clinic. It wasn't until the second scan that an issue was identified. (The extent of the narrowing can't be determined until they go in for the procedure.)

I traveled to the Hospital Clinica Biblica in Costa Rica for the procedure through Passport Medical. The procedure itself was very quick. Patients are put under anesthesia. A small incision is made in the groin, and they go in with a camera to see the extent of the narrowing. Then, a balloon is inserted to open the vein. In many places, it was a simple same-day procedure. I purposely selected the procedure in Costa Rica because you were kept in the hospital overnight for observation. Then, ten days of physical therapy were completed at the hotel patients stayed in. It was an amazing experience. The hospital and hotel staff were all incredible at making sure you felt comfortable and were getting what you needed. It is costly; the procedure and accompanying therapies were about $16,000. Fortunately, my friends and family held a benefit for me to help raise the funds.

The following is an excerpt from the report following my surgery:

"During the procedure, a 75% stenosis of the right internal jugular vein was seen, as well as a 90% stenosis of the left internal jugular vein. The lesions were dilated through the placement of a 14 x 50 mm Boston XXL Balloon and an 18 x 50 mm Boston XXL Balloon. Following the dilations, improvement of both vessel caliber and blood flow was observed."

My jugulars were 75% and 90% blocked; I was getting almost no blood flow! Following the procedure, the surgeon showed me images of where my body had created new veins to compensate for the lack of blood flow through the jugulars. The body is truly remarkable!

Following the procedure, I noticed an improvement in my remaining symptoms. I had more energy, my balance seemed better, and I had a reduction in headaches. It was interesting to observe others who were there for the treatment. In my case, I'd been managing MS through a healthier lifestyle for two years with minimal symptoms. Others who arrived for the surgery had progressed quite a bit. As a result, some of their improvements were even more noticeable.

Since 2011, CCSVI has fizzled out. You'd be hard pressed to find anyone offering the procedure today. Although some responded very well, over time, many who'd undergone the procedure had re-stenosis of the veins, meaning they'd need the procedure again to re-open them. There was additional controversy; in some cases, the procedure was completed using stents instead of an angiogram, as Dr. Zamboni recommended. Many clinics were using doppler ultrasound to detect stenosis but were not following his protocol.

CCSVI led us to many more questions about a potential vascular connection to MS. Why do so many MS patients have problems with these veins? Does MS cause the narrowing? Does the narrowing result in the presentation of MS symptoms for some? How does impaired blood flow affect the brain's ability to drain/clear toxins, etc.?

While opening the veins was by no means a cure for MS, and results of the procedure varied for many, I'm grateful I was able to have it done. Having blood flow impaired to that extent is NOT a good thing— whether you have MS or not! Was I just supposed to leave them blocked? I'm grateful that Dr. Zamboni and other researchers continue to challenge the status quo and investigate these findings. There are researchers still pursuing the potential vascular connection to MS, despite the fact that many others have dismissed it entirely.

One of the most challenging aspects of MS is not knowing how it will affect you in the long-term. What does the future look like? It can also be difficult determining when to disclose chronic illness to someone you are dating. People are often diagnosed in their early twenties, a time when they may begin to think about their long-term family planning, etc.

When I met my husband, he knew that I had been diagnosed with MS but really didn't know much about it or what it meant. Although we had been acquaintances, we didn't start dating until about a year and a half after my diagnosis. Initially, he thought my lifestyle was a bit drastic and that I had some crazy ideas. He was trying to understand why I chose to treat MS without medication, but knew I was well informed and could determine what was best for my body. Not only was he supportive, but he became invested in learning how the same principles might apply to his own health. The eye rolling and sarcastic comments in social settings were a regular occurrence, but he never made me feel like my choices were silly or a burden. Remember, this was nearly fifteen years ago when going gluten-free was NOT mainstream. I recognize how blessed I am to have had his support.

I'm sharing this because after speaking to many others with MS, I know one of the biggest challenges is partners or family members not agreeing with the changes being made. Having a chronic illness can be overwhelming, but it's amplified when thinking about how pregnancy and caring for children can impact your health.

For many women with MS, pregnancy seems to be protective. There is a much lower risk of a flare during pregnancy itself. This was my experience, aside from typical pregnancy symptoms, such as morning sickness, etc. For many, the postpartum period is where they are most at risk of a flare. This was my experience, as well.

While seven months pregnant with my first child in 2014, my dad passed away unexpectedly. After my daughter's birth, grief, coupled with being a first-time mom, took a toll on me. My healthy eating began to slide, I wasn't sleeping or working out, and MS symptoms quickly began to flare-up at about six weeks postpartum. I had joint pain (especially in my fingers and knees), my balance was off, and I struggled to get up with my daughter at night. After tightening up my diet, identifying some new food intolerances (pregnancy can change us), I was able to get things under control within about eight weeks.

I had gone into pregnancy in the best health of my life. My husband and I had been planning to get pregnant, so my body was able to rebound pretty quickly. I'd really focused on upping my nutrient status. I was avoiding processed foods, focusing on food quality, and taking prenatal vitamins (plus a variety of other vitamins) to ensure I was well-nourished. In 2012, I had adopted a vegetarian diet, but when it came time to get pregnant in 2014, I began craving meat. I truly believe the body tells us what we need, but it is up to us to listen. I incorporated meat back into my diet and consumed cod liver oil. I felt revitalized. I had more energy, less brain fog, and could feel there was something my body wasn't getting on a vegetarian diet. I needed more bioavailable protein, good fats, and other nutrients coming from pastured meats. I revisited Terry Wahls's work, given good quality meats and organ meats specifically were an integral part of her program. I ended up revising my diet to more of a paleo-style, limiting overall grain/legume consumption while prioritizing meat, berries, and a wide variety of vegetables.

I became pregnant again in 2019. During this pregnancy, I didn't feel well right from the start. It wasn't really MS symptoms that were flaring, but I just didn't feel great. Sure enough, I lost the baby at three months. I didn't notice a return of symptoms after the loss but felt very rundown and tired. It was extremely traumatic. The miscarriage occurred at the same hospital my dad passed away in, triggering a lot of big emotions. We had no issues with our first pregnancy, and I was almost out of the first trimester with the second, so it really caught us off guard. We had waited almost five years after our first baby to have a second; I was worried that my body had changed, and I wouldn't be able to have a healthy pregnancy again.

Several months after the miscarriage, we got pregnant with our rainbow baby. Little did we know what was about to transpire. COVID hit, and the world as we knew it was forever changed. Being pregnant during a pandemic is stressful: lockdowns, masks, not being able to take my husband with me to appointments; no social interactions, baby showers, or maternity shoots. I knew that I was likely going to feel good throughout the pregnancy itself, but the stress of it all, plus getting pregnant so quickly after the miscarriage, would likely put me more at risk of a flare in the postpartum period.

After my second baby, I did NOT have a flare because I found out I was pregnant again when she was five-and-a-half months old. What can I say? We were in lockdown! Being pregnant while caring for a newborn baby and simultaneously helping an older child with remote learning is a lot. It's even more daunting during a pandemic when you can't go anywhere, leverage community resources, or have any social interactions.

I started to have small symptoms six months after the birth of my third child in 2021. My father-in-law had just passed, my husband was going through major transitions at work, we had two kids under the age of two, an older child doing remote learning, plus we were still dealing with lockdowns and restrictions. I hadn't had time to build myself up in preparation for a fourth pregnancy. It was a good pregnancy, but truthfully, it was a blur.

Growing humans is MAJOR work. Many nutrients are passed on to a growing baby. Then, after birth, you may continue to pass nutrients on through breastfeeding. Not only did I breastfeed, but I tandem breastfed my littles simultaneously. All my kids have been nursed until at least two years old. I think this has been very beneficial but also depleting. Between pregnancy and breastfeeding, I have been giving away my nutrients to little people for over three years! If you've done this back-to-back, you're 100% going to need some major tender love and care to optimize nutrient levels. How many women do this though? Most of us grow and deliver our babies, then put 100% of our attention into the baby, older children, maintaining a household, WORKING, and any other life task that falls on our plates. Building ourselves back up is at the bottom of the priority list. What MS has taught me is that slowing down and caring for myself is not selfish—it's necessary. If you don't make time for it, your body WILL do it for you, and it won't be when it's convenient.

When my two youngest were thirteen and twenty-eight months, I learned this the hard way. I went into the largest MS flare I'd had since diagnosis. I was completely depleted. Three back-to-back pregnancies within eighteen months, breastfeeding continuously for two-and-a-half years, lack of sleep, a pandemic, and major postpartum hormone/immune shifts all caught up with me. I went grocery shopping one day, and upon returning home, found I couldn't get out of the car. I had no ability to hold myself up, let alone unload groceries and get my kids inside. I had to call my husband to come home from work and help us in the house. The next several weeks were hell. I was in denial that this could be happening to me after all these years. Did this mean I had failed? I tried to hide how bad things were, but my legs were covered in bruises from crawling around to care for the kids. I finally agreed to be admitted to the hospital.

This journey has taught me that not everything has to be "all or nothing". I had stated previously that I would never use intravenous (IV) steroids in a flare. It's one thing to say that when things are going well, but entirely different when you haven't walked in close to a month and have small children relying on you back home. I made the decision to use IV steroids, hoping they would jump-start function, so I could get home to my babies. From there, I could focus on giving my body what it really needed to heal. There was no guarantee they would work, but I was willing to try. It wasn't what I had wanted or planned, but sometimes we are faced with tough choices. Once I made the decision, I realized I had to be okay with it. I couldn't feel guilty; I couldn't stress over potential side effects. The mind is powerful, and I chose to believe the steroids would do what I needed them to do. And they did. I'm grateful that I had the option and ability to decide which tool and modality was best for me at that time.

Even though I've been on this journey for over a decade, I'm still learning new lessons. This last year, I've learned that as much as my young kids need me, they need me to care for myself MORE. I can't do everything for everyone—I need to ask for help. It's okay to say no, to have a movie day on the couch, and to have dishes piled in the sink. I've learned to lower my own expectations and to address the nervous system work I've been avoiding by constantly running from one stressful/ traumatic event to the next. My kids taught me that managing MS looks different at various stages in life. The way I did things while twenty-four and single looks much different than how they do now, at thirty-eight, with three kids. I have less time for myself, but it needs to happen. The balance between motherhood and chronic illness isn't always easy, but the more your lifestyle changes become a habit, the easier it becomes (for everyone). Thankfully, in the six months since my flare, I've regained full mobility. I continue to work on building myself up and am learning to "mom" while still prioritizing/meeting my own needs.

MS has been my greatest teacher. I'm grateful for the wave of change it brought into every aspect of my life, and the role it played in shaping who I am today. Prior to 2009, I wasn't taking care of myself, and MS was the alarm bell I needed. Had it not been for a diagnosis at twenty-four, I'd likely still be eating crappy food, burning myself out, and practicing unhealthy habits. I also wouldn't be passionate about helping others take control of their health. In 2015, I felt called to pursue further education in the field of health and became a Holistic Nutritionist. Now, I facilitate group classes, online workshops, and co-host the *Tipping Point Nutrition* podcast with my husband.

Throughout my journey, I've had periods of amazing health, followed by times where life challenges have led me off-track, causing symptoms to manifest. MS or not, is it surprising to display signs of poor health when not taking care of ourselves, physically and emotionally? We can eat the best organic, gluten-free foods, take supplements and exercise, but if we're constantly stressed out and not supporting our nervous system, we can't truly heal. Going the natural route doesn't mean MS will magically be cured or that you will never experience an MS symptom again. It's about building your body up, so that it has the nutrients and resources to most effectively combat the emotional, physical, mental, and environmental stressors that we face today. It also helps us learn how to "get to know" and listen to our bodies, something so many of us have lost the ability and the confidence to do. By focusing on prevention, following the latest research, and making better choices, I believe that I am adding less fuel to the fire and there is an element of health that is within my control. I often hear people complain about aging, but truthfully, thirty-eight-year-old Joanne feels a hundred times better than nineteen-year-old Joanne did.

If you're currently in a place of fear and uncertainty, know that you're not alone. It doesn't mean there won't be difficult periods but take things one day at a time. There are so many incredibly supportive people within the MS community who are willing to share what they've learned along the way. Invest in yourself, not because you are sick with MS, but because you want to THRIVE. I promise you will never regret it!

We are all different. What works best for me might not be what's best for you. We have varying health histories, environmental exposures, food intolerances, and nutrient statuses that all affect how our body functions and responds. If you're just starting to make changes, there's a good chance people in your life will begin to comment on your choices. You do NOT need to justify them. Often others are threatened when someone close begins making positive changes. That's their issue, not yours.

Focus on whole foods, containing anti-inflammatory and therapeutic properties. Lots of ethically sourced, grass-fed meats, deeply colored fruits and veggies, leafy greens, and spices, such as ginger, turmeric, and cinnamon. Remove gluten and dairy. Both have been identified as a trigger for many with MS/autoimmune disease. This has to do with how it contributes to leaky gut and systemic inflammation. Limit consumption of grains due to anti-nutrients that can aggravate the gut (even gluten-free varieties). Oats are a very popular gluten-free alternative. Many people with gluten sensitivity may also react to oats due to avenin, a protein that presents in a similar way to gluten (a process called molecular mimicry). Shop for organic food to avoid excess pesticide exposure. If you can't afford everything organic, use the Environmental Working Group's "Dirty Dozen" list to prioritize organic versus conventional purchases. Consume good quality fats from avocados, coconut, wild fish, etc. The brain is primarily made up of fat! Low fat typically means high sugar. Avoid unhealthy fats. Vegetable oils, such as canola and margarine, are heavily processed and highly inflammatory. Avoid deep fried food and hydrogenated oils. Shop the perimeter of the store, read labels, and purchase foods with minimal ingredients. Eliminate inflammatory foods that wreak havoc on the gut lining (gluten, dairy, soy, corn, and sugar). Consume fermented foods daily as a natural source of gut-friendly probiotics. Drink lots of clean, fluoride-free water. Herbal teas have been very beneficial to me, as well.

The beginning of my MS journey was all about food. When I became pregnant with my first baby almost nine years ago, I started to learn how the many home and personal care products we use today could be impacting mine and my developing baby's health. The skin is our largest organ—anything you apply or smell, you're absorbing! Many of the chemicals in our products do not have to be labeled due to "trade secrets". In recent years, researchers have been sounding the alarm on all these products containing known endocrine disruptors that affect fertility, cause cancer, and wreak havoc on our hormones. In the last hundred years, nearly 100,000 industrial chemicals have been introduced in consumer products. An example is fragrance—an umbrella term, consisting of over 3,100 chemicals. Fragrance can mean a combination of any number of chemicals. How are these all affecting us? Epigenetics has taught us that while it's genes that load the gun, it's environment and lifestyle choices that pull the trigger. These exposures literally have the ability to turn genes on and off.

Today, I attempt to live a low-toxin lifestyle. I use and teach others to leverage therapeutic grade essential oils for home, beauty, and personal care products. We are the gatekeepers to what is brought into our homes and vote with our wallets every single day.

Daily movement is imperative. If you don't use it, you lose it. This is especially true with MS when muscles tend to weaken and atrophy. I've learned focusing on foundational movements and proactively working the muscles that are weakest for me (hip flexors, ankles, etc.) helps keep me mobile and my brain feeling sharp. My favorite activities are rebounding, swimming, yoga, and hiking. The MS Gym and Dr. Gretchen Hawley both have amazing resources/exercises to help address some of the most common MS issues, mobility challenges, and more.

Over the years, I've taken many different supplements. Some are taken on a regular basis, while others are leveraged when I need additional support. The supplements I take most regularly include: magnesium (I prefer bis-glycinate or threonate), B Complex, cod liver oil, alpha lipoic acid, lion's mane, vitamin D, vitamin C, and essential oils—DiGize, peppermint, marjoram, frankincense, R.C., Progessence Phyto Plus, and Stress Away.

I use a ton of essential oils for both emotional and physical support. Some are used on a regular basis, and others are used when I need help with something very specific. Some of the oils I have found most success with are:

- Frankincense - for reducing inflammation and supporting the immune system (applied to the brainstem, added to an Epsom salt bath, applied to bottoms of feet, or specific areas of pain).DiGize - applied over the abdomen for digestive support/ upset stomach.

- Progessence Phyto Plus - includes vitex and wild yam, which have been traditionally used to naturally bring estrogen and progesterone into balance. We know that estrogen dominance can be prevalent in MS, evident by the fact that majority of people affected by MS are women. I apply this over the throat area twice a day.

- Peppermint - applied over the forehead for headaches. Used in a spray bottle with water to keep cool on a hot day (heat is a big trigger for my MS).

- RC - contains three different types of eucalyptus, plus some other powerhouse oils to support the respiratory system. I put this in a roller with some carrier oil and apply it along the side of the nostrils, brow line, low cheekbones, and around the ears to help alleviate sinus pressure. I also spend time each morning washing my face with ice cold water (good for the vagus nerve), then do some massage techniques, using my oils to help promote drainage.

- Marjoram - I have found marjoram to be particularly grounding/ calming and supportive of the nervous system. I simply like the way this one makes me feel and often feel called to use it.

- Cypress - helps me to reduce swelling/edema in my feet and lower extremities. I apply this to my legs and feet in the morning, and again before bed, if I have any swelling.

- Joy - this was the first oil I began using. After my dad died, I'd apply a drop over my heart each morning. It's amazing how much calmer, uplifted, and supported I felt when using it. It truly helped me to process and work through my grief. I was initially drawn to oils because of all the physical ailments they could assist me with (especially as a new mom), but I was not expecting them to be so effective as calmatives, supporting the nervous system and my emotional state.

- Rosemary - historically has been used for memory, focus, and overall cognitive function. I diffuse this with an uplifting citrus oil any time I really need to concentrate.

With my flare at the end of 2022, I saw another neurologist for the first time since being diagnosed. It was a better experience than fourteen years ago, but she still reiterated that if I wasn't going to go on medication, there really wasn't much she could do for me. I mentioned how I'd been successfully managing things for over a decade through diet, and she continued speaking as though she didn't hear me. I'm always amazed that there isn't more interest in learning about what's working for patients.

I choose to focus on the present. There is no point in stressing about unknowns or hypotheticals. I'm fourteen years into my MS journey, and while there have been setbacks along the way, I've also seen how incredible the body is, and what can happen when we support it. I have absolutely no regrets. I believe every experience has led me to where I am today. I want those who are in their darkest moments to have hope and know that they can still be empowered to take control of their health. Your mindset will 100% affect your state of health. It doesn't matter what changes you make—if you don't believe you will see your health improve, then it won't. MS is hard. But like everything in life, it becomes harder when we allow ourselves to go to a place of hopelessness and despair. This journey requires you to become your own biggest advocate. It also requires you evaluate relationships with those who hold you back or don't recognize the need to do what's best for your health. In the words of Michael J. Fox, "Gratitude makes optimism sustainable."

19

Story by

HELENA KNIGHT

Diagnosed in 2000
Currently 63 years old
Lives in Redditch, United Kingdom

My story—where to start? As Julie Andrews from the *Sound of Music* would say, "Let's start at the very beginning…a very good place to start."

I have many memories of me as a young child. I was vibrant and bursting with energy. At the age of eight, my potential as a gifted swimmer was acknowledged, marking the start of my path as a competitive swimmer. I trained seven days a week, both in the pool and at the gym. I enjoyed competing and won many awards. I even competed overseas at the club level and represented my county (Yorkshire), just missing out on the trials for the 1976 Ontario Olympics. My best event was 100m butterfly, and I last swam competitively at the age of thirty-six! I was super fit then, and that was only four years before receiving my multiple sclerosis (MS) diagnosis. In addition to my swimming skills, I had a talent for art. I wrote poetry and performed it on stage. I was even published in the local newspaper multiple times. I also enjoyed other artistic activities like painting, drawing, and working with clay. Looking back, even at the age of thirteen, my writing was quite political.

In 1991, I spent the year traveling around the world for thirteen months with my then partner Chris. We traveled to India, Thailand, Malaysia, Singapore, Indonesia, Australia, New Zealand, Mexico, USA, and Canada. Looking back, I suspect that I experienced the initial signs of MS during that time, but it's difficult to determine as the whole journey was challenging. Perhaps my fatigue was due to the physical strain of travel, lack of sleep, walking, climbing, etc. I know I wouldn't have changed anything, but considering my diagnosis in 2000, I'm glad I traveled when I did because I know I wouldn't have been able to do it afterward.

Upon my return to the UK in February 1992, I fulfilled another wish from my bucket list by starting and successfully establishing a tearoom in Kenilworth, Warwickshire. I loved baking all the cakes, something I still love to do, even though I don't eat cake myself! Within the first two years, Time for Tea was nominated for "Tea Place of the Year", and I had the privilege of being interviewed by Bruce Richardson from the US for his book, *Great Tearooms of Britain*. It was a beautiful hardcover book that dedicated six pages to me and my business. It was truly an honor!

In 1997, fate brought my ex-husband into my life when he visited my tearoom as a Food Hygiene Inspector. The rest is history! I never wanted to marry or have children, but I'm afraid the universe had other plans. Before I knew it, I was pregnant (planned). I met my husband just a few days after he had separated from his wife and daughter. He appeared very sad and carried emotional pain in his eyes. Interestingly, I later heard from others that he started telling everyone about meeting an incredible woman (me). At that time, he had made a personal promise not to seek or engage in any relationship for at least two years. So, it's puzzling why, after six weeks, we started our relationship.

We got married in early April 1998—a lovely day with family and friends, but deep down, I knew that I'd made a big mistake. It took me a long time to realize that I married a narcissist. I was pregnant when we got married, and despite not wanting to, I felt that I owed it to my parents. We had discussions about having a child because he had already left his daughter, and as I approached forty, I felt it was my last chance. I genuinely wanted our child, Bertie. I'm glad I had him when I did because I went through menopause at age forty-two! The day of our marriage marked the beginning of a pattern where he didn't engage in meaningful conversation.

Not long after we married, we moved to another city (Worcester) where we bought our first marital home. Three weeks after moving, I gave birth to my beautiful son Albert (Bertie) by C-section. Once again, my husband showed no sign of affection or empathy for what I was going through!

Nine months later, while on holiday, I experienced my first recognizable signs of MS: tingling in my hands, feet, and legs, as if ice water was running through them. When I returned home, the symptoms had subsided, and I chose not to take any action.

I'm sure you can tell by now that I felt incredibly lonely in my marriage but held on for seventeen years. Eventually, after he left me and took my son, I had a well-deserved emotional breakdown. But let's not get ahead of ourselves.

One day while walking my son in his stroller, I passed by a building with a sign in the window asking for volunteers. I went inside and shared my information. The organization was called the Worcester Association for the Blind. They matched me with a lady named Margaret, who both Bertie and I knew as Auntie Dimp. We loved her and were more than happy to visit her on a regular basis until her passing, a couple of years later. I wanted to continue working with the organization, and they asked me if I could work with members and help teach them to cook and bake. I happily accepted…until something unexpected happened.

My eye became very painful, and I suddenly lost sight in that eye overnight. Even though my legs were stiff due to my MS acting up again, I managed to walk to the town. There, I visited an optician's office who was kind enough to take care of my son Bertie while I was there. The optician gave me a letter to give to my General Practitioner (GP). As I was walking to see my GP, guess who I bumped into? It was my husband, who had just come home for lunch. Reluctantly, he accompanied me to see the doctor, showing his unhappiness. The doctor gave me another letter to take to the eye hospital. We went to the hospital by car, but my husband, being himself, didn't want to pay for parking. He parked somewhere else and insisted that I hurry because, in his words, I wasn't dying. Can you believe that? How did he know?

I explained all my symptoms and the timeline to my GP. She sat me down and said, "Well Mrs. Knight, you've told me all about your symptoms. What do you think you've got?" My immediate response was that I either had a brain tumor (which I thought was highly unlikely), or I had multiple sclerosis!

She responded with, "Yes, you probably have MS."

It was the first time I'd ever spoken those words, and as you can imagine, my husband's face went ashen! I thought it was multiple sclerosis because of a poster I saw years ago. The poster showed a woman with a body/back shaped like a cello, with her spine ripped out. That image stuck with me for many years.

After seeing two young medics who were reluctant to answer my questions about what they believed was wrong with me, they passed me off to another doctor. This doctor arranged for me to see a neurologist at Redditch Hospital.

My diagnosis became official following magnetic resonance imaging (MRI). I drove myself to Redditch to see Dr. Spilane to receive the news. I went alone, and after receiving the diagnosis, I said, "Thank goodness for that!" I'd rather know what I've got than face more testing!

My husband wasn't with me the day I received my official MS diagnosis. Honestly, I think my husband was also scared, but he never discussed it or talked about our future. My biggest concern after my diagnosis was regarding a lady from my hometown of Bradford who made national news because of her MS. Her situation was severe, and she became concerned about her future to the point of considering assisted suicide. Her husband was supportive until the end. If she had chosen to proceed, she would have had to go to Switzerland. However, while the legal issues in Britain were being scrutinized, she passed away naturally. Hearing her story was incredibly sad and deeply affected me.

Throughout my life, I've been surrounded by amazing friends, most of which I'd only recently met following my move to Worcester. They were incredible. In the meantime, my life went on. Not only did I look after my own son, but I also looked after my new friend Laura's son two days a week. I took on a part-time job, too. In my earlier years, I worked in Sales as a Sales Manager for a brick company. In my later years, I transitioned to realty as an Estate Agent. I found great success and equal enjoyment in both roles!

I had always followed a vegetarian diet. My ex-husband worked in the meat industry, so I went back to eating meat once I got married—wrong decision. When I received my MS diagnosis, I became vegetarian again. I have what I call a "clean" diet. Having read more about MS, I now know I made the right decision! I've always had a good diet. As a swimmer, it was imperative that I looked after my body. Although it wasn't quite as clean as it is now, looking at Dr. Jelinek's book *Overcoming MS*, I realized my diet was exactly what he recommends.

After I connected with Talia Halberor in January this year (I found her on social media), my diet became even cleaner. Combined with my focus on positive energy and quantum physics, I experienced a remarkable improvement in just a few weeks. In the past, I have used a cane or a walker, mainly for my vertigo, so that I wouldn't appear drunk while walking. The walker also provided a way for me to rest when I felt tired. However, since working with Talia, I've ditched both! Talia has been a godsend for me, and I will always be indebted to her. She also has MS but has totally reversed her symptoms.

When it comes to my diet, I have made significant changes. Nowadays, I only eat fruits and vegetables, often in the form of smoothies, excluding potatoes. To get my vegetables, I rely on deliveries from a local farm shop. I also go to the supermarket for groceries. I no longer eat eggs, dairy, or sadly, cheese. Sometimes I find vegan alternatives and always use oat milk or another alternative for dairy. I used to put photos of my vegetable deliveries on Facebook/Instagram and the dishes I made from them. People loved it! But that was before I met Talia, so my diet wasn't quite as strict then. I've always enjoyed cooking, but these days, I have to search for and adapt recipes to suit my diet. I stay away from processed food, meat, and saturated fats. I avoid carbs like pasta, rice, etc. I use flax and chia seeds for protein. I also drink three liters of water per day and take vitamins D, B12, magnesium, omega 3, and turmeric supplements. In addition to maintaining a clean diet, I do my best to go to the gym at least two to three times a week. The biggest change in my life is that I've had to give up working.

My sleep has improved compared to before my diagnosis, although it still tends to be interrupted. I find that going to the gym and taking walks helps improve my sleep. I do my best to live a stress-free life; however, if I decide to relocate to beautiful Hereford (where my son lives), then I'm sure my stress level will go through the roof! Hereford is a very flat city, unlike where I live now. During my visit there, I walked many kilometers, covering seventeen in just the first three days! My son, Thomas Albert, has a great job at the university in Hereford and is on the verge of being promoted to Assistant Professor. He teaches Mathematics at NMITE, a specialized university for engineers. His first master's degree was in Chemical Engineering. While I may not think about his father very much, it's evident that he has inherited good genes. Recently, his daughter also got her PhD!

People say that MS is caused by trauma. When asked what my trauma is, I always said, "I got married." I thought I was only joking until I worked on my history with Talia, and then I really did know that it was not a joke —it was fact. I knew my ex made me physically ill. The very last time I saw him in person, I instantly got double vision. We were supposed to be going on a family camping holiday to Europe with the two kids, but once the car was packed, there wasn't room for me. I was quite relieved if I'm honest. I think it would have been far too stressful for me as every previous family holiday was. The same double vision happened when I knew he was coming home. My son even wrote to his university at the time of his graduation saying that under no circumstances should his dad sit anywhere near his mum.

The symptoms that bother me the most are vertigo and fatigue. But since I started working with Talia, my fatigue has dropped drastically. I've also had issues with swallowing/choking, but even that seems to have stopped. However, my speech can be slurred, especially when I'm tired or stressed, and it hurts me more than anything because I used to give public presentations and speeches. Something I forgot to mention was that I ventured into local politics around 2010-2011. I ran for elections twice, once for District council and once for County council. Although I didn't win, I came in second place with a 40% improvement compared to the previous candidate. It's an accomplishment I'm still proud of!

Despite having had MS for twenty-three years, I've only had three MRI scans, with the last two in the past five or six years. Apart from two years ago when I last saw my neurologist, I have never been offered drugs. The doctor gave me details of a new drug for secondary progressive MS, telling me that I could research it online. He then sent an MS nurse to my house to see if I wanted to take it. I think she already knew the answer: "No, thank you!" At the request of my neurologist, I had two more recent MRI scans since he noticed that I had only previously undergone one. The lesions are located in my brain, but he tells me I have too many to count!

I've always done my very best to live my life as if I don't have MS, but at sixty-three, I guess we all slow down. I've never taken drugs for my MS. I'm sure some people don't understand why, but it works for me. I have an issue with "big Pharma", so I prefer to take a more holistic route. I choose to rely on nutritional supplements.

Thanks to the internet and my local MS Society group, I've connected with many people who also have MS. It took me some time to feel ready to join the society, but around seven or eight years ago, after moving back to Yorkshire, I finally joined. It has been a wonderful opportunity to make new friends who understand the challenge of living with this disease. Sadly, I've lost some friends along the way. But on a more positive note, I have a friend named Tommy who has MS. He is an incredible person and last year, he captained the Physically Disabled World Cup England Rugby League team to victory in the World Cup. How cool is that? I make sure I surround myself with only positive energy, especially when it comes to my choice of friends! I have a "tribe" of my own.

Another friend of mine I'd like to mention is Tracy Dawn, who I met for the first time when she came to an MS Society meeting. At the time, she hadn't received a diagnosis, but it was clear that she had MS. It took several months before she finally received an official diagnosis, and by that time, she was told that she'd probably been living with it for fourteen years. That was over four years ago. Since then, she's written her story in a book titled, *I'm Still Smiling*. I take my hat off to her. Sadly, she's a single parent for her nine-year-old son with autism. Dealing with these challenges is a struggle for her every day. Despite her difficulties, she is a seriously talented musician, although she can no longer perform. I have great respect for her. If you were to read Tracy Dawn's book, you would discover the traumas she has faced in her own life. Her story shows the connection between trauma and the effects it can have on people with MS. Stress made my MS symptoms worse, causing double vision. Stress also gave me anxiety and depression, something I'd never experienced before.

My advice to those who are newly diagnosed is that MS is not a death sentence. Trust your own body's signals and remember that neurologists don't have all the answers. In my opinion, those who truly understand MS are the ones living with this condition. Stay optimistic, practice meditation, engage in physical activity like yoga, and most importantly, never give up!

20

Story by
SAM PANKO

Diagnosed in 2015
Currently 28 years old
Lives in Dauphin, Manitoba, Canada
Instagram: @prairie_momma_essentials

My story is dedicated to Shelley Hood. Thank you for being my first introduction to living a life with multiple sclerosis (MS) drug-free. Even though I didn't know it at the time, you opened my world to the possibility of not needing medication, and I'm forever grateful. You are missed and loved always.

Imagine: you're eighteen, fresh out of high school and ready to take on the world. You have been dreaming about becoming a teacher since you were in kindergarten and can't wait to get started on your education degree. One day, you wake up, and something just feels off. You can't place your finger on it, but something is wrong, and you know you must go home. So, you pack up and move (which is an entire province away) after being there for only two weeks. The first week back, you wake up with minimal hearing, no taste, and messed-up vision. That was my reality back in September of 2013.

Hi! My name is Sam Panko. I am twenty-eight, a mom of two, and I live in Dauphin, Manitoba, Canada.

It was August 2013; I was preparing to move to a school located in a different province and live on my own for the first time. My summer had been rough between accidentally becoming pregnant, losing twins at thirteen weeks when I was in a car accident, and finding out that a dear friend from high school had lost his life in a car accident that same summer. The grief from suddenly losing a friend seemed unbearable, especially as I was moving away. I felt the best way to honor him was to chase my dreams and live my life to the fullest in his memory, so I planned to do just that. Because the stress and trauma I was going through felt so heavy, I was looking forward to escaping from my hometown and "starting fresh" in a new city on my own, where I didn't have reminders of these events everywhere I turned. I avoided dealing with these traumas and believed that if I didn't think about them, they would go away.

I had just moved into residence at the University of Regina, where I was going to start my education degree and was so excited. I was finally out on my own and couldn't wait to see what life had to offer. I was at school for less than two weeks when something just started to feel off. It's so hard to explain because I didn't feel sick and I wasn't experiencing any "symptoms", I just knew something wasn't right; I could feel it in the depths of my soul. I called my parents, terrified that they wouldn't understand and tell me to tough it out but thank God they didn't. They listened to me and started planning to come pick me up—no fighting, no anger, nothing. They just completely trusted me, and I will forever be so grateful for that. Thankfully, I was within the time frame that I could still withdraw from school without losing all my money, so I repacked my stuff and went home. Now that I was heading home, it forced me to face the traumas I had experienced over the summer with the added feelings around "failing" and moving home from my dream school. I was trying to figure out what my next step was now that I had just abandoned school on a whim because I was feeling off.

I have a long history of participating in musicals with a local production group, and they had a show happening the week I moved home, so I decided to jump on their backstage crew to distract myself from everything that had happened.

It was late September and show week was ramping up. I was so excited to have something to distract me from all the trauma that I didn't want to deal with. I woke up on the first day of the show, filled with excitement and ready for a great week. I was surprised when my dad came in to wake me when I had set an alarm. I realized that my alarm was going off, but I just couldn't hear it. I tried to find my glasses, and when I put them on, I realized my eyes were struggling to focus. I thought maybe I was just tired, and it would fix itself if I showered. I was seeing three of everything—moving up and down, side to side, and in circles—all at the same time. I continued to get ready, not knowing what I should do next. When I sat down to eat breakfast, I also realized that I couldn't taste anything. It was like eating lard. Trying not to freak out, I decided to ignore it and keep it to myself. I knew if I told my parents, they wouldn't let me participate in the show, and I wasn't going to let that happen. So, I spent the week driving to and from shows and rehearsals, getting by as best I could. At the end of the week, after our final Sunday Matinee (October 20), I decided to ask my dad if he would take me to the Emergency Room (ER).

To say he was angry at me for not telling him what was going on is an understatement. When I think about it now, I could have very seriously hurt myself or someone else while driving with impaired vision and minimal hearing. I thank God that nothing happened. When we walked through those hospital doors, I had no idea the journey that awaited. They looked me over and told me it was probably stress from the traumatic couple of months I had been through and told me to go home and sleep it off.

I knew that something more was going on, so we decided to seek additional opinions in hopes something would make more sense. We went to our family optometrist who told me that my eyes were perfectly healthy. He said that because of the symptoms I was experiencing, he believed it was neurological. We also went to a physiotherapist because of the accident I was in. She wouldn't even touch me because she also agreed that it was neurological and didn't want to make anything worse. Since they didn't take me seriously the first time we went to the ER, we decided to try the walk-in next. We saw a doctor that performed tests on me and was shocked that someone hadn't caught this sooner. He sent off a requisition to the local neurologists. Dr. Tamayo was luckily able to squeeze me in on October 23rd. He didn't usually deal with anything outside of strokes, but the other neurologist was on holiday, so he decided to fit me in when he heard the urgency of my condition. After his assessment, he immediately consulted one of his textbooks. He had his hand on his face and explained to us that in all his years as a neurologist, he has only seen what was happening to me in textbooks—never in person. He explained that my eyes were moving separately from each other, and they were also vibrating.

To investigate further, he sent me for magnetic resonance imaging (MRI). The MRI came back before we had even returned to the office. I remember looking at the screen and seeing fifteen lesions and feeling sick to my stomach when, in reality, there were three. Because of my vision, it looked way worse. I didn't find this out until many years down the road. He told us that he suspected it was multiple sclerosis, and my stomach dropped. I remember my father, who I had never seen cry in my life, burst into tears. He told us he would give us a minute before he came back to talk about where we should go from there. My mom and I left the room and went to use the bathroom. I remember standing in the bathroom, looking at myself in the mirror and trying so hard to focus, but my vision was too bad. My first thoughts were, "I'm only eighteen. I thought MS was an old person's disease. How did I become so unlucky to develop an old person's disease?" I remember thinking about all the life that I had in front of me and how worried I was that my life was over.

We came back to the room, and Dr. Tamayo told us that he was going to admit me to the ER, so they could run some tests to confirm what he suspected. They sent me for another MRI with contrast this time, blood tests, computed tomography (CT) scans, and finally, a spinal tap. When they performed the spinal tap, it was done incorrectly and went straight through my spine instead of stopping in the middle to retrieve the spinal fluid. They accidentally drew blood, which contaminated the sample, making it unusable. As a result, they had to take more than necessary. They advised me that I would likely have some severe headaches afterward since they had taken everything they could for the tests, but it should only last twenty-four hours. I stayed the night in the ER and went home the next day after all the tests were completed. They told me that it would take a couple of weeks to get the results from the spinal tap.

Over the next five days, I came back daily for two hours to receive my steroid treatment at the outpatient unit. It took me almost three weeks to fully recover from the spinal tap. I was too weak to walk, so my dad had to carry me everywhere. I couldn't sit upright, that's how weak I was. I needed help with everything from bathing to eating to using the washroom.

Finally, I got the call with my results. When I picked up the phone, they told me that all the test results had come back normal. They also informed me that the only test result they didn't receive was the test that would clarify whether or not I had MS. It was lost in the mail (these tests had to be mailed a couple of provinces away to be analyzed). I was devastated, angry, and frustrated. I'd endured all that pain just for them to lose it. I remember the doctor telling me that I could come in that weekend to redo the testing. Alternatively, I could wait until I had another relapse that met the criteria of a new symptom lasting for more than twenty-four hours—which could be years—to qualify for a diagnosis. I made it very clear that I was not going through that pain again, especially after they did it wrong the first time. The neurologist gave me the diagnosis of Clinically Isolated Syndrome (CIS), which is just a fancy way of saying they have no idea what is wrong and sent me on my way. I was also informed by another doctor that I would most likely be in a wheelchair by twenty-five, never be able to have kids, and probably wouldn't live much past thirty because of the severity of my lesions.

I spent the next two years just kind of floating by. I couldn't hold a job because of my symptoms, and I didn't have enough energy to go out and do things with friends. I was in pure survival mode. My parents split in March of 2015, something I didn't realize I took so hard until I look back now. At the same time, I was struggling to feel like an independent person because of how sick I was and how reliant I was on my parents for everything. I watched as all my friends were finishing school, finding partners, and traveling the world, while I was stuck at home because I needed help with the most basic tasks, like using the washroom. I was humiliated, ashamed, angry, heartbroken, and scared—I felt like my life was over. At the time, getting a diagnosis was my main focus; it was all I could think about. I wished for a relapse just so I could get the formal diagnosis. It was so important to me because I felt like I was isolated on an island. Without it, I didn't feel like I fit anywhere. I couldn't apply for any funding or help through the MS society, I couldn't attend MS camp, I couldn't even explore medication options. I believed that a diagnosis would give me the clarity I was searching for and was the only way for my struggles to feel valid and worthwhile.

I have been attending church for as long as I can remember. I was there every Sunday, followed all the "rules", like no swearing, being kind to everyone, and always including others—especially those who were left behind. I did outreach and helped the needy. I felt like, for the most part, I was your typical "good Christian girl". So, when I was dealing with the looming diagnosis of what I thought was a chronic, life-long illness that would be debilitating, I was angry. I felt like God had betrayed me, that I was being punished for something that I didn't deserve. I had done everything I thought I was supposed to do as a good Christian, and here I was being punished and having all my dreams taken away from me. I was filled with aspirations to get a good career, travel the world, have a big family, and live a very big, full life. I completely fell away from God and Christianity. I stopped talking to my friends from church, stopped attending church and all the associated groups, and removed it from my life in every aspect. I believed that this was proof that God didn't exist. Why would he punish someone that was doing everything "right" when there were much worse people in the world who were going unpunished?

During this time of limbo and being distant from God, my self-esteem and self-worth was at an all-time low. I truly believed that I would never find someone who would want to be my husband. Why would any man want to marry a woman that he would have to look after and would be around for less than ten years, according to the doctors? I'd become numb and started looking for anything to make me feel something. I started a relationship that was not good for me. I knew in my heart that it was toxic, but I believed I didn't deserve better and if I left him, I would never find anyone else. I believed that staying in an abusive relationship was better than being alone. I fought hard to keep the relationship from falling apart. Eventually, he ended things, and I was devastated. My worst fear of spending what little life I had left alone had come true. In hindsight, I'm glad that my ex broke up with me because looking back, I probably never would have done it myself. I moved back in with my parents and spiraled even more. This was the same time that they split, so I was returning home to only one parent. My childhood cat, who I'd adopted when I was five as my "big girl present" for starting school, was very sick and passed away only a couple of months after I moved home. This was the biggest loss I had experienced up to that point and the most painful experience. She was the one I would turn to when I felt no person understood me. She was always there to comfort me when I was feeling down. I never had to worry about her judging me or not loving me. She was my best friend, especially since I'd pushed everyone away. Losing her felt like I lost a huge part of myself.

I felt so lost. I would attend groups at the MS society, but because I didn't have the MS diagnosis, I didn't feel like anyone understood me. The youngest person in the group was a couple decades older than me, so I felt very alone and isolated. It felt even more devastating because I saw all these older people living with MS just fine, and I was using a cane, couldn't drive, and was told I wouldn't live to see my thirtieth birthday. I felt like everyone was mocking me with their health and wrinkles. I was desperate to have gray hair, a wrinkly face, beautiful children and grandchildren, and celebrate wedding anniversaries that made it to the double digits. Everything seemed pointless when I had an expiration date. I was just waiting to die.

I had no reason to do anything because I believed I wouldn't be around long enough to enjoy the rewards. I felt lucky when asked to be the ambassador for the MS walk in my town in 2015. They wanted to focus on a story of someone that was in the "limbo" stage who hadn't received a diagnosis yet. They believed that it was an important side of the story to tell. It felt great to be able to share my struggles with the hope of helping someone else.

I felt that maybe I could make a difference with the short amount of time I had left. From my first relapse in 2013 up until June 2015, I relapsed on average every three months. Most relapses were vision-related, so they weren't classified as a new symptom and didn't make me eligible for a diagnosis. Every time I relapsed, I was put on steroids for five days and told to go home. During one of my many relapses in June 2015, my mom took me to an appointment. This relapse was more related to weakness in my legs, so I was hopeful that it might be the one to get me the diagnosis I was so desperate for. My neurologist wanted to see me for a follow-up to discuss the routine MRI I'd recently undergone. The office was in a city that was two-and-a-half hours from where I lived, making it an all-day trip. On the way there, my mom was trying to check in and help by asking questions. Most of them were related to my faith and the feelings I had around God. I told her how I felt betrayed by him and didn't believe that he was real anymore. If he was, he wasn't someone I wanted to know. She said something along the lines of, "We know there is sin in the world. God didn't create sin to punish us; sin was brought about when Eve betrayed God. But I believe even though God did not create sin, he uses it for good. Just like when a mother doesn't stop their child from climbing on something like a short box; she knows that the child will probably fall but will also learn a valuable lesson from the scraped knee. She wouldn't let her child climb to the top of the deck where they could be seriously hurt, but a small fall might be what the child needs to grow into a better version of themselves." I had never thought of it from that perspective before. Maybe God did have plans for me that I couldn't see yet. God loved me and was with me the whole time, even when I tried to push him away; He was there protecting and guiding me because of his undying love.

During my appointment, something happened that changed everything for me. My neurologist pulled up my MRI and said because this relapse involved different symptoms than the others, he could now confirm it was MS. I finally received the diagnosis I had been waiting on for two years! But something else miraculous happened. When he pulled up the scans, one of the lesions he'd been most worried about had vanished. He looked over the scan multiple times and couldn't figure out what had happened. He said that it was odd, and he'd never seen one disappear like that. The lesion was nowhere to be found. He told me that it must have been a machine error, or I must have moved during the scan because lesions can't just disappear. He said that it would probably show up again in my next scans, but it never did.

At that moment, it clicked. God had healed one of my lesions even when I was the farthest away from Him that I had ever been. That's when I realized I had never been alone; I had a huge group of people I didn't even know that were praying and walking this journey with me. Even though they didn't physically know what it was like, they were still there for support. Most importantly—I had God. He never left my side, even when I tried to distance myself. He was there, guiding me the whole time. I realized that through all this pain and suffering, I was now able to help others who were in a similar situation. I walked out of that office with a new diagnosis, a plan to start medication, and a new lease on life. I was ready to take my struggles and help others, so they never had to feel as alone and lost as I did.

I found out about a camp that was held in Ontario for young people with MS, and I was thrilled that I would finally be able to attend. I was scared to be traveling so far away from my family when I'd been relying on them so heavily, but knowing I would be surrounded by others who were not only going through the same things as me but were also my age made it so exciting and worth the risk.

I had no idea how much camp would change my life. I went feeling lost, alone, and hopeless about my future, as if nobody understood me. I had very low expectations but figured it was better than sitting at home and feeling sorry for myself. I'd started on Copaxone shortly before I set off for camp, adding an extra layer of complexity to my journey. Not only was I traveling alone, but I also had to navigate the challenge of keeping the Copaxone at the proper temperature and finding a way to travel with needles.

My week at camp was nothing short of life-changing. I got to spend a week with people my age, who had been through similar situations (sometimes even worse), and yet, they were still living their lives and enjoying every moment. It was at camp that I realized the doctor who told me I had a life expectancy of thirty was completely wrong. MS does not necessarily mean you have a shortened lifespan. I left the camp with new, lifelong friends, like my dear friend Kadesha (you'll read her story in here, too!), a new way to look at life, many new coping skills, and so much more information about what MS was. I no longer had this looming "death date" over my head. I was so much more positive about all the possibilities my future held, and for the first time in two years, I finally felt like I wasn't walking this journey alone.

My experience with Copaxone was not great. I have always been DEATHLY terrified of needles. Ever since I was a child, I had to use numbing cream to be able to receive any shot at all. But I decided to try Copaxone first because, even though it was a daily injection, they said it was the least damaging to my body. Looking back now, I realize that even amid my intense fear for my life, I had the instinct to seek the least damaging route.

When it comes to disease-modifying therapies (DMTs), you are required to be on them for a minimum of four months before they will switch you to a new one. I was on Copaxone for less than three months when I went back to my neurologist and requested to change medications. I was getting bad bruising, terrible cellulite, and the injection sites were constantly sore even when I rotated sites properly. I decided to switch to Aubagio. It was a much-needed break from the needles, but it also meant that I needed to get routine blood work to monitor my liver levels. They also told me that I had the JVC marker, which means that I didn't have as many options for medication because it could trigger a deadly brain infection.

I was still struggling with symptoms from my relapses and was looking for a way to manage them as naturally as I could. One of my friends, Jordyn, was hosting a class at her house for an essential oil company she'd started using called Young Living. I decided that I would go and listen to what she had to say. I'd tried every other avenue, and nothing was working, so I figured I had nothing to lose. When I first got my kit in the mail, I was very overwhelmed but excited to hopefully find some relief. I started using the oils that were suggested to me to relieve my muscle spasms, migraines, brain fog, weakness, and fatigue. I found some relief, but I wasn't using them consistently enough to see noticeable changes.

My daily symptoms were extensive, but I had finally stopped relapsing every three months. I had no feeling in my hands to the point that I would cut myself without noticing, hypersensitivity in my thighs, almost all fabrics caused me pain, daily migraines, light sensitivity requiring me to always wear sunglasses, little to no appetite, constant vision issues, brain fog, memory issues, trouble forming thoughts and articulating them, difficulty finding words or engaging in conversations, sleeping a minimum of fifteen hours a day without feeling rested, extreme chronic fatigue, and being in a constant state of sensory overload. Looking back, I realize that a lot of the "MS" symptoms I was experiencing were related to the medication—not caused by my lesions.

Fast forward to August of 2018, I went to a bible study at a friend's place, and I met my husband there. We started dating in November 2018 and fell in love fast. In January 2019, he came with me to my neurology check-up at the MS clinic. This was our chance to ask questions about family planning and how this would affect us as a couple. Now, if you know my husband, you know he researches EVERYTHING. He'd put tons of time into researching MS from what it was, to how it's treated, to what it means for him, and every way he could help to make me better. My neurologist told us that my clock was ticking; the longer we waited to have kids, the less likely I would be able to get pregnant and have a healthy baby. He told me that to get pregnant, I would have to go off Aubagio. To do that, I would need to either wait two years for my body to naturally detox, or I would have to do a fourteen-day detox by drinking powdered charcoal three times a day.

On the drive home, we talked about our options. That is when my husband said, "Well if we want to have kids, we should probably do it sooner than later, and we need to get married." I asked him if that was his way of proposing to me, and he replied, "Yeah, I guess so." We started planning our wedding for June 2019, so we could begin building our family before I started working again in September. I was in school for the third time, this time to be an Educational Assistant. I was scheduled to start my first position in September, and I wanted to have the charcoal detox done before then. So, that's exactly what we did! We got married on June 22, 2019, and I found out I was pregnant with our daughter on October 8, 2019.

My husband had already been living a much healthier life than I was when we met. He only ate food with one-word names: apples, potatoes, steak, etc., that had no ingredient list. He'd cut seed oils out and added extra healthy fats, such as grass-fed butter, to his diet. He was adamant that changing my diet would make a big difference in the way I was feeling and would help with symptom management. He also brought up vaccinations, showing me the research that he'd found supporting the fact that vaccinations do more harm than good. I thought he was insane and fought back hard. I truly didn't believe that changing my diet or abstaining from all vaccinations would make any difference. He told me that he would not allow our children to be vaccinated, and I almost left him three months into our marriage. I was confident that if our children weren't up to date on their vaccination schedules, then their risk of getting sick and dying from preventable diseases was uncomfortably high.

I truly believe that the charcoal detox not only drew out the Aubagio, but also helped to remove some of the toxic burden my body was experiencing. My pregnancy with my daughter was extremely difficult. I had to quit my first Educational Assistant position only two months in because I was so sick. The doctors wrote me a note recommending that I take a leave from work for the remainder of my pregnancy. They prescribed "light bed rest", which meant refraining from any strenuous activities. During the first trimester, I experienced constant sickness. I would throw up multiple times every day. My appetite suffered as I felt too weak to get up, resulting in barely any eating. It was a miserable time for me. Thankfully, the morning sickness went away during the second trimester, but I didn't receive much reprieve before the crippling anxiety set in. My father was traveling two hours one way to spend the days with me because I couldn't be left alone. I couldn't sleep, and I had anxiety attacks multiple times a day. On top of that, I was experiencing what I believed to be a relapse where my vision started to worsen. Thankfully, the third trimester was better. I experienced only the typical pregnancy symptoms like sore bones and being tired, but I swore that I would never get pregnant again. My birth experience was far from pleasant. I was told because I was "high risk", I couldn't have a midwife and had to give birth at the hospital.

At three o'clock in the morning on June 6, 2020, my water broke. They refused to let my mother into the birthing suite due to COVID restrictions and the limitations of allowing only one support person. I was devastated and didn't know how I was supposed to do this without her. After the doctors induced me, the progress was slow. I was induced a second time because nothing was happening. While I was there, the government changed the restrictions from one support to two. My husband called my mom, and she came straight to the hospital. I have never been so relieved to see her. Once she was there, things started moving. After they induced me a third time, I finally began having contractions and dilating. The pain was so bad that I couldn't move, I couldn't talk, I couldn't even open my eyes between contractions.

The doctors told me I could push for two more hours. If nothing happened, then they would need to do a cesarean (C-section). One of my biggest fears in life was getting surgery, especially a cesarean. I was going to do everything I could to make sure that didn't happen. Suddenly, her heart rate dropped. She was stuck, and they had to prepare me for an emergency C-section. The room was swarming with nurses and staff, preparing me for the surgery. I'd never been so terrified in my life. They took my husband to get prepped and whisked me away to the operating room, leaving my mom behind. At this point, I had been in labor for close to thirty-six hours. I was so tired that I couldn't keep my eyes open, even if I tried. I remember lying on the table while they told me they were going to start, asking if I could feel them touching me. I told them I could, but another doctor said they couldn't wait—they had to start cutting. I felt the first half of the surgery, but luckily, my daughter came out healthy. They took her away to the NICU because she wasn't breathing initially, and she was three weeks early. I was left on the table alone. I told my husband to follow her and make sure she was okay. They left me in recovery for over four hours. I begged them to bring Sophia to me, so I could meet her and feed her.

I finally got to meet her five hours after she was born, and suddenly, my life had new meaning. I had the most perfect little girl that relied on me being my best, healthiest self, so she could thrive. I was going to move heaven and earth to make sure she had the best mom possible. I now had a reason to be as healthy as I could, so I could live as long as possible to see her grow up. I could no longer say, "Well, if I don't live that long, then it's not a big deal. It won't impact anyone that much." The pain I felt when I thought about not being around to see her grow up was unbearable. I wanted to show her that no matter what life threw my way, I would fight as hard as I could to be my best self for her.

Something in me clicked after she was born. I finally understood where my husband came from when he talked about how important diet was. It was like the veil was lifted, and I was no longer blind to what was happening in the world. I finally understood how corrupt the systems were from the crap they put in our food to the forced vaccination schedule. By realizing the harmful ingredients in these shots, I became aware of the importance of detoxing our lives and making conscious efforts to improve our body's natural healing ability. This realization led me to question the necessity of vaccine schedules and to prioritize preventive measures to avoid further damage. After all, God made our bodies perfectly; God doesn't make mistakes. He made it so that we could naturally heal and gave us the tools on earth from the beginning to do this.

I reached out to my friend, Jordyn, who'd hosted the oil class back in 2015 to talk about how I could get started making healthier choices. I'd researched all the top companies that offered oils, and Young Living kept coming out on top. They were the only company that sold 100% pure products. I could visit the farms to see where and how my products were made first-hand, so I knew the quality was amazing. Transparency like that is very hard to find. I discovered that despite being labeled as green and eco-friendly, many companies claiming to sell 100% clean products actually include synthetics, fragrance, and other chemicals known to be linked to health issues. It became clear to me that avoiding these substances was crucial if I wanted to regain my health. That's why I started with the cleaning line this time, and it was a game-changer. I noticed improvements immediately. I understood that I needed to reduce the stress and toxic burden on my body and drastically change my environment to address the root cause of my symptoms, whereas before I was just using natural remedies to chase symptoms as they came.

I also changed my diet; I went from eating mostly processed food to now eating all whole foods with the occasional treat. Additionally, I stopped using toxic household products from the grocery store that were full of endocrine disruptors and carcinogens. I created an environment where my body could begin to function optimally again. This was the beginning of shifting from survival mode and symptom management to thriving and root-cause healing. I believe that removing the toxins from my home was the key to no longer relying on medication. My specialists were trying hard to get me back on DMTs as soon as I was done breastfeeding. But just before Sophia's first birthday, I became pregnant with my son.

This pregnancy was such a breeze compared to my first, and I believe that it was because I had changed my diet drastically and removed all the toxic products that were making me sick. We decided that we weren't going to vaccinate our daughter, and I stopped receiving all vaccinations, including the flu shot, which was something I was so adamant about in the early years of my diagnosis. I believe that this made a huge difference not only for myself, but also for my children. I had no symptoms at all, and at points before I started showing, I forgot I was pregnant; it was so easy. I had the oils and other products to help me. I was able to handle any issue in this pregnancy strictly with oils.

Because of the traumatic birthing experience with my daughter, I wanted to investigate alternative methods for my son's birth. I was told by my OBGYN that he was going to schedule me for a C-section because my pregnancies were less than three years apart. He told me that I would also certainly rupture my incision, and there was a high chance that I would kill either myself, my son, or both of us if I tried to have a vaginal birth after cesarean (VBAC). He told me that a cesarean was also easier for him, so he wanted to go that route. When I heard him say this, it triggered something in me; I was determined to find an alternate option. I started looking into home birth and was amazed at what I learned. The more I researched and talked to others that had VBACs, the more I realized what I had been told by the doctors was simply not true. What they were taught to believe was not based on science at all. I realized that my body was built to birth babies. I realized that the trauma I experienced in my daughter's birth was a direct result of the lack of education on my provider's part. All the things that contribute to a natural birth were not present at the hospital. Women are mammals and therefore, we need the same thing any other mammals needs to birth: a quiet space we feel safe in, only people we trust to be with us, darkness, and to be undisturbed. My experience at the hospital was the exact opposite. So, I decided to trust my body and have a home birth, alongside my birth attendant, who'd been present for hundreds of births, and my husband. I stopped attending prenatal appointments after my anatomy scan at twenty-one weeks because they tried pushing tests and immunizations that I did not want. They threatened to terminate my prenatal care if I didn't get what they were "suggesting", so I decided to stop going.

My water broke on January 23, 2022, which was a month early, but labor didn't start until noon on January 25th. I was able to lay in my bed and watch my favorite movie while labor started. Once things got a bit more intense, I moved to the tub and continued to do the hypnobirthing techniques I had practiced. When my birth attendant arrived, she set up the pool, and I finished my labor there. From the start of labor to when my son arrived was only five hours, and I was only in pain for the last fifteen minutes.

This birth was so transformational for me. It was the first time since 2013 that I trusted and worked with my body. I'd spent the last nine years feeling like my body was working against me and feeling so disconnected from it. I finally felt like my body and I were on the same team again; I wasn't as broken as I thought I was. This was huge because it showed me that just because a doctor says something doesn't mean it's true. It proved to me that I know my body best—no one else should be making any decisions regarding my health but me.

When I started taking my health decisions back into my own hands, I realized that we are all unique and experience our symptoms and triggers differently. The great thing about natural alternatives is they can be tailored to benefit us in the way we need and can be adjusted until we find something that works best. I found when I was looking at medications that they always came with a long list of side effects. To me, this defeats the purpose of taking the medication. Why would I take a pill to stop one issue if it was going to potentially cause fifteen others? I didn't want to spend my life managing side effects. I knew there had to be a better way and that is why I turned to plant-based products that work with my body the way God intended.

After my experiences with the medical system, I committed to learning as much as I could about the changes I could make to reduce my reliance on it. I continue to monitor with annual MRIs, but I have stopped receiving the dye because of the impact it has on my health. To stay proactive, we are doing other things, such as eating a diet focused on whole and fresh foods and reducing our consumption of packaged foods with long ingredient lists. We get our eggs from a local farmer, and we have started buying our beef from my friend (a local farmer who grass-feeds his cows). We very rarely buy meat from the store anymore because we felt we couldn't trust what was in it. Of course, we still splurge occasionally, but nothing compared to the way I used to eat. We cook 98% of our meals at home, and we very rarely eat out. I make the majority of the kids' snacks from scratch which cuts back on the damaging ingredients found in packaged foods. By doing this, we can stay away from seed oils and artificial dyes as much as possible, especially red dyes and canola oil that fuel inflammation and disease in the body. We have noticed the biggest changes in the kids: they throw far less tantrums, they can communicate clearer, they sleep through the night, they have bigger appetites, and they can focus on tasks easier. I personally saw an increase in my energy, focus, quality of sleep, and mood control.

In my experience researching chronic illness, it is the result of two things: either too much of something toxic and/or not enough of something vital, like nutrients. Every illness can be attributed to either factor. By focusing on improving these, you will see big changes. You cannot heal in the same environment that made you sick. To shift your body back into balance, you need to clean up your environment. Your environment is classified as anything you breathe (chemical compounds in the air from cleaning products, pollution, mold, etc.), anything you consume (food, water, the news), and anything that touches your skin (soaps, lotions, makeup). It took me a long time to realize that our daily habits contribute to either disease or wellness. Once I decided to embark on a journey of healing and allowed my body to detox, I started seeing improvements in my health.

Do you know how many known toxins are allowed in our everyday products? These products interfere with our hormones, suppress our immune systems, interfere with our nervous systems, and negatively impact virtually all body functions. When our bodies are out of balance and struggling to filter out these toxins, we experience things like difficulty sleeping, poor energy, mood fluctuations, fertility problems, weight gain, fatigue, muscle weakness and aches, decreased sex drive, depression, anxiety, and so much more. These symptoms are really like a warning sign from our body that we must make a change. Sadly, most of us are taught to take a pill for each individual symptom rather than addressing the root cause of the issue. More toxins mean more stress on our bodies, causing more severe symptoms. Most people stay stuck in this loop until they eventually get diagnosed with a chronic disease.

Fragrance is a term that companies use because it means they don't have to disclose what ingredients they include to make your products smell "nice". It's chalked up as a "company secret" when it's just a dumping ground for toxins. Did you know that there are over 3,000 chemicals that can hide behind that word? Most of them are known to be endocrine and immune disruptors, carcinogens, and much more. Fragrance is linked to asthma, eczema, cancer, neurological conditions, birth defects, migraines, irregular menstruation, worsening of menopause symptoms, and so much more. Common culprits that have fragrance include wall plug-ins, candles (yes, even soy-based), room sprays, fabric softeners, laundry detergent, dryer sheets, scented cleaners, sunscreen, lotion, soap, etc. These products are wreaking havoc on our bodies. When I ditched these for an all-in-one cleaner that smelled amazing and didn't carry any toxins, that's when I noticed a massive change in my symptoms; my relapses stopped.

The biggest lesson I learned during my switch to healthy living is that the products you use matter. Is it better to buy a cheaper, more convenient product that might save you a bit of money and time, or is your health worth investing in? After all, if we don't have our health, what do we have? It's the most important investment you can make not only for yourself but for your family and the generations ahead of you. The decisions you make have long-term effects, especially if you are a woman.

What made the biggest impact and shift in my health were the daily practices I implemented to start living a healthier life. Switching out over-the-counter drugs I used for symptom management to products that are clean and benefit my body instead of adding to toxic overload but also provide the same relief has been a game-changer. I started addressing the root cause of the symptoms I was experiencing. For example, I have always struggled with headaches and migraines. I used to take Advil, which took the pain away temporarily, but once it wore off,

I would be dealing with another headache. Once I changed my mind set and started looking into what could be causing the migraines, I realized that I was extremely deficient in minerals and electrolytes and usually dehydrated. Now, instead of popping a pill, I drink water with added electrolytes and minerals, I eat foods high in antioxidants, and consume a drink with added antioxidants daily. Since starting this routine, I went from having a headache/migraine daily to getting one every five months.

I now know what it truly means to be healthy! I have learned the true markers of health: high energy, restful sleep, pain-free periods, easy to maintain weight, clear skin, strong immune systems that can fight off illness quickly, balanced mood, consistent appetite, regular bowel movements, healthy pregnancies, and so much more. Regarding the essential oils that I use daily, it took a lot of trial and error to figure out what worked best. Once I found the best oil and supplement routine, it became my favorite part of the day. I used to spend my days in bed, sleeping constantly. If I was awake, I would eat food that was convenient and didn't need any energy to make, and I watched TV. I never did any housework because I was too weak to stand for longer than a couple minutes. Now, I get up with my kids every morning, take them for walks, do activities with them, cook them homemade meals, do most of the housework and errands, and truly enjoy the day with my beautiful kids.

Working on life changes helped me the most. Adding the essential oils just sped up the process. When I switched to healthy living, my eyes were opened to how many other people were also struggling, feeling lost, overwhelmed, and alone with no one to turn to for advice. After experiencing my transformation, I used the knowledge to help others figure out what their bodies needed to be able to live life to the fullest.

I avoid making generalized recommendations in terms of supplements and products because every person is very different. I believe that health should be individualized. When we take this approach, we see the best results. When I work with individuals, we dive into their personal history and thoroughly explore the areas they want to address, along with their desired outcomes. I have a questionnaire that we will fill out together. This helps me to create a specialized, individualized plan to help you meet your health goals. Then, I can work with you to figure out a routine that is tailored to exactly what your body needs; we can adjust accordingly to make sure it's a perfect fit. You can learn more about the changes I have made and the incredible products that changed my life on Instagram and Facebook at @prairie_momma_essentials. If you are just wanting to browse products, you can check out the Young Living website. Use my referral code, 3451893, when signing up, and you will receive a special welcome gift from me!

I am so lucky to have an entire community of like-minded individuals that I get to walk this journey of true health with. Feel free to reach out to me, and I will introduce you to this huge community with endless resources. We band together, cheer for each other, sit with you through your struggles, and help you to find a way out.

My advice for someone newly diagnosed is to advocate for yourself— don't let anyone tell you what is best for your body. You know what is best for you and your body, and if you feel that you don't, sit back and really listen to the signals your body is sending you because I promise it is trying to communicate with you. Don't feel like you need to know it all right away. You will find your flow and figure out what works for you as time goes on. Resting is more than okay. NEVER feel guilty for taking the time to rest. You are no good to anyone if you are burnt out, over stimulated, and at your breaking point. Resting is just as productive as anything else. And don't feel bad if you get things wrong. Failure is the most important part of learning. If something doesn't work, just pivot, and try something else.

MS has taught me more about myself than I ever thought it would. I have learned to listen to my body, treating it with respect and care. It has taught me that I am so much stronger than I give myself credit for. MS taught me how to prioritize my health and how necessary rest is. I used to feel extremely guilty if I wasn't always doing something. MS forced me to slow down and focus on listening to what my body needed and resting before I burnt out. Because of MS, I found my purpose in life. I struggled as a young person, figuring out what I had to give to the world and how I could help. I finally realized that my purpose is to help others realize the importance of getting back to the basics, like cooking our own food, relying on plants for healing, being part of a community, and teaching others how to listen to what their bodies are telling them.

21

Story by
ALICIA
Diagnosed in 2018
Currently 39 years old
Lives in New England, United States
Contact: alee132@yahoo.com

Hi! I am one of the 2.1 million people worldwide who have been diagnosed with multiple sclerosis (MS). I was asked to write a chapter in this book by a purely innocent dose of inspiration that happened in August of 2019. A big part of my life at that time was research, social media, support groups, etc. That's when I started reaching out to people to discuss their opinions on alternative ways to help feel our best while managing this difficult disease.

It's not often mentioned that there are many things we can do to help heal our symptoms by altering our lifestyle. I've heard many stories in support groups that weren't so supportive. I felt like the certain few I joined were geared toward hopelessness. I'm absolutely sensitive to the people that are having a hard time sustaining a positive attitude through this journey. It's no fun hearing you have a disease that is unpredictable and has no cure; I know that because I have experienced it. I was an emotional wreck as anyone would be to find out they have a clinical diagnosis. I sympathize with everyone afflicted, and for once, I wanted to read, "We can do it!" or, "We got this!" But there wasn't as much of that out there, unfortunately.

We all have a different story to tell. The purpose for mine is to give true hope and inspiration to those who are just as scared as I was when I was stumped by symptoms that appeared unsolvable. For as long as I can remember, I have never really felt right. I grew more concerned as time went on. I was previously diagnosed with Hashimoto's Thyroid disease in my early twenties. From that point on, any concerns that I explained to my doctors were blamed solely on that—Thyroid disease. I accepted that answer for much longer than I should have and went on with my life, persistently aware that the way I was feeling every day was not right.

My name is Alicia. I reside in New England where I was born and raised. I live with my fiancé and our two beautiful boys, ages five and seven. I was diagnosed with Relapsing Remitting Multiple Sclerosis (RRMS) on June 11, 2018. It was the day before my youngest son's first birthday and just about three weeks before my fortieth birthday. I, like many others, fell into major stressors. Looking back, I believe they led to more serious symptoms that became concerning to me. Stress does play a role in this disease!

I needed brain surgery in 2008. I was helping decorate for my goddaughter's birthday party one summer morning and became extremely tired. I remember leaving to go home and take a nap. My dad found me on the floor, having a grand mal seizure in his home. It was later discovered that my brain was hemorrhaging from a cavernous malformation. There was a cluster of blood vessels that popped, causing the seizure and very bad headaches. Thank God I had just moved back home with my dad after a difficult break up. Nobody at my previous residence would have found me for hours. I am very lucky to be here today.

Doctors said there was a good chance that the hemorrhage wouldn't happen again, but unfortunately, it continued from July through October. There were a lot of emergency visits during those months. I remember medical staff wanted to send me home, but I insisted on staying until they performed a scan and reassured me that I wasn't hemorrhaging again. I was, in fact, having more active bleeds. Because I wasn't presenting with the same severe symptoms, it was almost dismissed. The doctors and I then decided to schedule a craniotomy for the second week of October. I will never fully recover from that experience. I have high anxiety in fear of something like that ever happening to me again. I'm currently learning ways to heal my anxiety, such as breathing and meditation.

Five months into my recovery from brain surgery, my fiancé had a heart attack. While he was in the emergency room, they took his vitals and performed an electrocardiogram (EKG). He insisted something wasn't right, but they told him his tests and vitals were normal, so they sent him back to the waiting room. He drove himself to another hospital. They told him there that everything was normal (EKG and vitals). So, he went to a THIRD hospital. When they were done taking his vitals, he had a heart attack in the waiting room. They performed surgery and found that he had blockages in three arteries and placed three cardiac stents. This scenario sounds like it could be exaggerated, but I promise you every word is true. He's okay now. My point here is to convey the importance of listening to your body; pay attention to the signs it gives you. Don't be dismissed. Pay attention to factors that make you feel both your worst and your best, and make small changes to improve your overall health. My fiancé was able to get off his high blood pressure medication and his cholesterol meds that made his joints ache so badly. He did that by making changes to his diet and lifestyle.

Years later, my dad experienced a major stroke that left him very disabled. I was six months pregnant with my first child. I spent much of my time in hospital rooms, on a recliner beside my father, going to rehab facilities to cheer him on while learning to walk again, and attending speech therapy sessions to help him relearn to speak (roller coaster of emotions), all while embracing my first pregnancy. It's a huge challenge to accept the condition that his stroke has left him in. The guilt of not being able to care for him is a huge stress for me to this very day.

I have an older brother that primarily takes care of him, who doesn't understand why I can't just "do more". I guess trying to act "tough" while raising a family and not feeling well all the time was misleading. I am often misunderstood because I "look fine" or "act fine". It wasn't until recently that I started saying "I'm not okay" to perform a certain task or show up for a plan I made earlier. I need to heal; I need to focus on things my body is telling me are necessary.

My pregnancy went extremely well, and I carried my baby boy to full-term with no complications, other than needing a Cesarean (C-section) at the end because the baby wasn't descending, and I have that history of hemorrhaging, so they wanted me to stop pushing.

A year and a half later, my second son was born, also with no complications. I remember breastfeeding him while watching television, and I was seeing two of everything. It was to the point that I had to shut one eye to see normally. I knew then that something was NOT right. I believe this was my first relapse, but I wasn't aware of it at the time. I made an appointment with my primary care doctor who suggested that the fatigue and double vision were because I had two small children, breastfeeding, getting little sleep, and potential dehydration. That all sounded like a possibility, but it wasn't enough for me to just accept it, so I insisted on bloodwork. After receiving the results, we learned that my vitamin B12 was very low, as well as my vitamin D. I started B12 injections weekly until the levels were maintained orally. A prescription of 1.25MG (50,000 units) of vitamin D was also ordered.

The double vision lasted about two weeks, which felt like months. As you can imagine, I was scared as hell. I made an appointment with an eye doctor right away. My poor vision was interfering with everything. I had an eye exam and underwent various tests. Although my eyesight was found to be good, I was diagnosed with diplopia (double vision). However, at that time, no specific medication recommendations were provided. The doctor was concerned and submitted orders for me to undergo magnetic resonance imaging (MRI) to rule out a possible tumor causing the vision issue. I scheduled the MRI and luckily got an appointment within weeks. The appointment was made for May 30, 2018. (The reason I am providing the date is quite ironic as you read on.)

My symptoms worsened, and new things started happening to me. For about a month or so, I felt like I had shards of glass stuck in both thumbs and index fingers. So bizarre, right? It was not painful but super annoying, as you can imagine. I found out later that it could have been caused by a B12 deficiency.

I was in the shower one morning, and I felt like I had ants marching up and down my back. It was a strange feeling, but I thought maybe it was just the suds from the shampoo rinsing off. It continued as I dried off, got dressed, and occurred a few more times outside of the shower. The numbness and tingling in my back persisted, as well as the horrible feelings in my thumbs and fingers. At this point, I found myself doing more and more research regarding my symptoms, trying to find answers.

I visited the neurologist who I followed up with after my brain surgery, and he was concerned I may have myasthenia gravis disease (MG). It is a condition that causes muscle weakness. This weakness tends to get worse the longer the muscles are used and gets better after the muscles are rested. It is caused by a breakdown in the communication between the nerves and muscles. Those tests came back negative, and he also tested me for Lyme disease. Good news, but what now? More bloodwork and an MRI.

I remember sitting in the waiting room for the MRI and on the overhead radio, they announced that it was World MS Day! I got such a feeling inside. I had never even heard of World MS Day, and it was honestly the strongest sign that I have ever received in my life. It was May 30, 2018. I had a gut feeling walking into that MRI appointment that my results were going to read multiple sclerosis. Did I mention the waiting process to get results from these tests? Talk about nerve-wracking. If you know, you know! It took a little over a week to hear back. My advice to you while waiting for these tests is to stay busy and try to stay positive.

The moment I received the phone call with the results from my neurologist, I stepped outside while celebrating my grandmother's ninetieth birthday. The doctor confirmed that the MRI showed lesions in my brain and gave me the diagnosis of multiple sclerosis. I remember needing to compose myself while walking back into the house, as if everything was okay. That evening was tough. I was in shock, I was sad, and I was scared. I couldn't contain my negative thoughts. To hear the words "multiple sclerosis" from a medical professional speaking to ME was incomprehensible, even though I had known something was wrong. I wasn't even scared for me; I was scared for my two small children who need their mom, and I was scared for the man I had plans to marry. Thoughts of possibly being in a wheelchair made me panic. Would I become a burden? My mind just kept spiraling with scary, crazy thoughts. It was a mix of so many negative emotions. It was all starting to make sense: the headaches, fatigue, numbness, tingling, double vision, and brain fog.

A few days later, I went to my best friend, Olivia's, place of business. She had a red binder full of papers she had prepared for me and asked me to come sit down. Now, I call my friend Olivia my "witch doctor" friend. She is always conjuring up some type of natural lip balm, serum, and even the most delicious, healthy recipes from her garden. As I sat beside her that day, she explained to me how important it is to take care of my body with healthy foods. Of course, we all learn that as children, but does anyone listen? I didn't listen as a child or as a young adult. My breakfast daily was a blueberry muffin and an "iced coffee extra extra" (for those unfamiliar with the term, it refers to a coffee with more cream and sugar than coffee itself). While this may be acceptable for some people, it proved detrimental for me due to my autoimmune disease.

Over time, I learned that such food choices were working against my health. It is reassuring that society has become more educated on how food and health go hand-in-hand.

Back to that red binder—it was full of recipes that slowly welcomed me into a healthy diet; recipes that included anti-inflammatory foods that she knew I would try and enjoy. She explained the effects that certain foods have on our bodies. She asked me to try it for a few weeks and see how I felt. I will be forever grateful for that conversation because it led me down a path that has helped me tremendously. I went home with some encouragement and started focusing more on research, healthy diet, and lifestyle changes that would help with my symptoms. The next few weeks were filled with concoctions of smoothies, supplements, and books. I was continuing with my vitamin D and B12, which was helping me feel less tired. My research was flowing, I was learning new things, and I was feeling better physically, mentally, and emotionally.

I finally got an appointment with a local neurologist. My fiancé came with me to help calm my nerves, as I didn't know what to expect. (I feel it is important to mention how supportive my fiancé is with my diagnosis, as it was a major insecurity of mine in the beginning.) The wait was long, making me even more nervous. Did I mention that I have really bad anxiety? I was finally called into the room where the doctor greeted me and introduced himself. He confirmed that I had a few lesions on my brain, which is something I read about in my research but was terrifying to hear. He was able to pull up the MRI on a big screen and point out where the lesions were located. I learned about words I'd read in my research, like white matter, myelin, demyelination, sub cortex, and peri ventricular parts of the brain. We discussed how I was feeling and what my symptoms were. He immediately started handing me brochure after brochure of the newest medications on the market for treating multiple sclerosis. This was my first visit; I was very overwhelmed. He suggested I book an appointment to have an aggressive infusion in his office the following week! He told me I should book sooner rather than later because the seats in the infusion room were hard to reserve.

I was newly diagnosed and still processing the whole thing. I didn't know if I was ready or educated enough to make these decisions. I explained to him that I had been conducting a lot of research on managing my health through diet for a few weeks, and I wanted to see if I noticed a difference in the way I felt. I didn't know a thing about the medication he recommended. I said that I would go home and read through the side effects and weigh them out. As I was leaving (I will never forget this), he looked at my fiancé and told him to "go get her a cupcake", while laughing at the approach I was taking with my diet and lifestyle. I never went back to that doctor.

In the meantime, I continued my research on the medication brochures that were sent home with me (Ocrevus infusions and Tysabri shots were two of them). I didn't feel comfortable with either one. I couldn't even leave them out; I hid them in my drawer. I was so uneasy about all of it. I went to neurologist after neurologist; I think I saw about seven or eight in the state of Rhode Island. All they wanted to do was start me on whatever medication was newest on the market. I remember being petrified as they handed me packet after packet, with unlimited side effects. My ideas of changing my lifestyle and diet were not considered in their plans. I don't remember any of them showing compassion or offering alternatives on how to deal with this unpredictable disease, other than aggressive medication. I did sit and listen to all the options, such as infusions, shots, pills, etc. They just never sat right with me.

I was eight months into my diagnosis, and I hadn't told my mother yet. I waited so long because I knew how heartbreaking it would be for her. We are very close, and she knew everything that was going on with me, as far as my health and symptoms. However, I was sugar coating all of it, and it was wearing on me. She deserved the truth, but I think telling her was harder than hearing it from the doctor. She was very emotional; she hugged me and reassured me that she was here and would help me with anything I needed. I felt so supported.

She found a doctor for me who was an hour away in Boston. I made an appointment, and she came with me. I finally found a doctor that I felt comfortable with! She was understanding and compassionate. She took her time with me and listened to every concern I had. I told her I was apprehensive to take medication. She told me to take my time in making whatever decisions I felt were right for me. If she felt my condition was worsening and required medication, then I would be open to that discussion. What a relief it was to actually hear that from a doctor! She gave me a thorough neurological exam while explaining, then went over the MRI with me and explained the different stages of MS. Mine is Relapsing-Remitting, and she explained what that meant, as well. I left that office feeling hopeful that I wouldn't be pressured and persuaded to go against my will, and most importantly, not be judged for it!

I could go on and on about how scary it can be getting diagnosed with multiple sclerosis, but I would rather talk about how important it is to take a positive approach. I get it! It's awful and hard and scary, and it took me years to find acceptance. I want to share the story that helps me get through. I will start by saying how happy I am that I chose to manage my MS by changing my diet and lifestyle. It is so important to surround yourself with a positive support group and to not feel judged for the decisions you make that feel right for you! Nobody knows your body like you—listen and be kind to it. I have consciously decided to explore alternative options instead of relying on medication, as long as they continue to work for me. I have had a stable MRI for the past two years, and my doctor recommends staying on the path that I'm on. She is not currently recommending medication.

It is imperative to have inspiration and encouragement in our lives no matter what the situation is. This book is a prime example of the power of support and positivity through real-life stories. It shares the trials and tribulations that, when faced alongside the right people, can help make your journey a little bit lighter.

My perspective was changing. I was beginning to think more positively, and it caused a rippling effect. My fiancé was able to manage his cardiac issues without medication because his blood pressure and cholesterol dropped to a healthy level with the right diet and lifestyle—doctor approved! The medication he was taking was making him feel terrible, and he was essentially just masking the issues he was experiencing. He tackled the root of the issue by eating clean and healthy. I would also like to mention that I have impacted my friends and family's diets and lifestyle changes. It has made my family, friends, and loved ones much more conscious of their food choices. I am proud to share that.

I started making smoothies for breakfast and learned that I actually like them! A few of my favorites are frozen organic blueberries, frozen banana, spinach, a teaspoon of peanut butter, some chia seeds, almond milk, and ice. Another is frozen banana with peanut butter, honey, ground flaxseed, almond milk, and ice with a sprinkle of organic cinnamon on top! Last is kale, pineapple, mango, ice, organic apple juice, and water. I also learned a lot about food and recipes to promote good health. I took a couple of classes on how to make fresh spring rolls, rice paper, fruits, veggies, and edible flowers by Food Fairy Ri. Nutritional tips and doctors are all over social media with recipes fit for everyone.

The symptoms I experience these days are mostly triggered by stress, the wrong foods, and in some cases, the weather. If I eat a lot of sugar or bread, I feel it! I try to eat mostly gluten-free and not a lot of sugar. Processed foods are the worst thing for me! I keep alcohol to a minimum (if any). I drink socially a few times a year, and when I do, I feel the effects from it for days. My fiancé built me a beautiful garden in our backyard. Not only am I growing healthy, organic food, but it's calming and peaceful. My boys have also learned so much through gardening!

When I get stressed, I experience numbness and tingling down my back. My vision gets blurry and "off". I get vertigo but not as frequently as the other symptoms. I'm still trying to find the trigger for my leg becoming stiff at night (part of the disease). My hips hurt some days, but I stretch and do yoga to help relieve them. I have a phenomenal massage therapist who helps me once every six weeks or so, and a physical therapist who will dry needle certain muscles that are bothering me. Look up dry needling—it does NOT hurt, and I highly recommend it.

It would be nice if insurance covered these much-needed resources! It would help if they covered Pilates and yoga class, as well (sigh). I find going outside helps with mood changes, something that affects me often. I'd like to make it known that although I've had a bumpy road with decisions that doctors may not agree with, I have the utmost respect for medical professionals who respect patients' choices and the journey they choose.

This journey has taught me so much already. I've become more aware of my body, understanding what causes inflammation, and how stress affects me. As a result, I've experienced reduced joint pain, brain fog, and fatigue. Feeling better has motivated me to explore various resources available to support my well-being.

If I can influence just one person's decision on how they treat their body, or even their mindset, I believe it will be a ripple effect. I was chosen to take part in this book by inspiration when this author reached out to me upon her diagnosis, and I'd like to think I am a little piece of her reason for writing this book. She asked me about drugs, treatment, diet, lifestyle, motherhood, and what I found helpful after receiving my diagnosis. We hit it off immediately, just through comforting each other without judgement on what the other was doing. It is about what works for you as an individual and gets you through. Don't give up on putting in the work to feel your best. If you can't manage to feel better physically, work on your mental health and mindset. Stay hopeful. There are so many reasons to look forward to another day. Again, it's a ripple effect, and I'm so proud of it.

When talking to myself, I say, "You've got this!" Listen to your body, as you are the only one who knows inside and out if something isn't right. If you don't get answers that make you feel at ease, move on to the next. Make sure you find a person who is willing to listen to you and actually hear you out. Do your research. Be hopeful. Stay positive. Live a healthy lifestyle. Stay persistent. Cry when you need to. Laugh as much as you can. Surround yourself with good people. Love yourself. Don't be afraid to talk about things and most of all, don't let it define you. You got this!

I want to thank my fiancé, my family, and my friends who support me every day. I am so grateful for their positivity and encouragement that surrounds me. Thank you for paying enough attention to realize when I'm not feeling my best without me having to say it, and even more for listening when I need to vent. Words can't express how much my children mean to me. My greatest accomplishment is being their mommy. They push me every single day and put the biggest smile on my face, effortlessly. Thank you from the bottom of my heart to my mom and my mother-in-law for giving me the much-needed breaks without me even having to ask. I'd like to add how proud I am to be the little voice behind some of the choices my loved ones are making because of my influence. It has been mentioned to me more than once that I've made an impact with the outlook I now have, and it makes me so happy.

22

Story by
DAWNMARIE DESHAIES

Diagnosed in 2012
Currently 57 years old
Lives in California, United States
Instagram: @dawnmarie_deshaies
www.dawnmariehealthyandfit.org

I was in my twenties when I started to lose vision in my right eye. The blurriness went in and out, and my fingers were constantly going numb. Doctors told me that I was basically just tired and put me on Xanax, Prozac, Zoloft, and recommended that I take a vacation. While I battled the disease, doctors continued to prescribe me more antidepressants. I struggled with incessant pain, miscarriages, and everything else in between. I tried to take care of my body and continue working, but I was fueled by penicillin and medication. I wasn't diagnosed with multiple sclerosis (MS) until 2012. That's when I was given MS medications to help me manage various types of tremors and the side effects from the previous medications. It was a never-ending cycle. I was having allergic reactions to them—even suicidal thoughts—so I finally decided to stop taking everything completely.

While I was learning about the disease, I met many other people experiencing similar challenges in managing their daily lives. This is when I learned that we are never alone. To get over our own challenges, we need to help each other with loving care and compassion, self-care, positivity, mental and physical health, and community support. These were all the areas I knew I could bring change, and that's what I've been doing for the past decade.

My personal health battles and emotional struggles were the fuel to start my company, Dawnmarie Healthy and Fit LLC, that offers multiple services related to health, self-care, mindfulness, restoration, and positivity. This was an idea that would allow me to share my journey with others and deliver a community platform for warriors alike to find their own path to healing and health. By helping others heal and paying it forward, I have found that it benefits my own healing journey, as well.

I also run a podcast called *Live with Dawnmarie* that shares stories of MS survivors and how they have dealt with the disease. I interview people from around the world, men and women who have decided to continue living life with their inspiring, personal journeys. The purpose of the podcast is to liberate listeners from the burden of "should-haves" that weigh them down, empowering them to confidently move forward on their path towards a brighter purpose.

Throughout my journey, I learned to let go of what I can't control. Finding peace wasn't easy. Over the years, I have found that I am stronger than this disease with God and Jesus on my side—I can overcome it all. There is no fear, depression, or pain with God.

These days, I focus on prayer, daily meditation, keeping all negative energy and thoughts away from me, and finally, giving it all to God. I no longer accept anything less than the highest love of God. My body is doing better; it doesn't hurt, and I no longer experience multiple sclerosis symptoms. Of course, keeping my diet as clean as possible helps a lot.

Many people with multiple sclerosis say they feel better when they eat healthy. I'm right there with you! A healthy, well-balanced diet, combined with daily exercise, helped to relieve my MS symptoms. It lifted fatigue, mood, improved my memory, gut health, and even my skin. It also helps control weight gain and weight regulation. Getting a good night's sleep is just as important as any diet.

As we know, there's no evidence supporting one specific diet, but there are potential benefits in several. My balanced diet includes the major food groups: proteins, carbohydrates, fats, fiber, vitamins, and minerals. Protein helps growth and tissue repair. Fat helps with energy, providing essential fatty acids and helping to absorb vitamins. Fiber aids in digestion. Vitamins and minerals are needed for different cell processes. And let's not forget to drink plenty of fluids because water helps transport nutrients to every cell in the body.

I eat fish high in omega-3 fatty acids, such as salmon, herring, mackerel, tuna, and sardines. For meat, I eat skinless chicken or turkey and lean meats, trimmed of visible fat. I try to include at least five different organic fruits and vegetables every day. I only eat organic eggs and gluten-free grain products. Foods that I try to avoid are red meat that is high in saturated fats, butter, cheese, and other full-fat dairy products. I do drink caffeine in moderation.

My first piece of advice is that this disease does not define you; it is your life, and you can take control over it. The bottom line is that you need to take care of yourself by consuming healthy food (not processed). If you do eat processed food, drink lots of water to help detox your body.

For decades, I lived with and suffered from this autoimmune disease; it impacted my life in many ways. This is why I chose to dedicate my life to helping and educating people by contributing to raising awareness. You don't have to believe in a religion to pray to the higher rounds of God. Stop listening to negative music and negative talks, and instead, focus on the positivity of your life and what you're doing in the moment.

You are not defined solely by your past; it is your present actions and how you handle them that truly shape who you are. Fear is not real; fear is man-made, and it comes from darkness. Moving forward is what matters. You need to leave the diagnosis behind, and start changing your life. Live a clean lifestyle, focusing on the positivity of what you can do, and everything will change.

23

Story by
CLARE McKENZIE

Diagnosed in 2019
Currently 50 years old
Lives in United Kingdom
Instagram: @ms_jellylegs

"Start at the beginning, continue on, and when you reach the end, stop."
-Lewis Carroll

My name is Clare, and I live in Burnham-on-Crouch, in the UK, with my partner, Gary, plus our cat, Cosmo. I hope you enjoy reading my story. I'm sorry to start on a somber note, namely, with my elder brother who took his own life at the age of forty-three. He had suffered from multiple sclerosis (MS) since he was twenty-six. I dedicate this story to his memory with the hope that it may make a difference to other MSers' lives and to avoid anybody feeling the need to take the same tragic path as Ian.

It was December 1994 when my brother was diagnosed, after a spot of double blurred vision. That was the first time I had really heard about the condition. My family never spoke about this with me again; nothing was said. Life went on. At that time, I was twenty-one years old and just starting out in my sales and marketing career in publishing in London.

When I turned thirty, my brother tried to take his own life. I received the news by phone. Nothing more was said. That year (2003), I took part in a charity called Moon Walk for Breast Cancer, walking twenty-six miles through London.

Fast forward to when I was thirty-five, and my walking became disrupted. I began to notice a significant decline in the distances I could cover, and I started experiencing increased fatigue. Despite those challenges, including the occasional trip and fall, which I managed to turn into a comedic act to make everyone giggle, I carried on…

On July 10, 2012, I attended a London Ambassador training event in London. I felt something was wrong, and I had a tear in my eye between 8:30am and 9:00am. My brother had taken his own life at the age of forty-three. I was thirty-eight. No one talked about this either, just like when he was diagnosed. In my family, illness was never allowed to be out in the open, nor was the MS support landscape as developed as it now is. The result was that my poor, poor brother got very little in the way of psychological help, and he struggled with severe, clinical depression for almost twenty years, from which he never emerged.

I am now forty-five, and I have just organized a charity walk, in aid of Cancer Research UK, for my team at Wolters Kluwer, in Canary Wharf. I knew this would be a challenge. I was barely able to walk thirty minutes by this point. Upon returning to the office, I face-planted onto the marbled floor of my reception. It hurt. That's when I thought I should make a doctor's appointment. This was during October 2018.

After three magnetic resonance imaging (MRI) scans, I was diagnosed with Relapsing-Remitting Multiple Sclerosis (RRMS) in March 2019, by my general practitioner (GP). As you might expect, my brother's tragic experience scared me, but not in the way you might think. I became acutely aware of the importance of being open about my condition and actively seeking out and accepting all the help that was available. I took it fairly well. I started conducting research on RRMS, focusing on exercise and diet. I had already been a pescetarian since the age of eighteen, and I also did not smoke or drink much. Yes, what a bore I am! I do have a fizzy personality though! In a nutshell: my supercomputer (my brain) does not always send messages down my superhighway (my spinal column), and my legs sometimes get in a muddle.

MS is considered an autoimmune disease, as the body's immune system attacks myelin. This is a fatty substance that insulates and protects the nerve fibers of the Central Nervous System. When myelin is damaged, it becomes difficult for the brain to send signals to the rest of the body and within the brain itself. The symptoms of MS vary from person to person. That's why it is known as the "snowflake" condition. I love that we are all special and unique!

According to the *MS Trust*, an estimated 2,500,000 people in the world have multiple sclerosis. Research suggests the proportion of women with MS is increasing; roughly between two and three women have MS for every man with the condition.

I have a penchant for the book *Alice's Adventures in Wonderland* by Lewis Carroll; it seemed that just like Alice, my MS journey would open many doors. Like Alice, I wanted to stay curious; I would have eaten the proverbial cake and drunk the contents of the bottle just to find out what would happen. Here's what transpired next. I discovered:

- Instagram – I set up my IG account @ms_jellylegs (see what I did there?!) to learn, educate, empower, and inspire others.

- Overcoming MS program – This lifestyle program resonated with me, and I was lucky to stumble upon it only three months post-diagnosis.

- Knives Over Forks documentary

- Mathew Embry's documentary *Living Proof* – A true inspiration. I was lucky to cross paths with Mathew when I reached out and booked him to collaborate with Dr. Gretchen, my MS-Specific Physical Therapist.

Information overload. But here is what I learned: when we give our bodies a break from digesting food all the time, our cells can then focus on other things, like cleaning out damaged cells, in order to regenerate newer, healthier cells. Gut rest can lead to a brain reset. We can also call periods of gut rest, with the intention to reverse chronic conditions, therapeutic fasting. Fasting has been gaining momentum *outside* of the weight loss community due to the multitude of benefits, particularly for the brain. Research in this area is expanding every month and has been indicating that periods of fasting can help reverse or slow down diseases, like diabetes, Alzheimer's, and cardiovascular disease. We now have early hope that fasting may benefit multiple sclerosis warriors, as well.

Preliminary evidence in animal studies has indicated that fasting, or caloric restriction, helps prolong lifespan, and improves MS, by bringing down inflammatory markers, bringing about positive changes to the gut microbiome, demyelination prevention, and axon protection—all while keeping the immune system function optimized. Human data indicating the benefits of fasting for the brain are on the rise, though studies of the effect of fasting on MS are still limited. However, a new study, released January 2022, offers us some hope of what's to come. In this study, thirty-six people with MS were followed for eight weeks and were randomly assigned to either a daily calorie restriction diet, an intermittent calorie restriction diet, or a weight-stable diet. The intermittent calorie restricted diet, similar to a fasting protocol, was associated with a reduction in memory T cell subsets. Though fasting can feel intimidating to someone who eats three meals and multiple snacks throughout the day, when we slowly compress our eating window, our gut has time to rest and repair, along with all the other cells in the body. If you can start with the goal of not eating after dark and completing a twelve-hour fast every day, it may make a huge difference for you.

I have suffered from non-chronic episodic migraines for years—long before I was diagnosed with RRMS. I do not recognize these migraines as a symptom of MS. Many would argue just that, but not everything is MS-related, right?! My migraines are always around my menstrual cycle, and I have two or three days where I am wiped out. Whether that be from fatigue, light, or food sensitivities—and that's before I mention the roaring migraines. I first discovered Susannah Juteau , a nutritionist and headache specialist, as a guest on the "Multiple Sclerosis Awareness" group via IG, presented by Ritu. I was eager to fix my monthly migraines, so I signed up for the Headaches Bootcamp that I have now completed. I was looking for strategies to relieve headaches without medicine, and understand how I could not only survive, but thrive!

Understanding not just *what* you eat, but *when* you eat is super important if you are embarking on an intermittent fasting program. When you fast, insulin levels drop and human growth hormone (HGH) increases. Your cells also initiate important cellular repair processes and change which genes they express. There are so many benefits associated with choosing an intermittent fasting regime, such as improving heart health, lowering blood pressure, cholesterol levels, and reducing other inflammatory markers. By fasting, your body will trigger a metabolic pathway called autophagy, which removes waste material from cells, improves your brain health, and may help to build new neurons.

Initially, I started with a 12:12 hour fast, and quickly progressed to the 17:7 fast; that's seventeen hours of not eating with a gap of seven hours to eat. I have completed two days of twenty-four hour fasting, which is not that scary when you consider most people naturally do a 12:12 hour eating program. I generally stop eating by 7:00 pm. If you consider relaxation, sleeping, and not eating until breakfast time—that is an easy twelve-hour window. The process has been super educational. Personally, I need to remind myself the reason "why" I am doing this—that's my motivation.

I strongly believe fasting is as much of a mental exercise as it is a physical exercise. Dr. Gretchen Hawley – MS Specialist Physical Therapist, always tells me to remember why I want to improve something about my mobility. Quite simply, it is because I want to enjoy myself with my friends, socialize, and feel empowered; that keeps me motivated to exercise. Dr. Hawley released her new book in July of 2023, *The MSing Link: The Essential Guide to Improving Walking, Strength, and Balance for People with Multiple Sclerosis*, which I highly recommend!

The next big thing I discovered was meditation! Did you know that meditation is for the soul? It helps improve your physical AND mental health. I am sure some of you will agree with me that there are many times where you find yourself rejecting the life you must now live; wishing that those weights and burdens did not exist. What if we all had a superpower? An extraordinary gift that you could tap into anytime, anywhere?

Enter mindfulness. In a world that's constantly forcing you to reach outward (work, fatigue, family, financial worries, illness, etc.), reach *inward* and check in with yourself, using the powerful technique of mindfulness. Meditation is all about relaxation and finding your inner peace. I certainly know what I could do with some inner peace to quiet my pontificating mind!

You need to create a place that works for YOU:

- Find a space with the perfect ambience! Maybe you're a complete silence kind of person, or someone who needs a little white noise. Taking ten minutes before I start my day does help.
- Get comfy! Grab a yoga mat, a fluffy blanket, or—if staying in bed does it for you—do just that! (Meditation naps are real!)
- Try a new position! Anyone who endures symptoms, such as pain, numbness, or muscle spasms, may have a difficult time focusing, so take the time to find the right position to minimize these symptoms, if possible.
- Keep the distractions to a minimum. Phones (and children) on silent mode, please!

Take a moment to recognize what makes you so extraordinary: your foundation of strength, resilience, and perseverance. Meditation takes practice, and finding the right space for your mindful practice might take a few tries. No space will ever be perfect, but don't let that stop you from trying today!

So, how did I miss MS? I ignored and brushed off symptoms that may or may not have led me to my MS diagnosis, such as migraines, trips and falls, tingly hands in the cold British winter, heat intolerance when living in Curaçao, tingly feet that I thought were caused by my sciatica (don't ask how I got that!), walking distance, and fatigue. They all seemed minor to me, so I just brushed them off and carried on.

Has the diagnosis made much of a difference in my life? Well, it has given me some answers. I am super lucky as my symptoms are mild. Generally, I am in full control of everything that I choose to do. MS has not stopped me, and I feel that I am living my best life right now. I have a lot of things I want to accomplish—one wonky step at a time. It's all about the way you frame it. "What if" can be changed to "even if"! I am super thankful for what I have today. Alice fell down the rabbit hole, as I did during COVID lockdown. But the difference is that I got back up and carried on. The only way is most definitely up!

I have always loved walking. Happily, I'm still a 20,000-steps-a-day person, despite my MS. However, my perambulations haven't been without their moments—some with quite hilarious consequences (in retrospect, at least). I strive to continue living life to the fullest, to not get down about what I've lost, and most of all, to have a jolly good laugh about the curve balls MS sometimes throws at me.

Lastly, I'm happy to announce that as I was writing my story for this book, I received a letter from my neurologist, whom I visited recently, with news that I have to share here. Let me quote: "She has Relapsing-Remitting MS and remains stable through the years, not being on disease-modifying treatment. EDSS score stands at three, and most likely her case, if we consider that the onset of her disease was many years ago, in benign." Hallelujah! Something we agree on—now that my doctor is retiring. So, in no particular order: exercise, diet, fasting, meditation, and not taking DMTs have worked out for me this far. Of course, we do not know what the future holds. Every day is different, and I'm taking it as it comes with a smile and a bag of positivity. My motto is to keep on keeping on; slow and steady.

If you, a member of your family, or a friend have been affected by multiple sclerosis, I highly recommend these sources as a great starting point to find out more:

- Overcoming MS – I am a global Ambassador and founding member of the OMS Essex Circle.

- MS-UK – I support the MS-UK Peer Pod for the Newly Diagnosed on Monday evenings at 7 pm. I am also a member of the Virtual Insight Panel, offering communications and marketing support.

- Doctor Gretchen Hawley – MS-Specific Physical Therapist - The MSing Link.

- MS-Selfie – I am a supporter of Professor Gavin Giovannoni's weekly newsletter that brings you the latest in scientific discoveries and observations.

- MS Awareness Week – It's a chance to raise awareness of multiple sclerosis and spread the word. #LetsTalkMS

- shift.ms – By people who get it!

- MS Trust – Great for MS Education.

- MS Society UK – Great for MS research and fundraising.

- talkhealth Partnership – Whatever health concerns you may have, talkhealth comprises a team of like-minded individuals, who are keen to provide the latest health information and support that is currently available. I have submitted articles for the MS Hub, and I am a regular contributor.

24

Story by

SOFIA COLESNIC

Diagnosed in 2013
Currently 33 years old
Lives in Raleigh, North Carolina, United States
Instagram: @sofiawalkingwithms

I am not my disease; I am Sofia. I need to separate myself from my disease. It puts up a daggum good fight, but I am strong, and you are, too. What should you focus on first? Not vitamins or therapy—although those are important—but POSITIVITY. Positivity is difficult at times, but it's so important.

I had to choose between a natural treatment or a disease modifying drug. Both were scary as heck but having a multiple sclerosis (MS) diagnosis, in general, is scary as heck. The medication had so many possible side effects, and it only lessens the number of flare-ups—it's not a cure. I had sixty-to-seventy lesions. I couldn't afford to just lessen the number; I had to get rid of the flare-ups and lesions altogether. Unfortunately, the medical community deems this impossible. To alleviate the symptoms, I wanted to try natural treatment options, but support was few and far between. That was scary. The stress of trying to make this decision was exacerbating my symptoms. I didn't know then how much the decision to seek natural treatment would positively change my life, quality of life, and my overall health.

In 2013, I experienced the first symptom. I'd brushed my teeth a thousand times before, but on this day, I just couldn't steady my hands when holding water to rinse with. My hands were developing tremors. Soon after, I started experiencing very bad headaches, occasional dizziness, and dry eyes. A few more symptoms appeared (numbness and tingling down the left side of my body), and with that, I went to get magnetic resonance imaging (MRI). I didn't expect a major diagnosis, but to my surprise, in 2013, I was diagnosed with MS at the age of twenty-three.

The lesions were located mainly in my brain, with some also found in my spinal cord. I was told I would soon be in a wheelchair for the rest of my life. I received this diagnosis while my mom and boyfriend were in the room. Before this diagnosis, I was an active, healthy girl who played soccer for my college. I loved playing violin, skiing, exploring nature, and all things movement and outdoors related. The symptoms became noticeable when I was a preschool teacher at a Children's Development Center. I absolutely loved that job, but as a teacher of two-and-a-half to five-year-old cuties, I often taught fine motor skills. I noticed that my fine motor skills were getting worse. I would write lesson plans every month and turn them in to my director, but those plans became less and less legible. This was embarrassing because my plans of teaching the children fine motor skills were evidence of my own fine motor skills going out the window.

If I had been serious about the disease in the beginning, then everything might have been different. It is not easy to be serious about something when it doesn't seem real. I advise not waiting for something bad to happen but to address it through healthy, natural treatments before things progress. If only I had prevented these additional flare-ups. My timeline seems scary, and it was difficult to write, but just know that there is a light at the end of this tunnel, as well as light all along the way.

In 2015, I married a godsend of a man who was with me through the diagnosis. I somewhat followed the Terry Wahls diet and took some supplements, but the MS was not bad yet. So, I didn't try as hard as I should have.

In 2016, my doctor recommended that I stop taking vitamin D because my levels were high, according to him. My level was 97 ng/ml, and I was taking 25,000 IU's. Dr. Mercola says we need 70ng/ml-100ng/ml for serious diseases, like MS, cancer, etc. I wish I had continued taking vitamin D, but it's important not to dwell on the past. Please know that some doctors are not aware of the importance of high doses of vitamin D for MS. Shortly after, I got food poisoning, and I was sick in bed for three days. This led to a horrible flare-up, with foot dropping and dizziness. I began using a wheelchair at times. I was also unable to drive safely due to my dizziness, so I stopped driving!

By 2017, my life had spiraled so out of control that my ability to walk, drive, or enjoy any freedom had been taken away from me. I tested positive for H. pylori, which I healed with Mastic Gum. I had several falls due to dizziness, and, unfortunately, landed headfirst on the granite countertop and the floor several times, leading to concussions. The dizziness I experienced was not vertigo—I had already dealt with that and successfully resolved it, using the Epley maneuver. However, this persistent dizziness is one of the big reasons I stopped walking well.

On top of the constant dizziness, my eyesight was also giving me trouble. Because of this, I was referred to The Mackowsky Visual Learning and Rehabilitation Clinic. This clinic is in Raleigh, North Carolina, where I live. I was referred to Dr. Mackowsky by Darcy Dane, a chiropractic neurologist that I see occasionally. I went through a series of visual rehabilitation, where I completed visual homework with eye exercises and had weekly appointments to check my progress. They discovered I had nystagmus, optic neuritis, blurred vision, and more. I got prisms in my glasses, learned about binasal occlusion, and went through a lot of visual rehabilitation. Through this healing journey, I no longer need the prisms!

This was a rough year for me and my husband; he helped me so, so much. Thankfulness is important, and I am so very thankful. My chiropractor recommended stem cell treatment, but my brain was too foggy to grasp the suggestion. I tried intravenous (IV) vitamin C, low-dose naltrexone (LDN), and horseback riding. These seem to help many people, but I was still having flare-ups. Looking back, I remember not being able to use my hands because of the tremors. Originally, I was right-handed, but when that hand got shaky, I was forced to become left-handed. For a while, both of my hands were malfunctioning. I was unable to do certain tasks safely, like applying makeup or drinking a cup of hot coffee.

I was working part time for my parents' real estate management company, so they were able to pick me up for work every day. Thankful. Most days it would be my mom, and she would help with my makeup, but some days my dad would come to pick me up. I already couldn't walk. At the very least, I wanted to wear mascara. My dad would stand behind me, with his arm around my neck, and ever so slowly, touch my eyelashes with the mascara wand. It was a very strange way of putting on mascara, but it worked.

During this time, I discovered that Hyperbaric Oxygen Therapy (HBOT) works wonders in healing so many things, such as concussions, inflammation, and more. I have read about people healing multiple sclerosis with HBOT alone. HBOT involves breathing 100% oxygen while enclosed in a pressurized chamber. While in this chamber, the air pressure inside rises to a level higher than normal air pressure, which significantly increases oxygen supply to your cells and tissues. This elevated air pressure in the chamber increases levels of oxygen in our blood plasma, speeding up our body's natural ability to heal. In 2018, I ramped up the usage of HBOT and had success. To this day, I use this modality of therapy when I am feeling inflamed or very unwell.

I studied electromagnetic frequencies (EMF), and their effect on everyone, especially sick people. Electromagnetic frequencies/fields are produced anywhere electricity is used. We are exposed to these invisible toxins every day from Wi-Fi routers, smartphones, Bluetooth devices, powerlines, cell phone towers, even dirty electricity in walls, and more. Unfortunately, these toxins are more dangerous than most people, including myself, ever realized. Having an autoimmune disease means that we cannot tolerate toxins because our toxic load is already very high. It is important for all of us to read up on this specific toxin and share the information with others. I wear a necklace called the Harmoni pendant, which has been tested and shows great results in, not only repelling harmful EMFs, but also neutralizing them. I keep my cell phone on airplane mode every night, I use speakerphone instead of holding the phone close to my ear, I went back to using a wired mouse and keyboard, I opted out of utility companies smart meter program, and I practice grounding/earthing (standing barefoot outside) to assist with equalizing to the earth's negative charge. Grounding is very beneficial for everyone. Being barefoot outside on the grass, sand, or even concrete is supposed to help with the electrical signals we are subjected to daily.

Then, the biggest take away, and most effective therapy, came along. My dad drove my mom and me, with my wheelchair in tow, from North Carolina to Florida, to start the Coimbra protocol of high doses of vitamin D. If you haven't already heard, vitamin D is important for everyone. Dr. Coimbra has been able to suppress disease activity in about 95% of MS cases. In addition to vitamin D, he also prescribes other supplements (depending on the patient), such as vitamin B2 (riboflavin), B12, magnesium, and omega-3 DHA. He recommends a diet excluding calcium, plus an intake of extra fluids, with a minimum of 2.5L/day. Doctors practice the Coimbra protocol all around the world, but there are only several practitioners in the United States. Because I live in the U.S., I am now a virtual patient of Dr. Scott Jensen M.D., in Arizona. Since starting the Coimbra Protocol, my flare-ups subsided, but I was still dealing with past symptoms. I had gone from wheelchair to walker, but my hands were still shaky, my dizziness was present, and I was unable to safely drive, or even walk well, with a cane!

When my brain fog began to lift, I started studying different ways of repairing the damage my lesions had caused. I watched a great Joe Rogan interview with Mel Gibson about stem cells and their healing, then I remembered my chiropractor's suggestion to receive stem cells to assist with my healing. My husband and I were eager for my healing to speed up because we wanted to have a baby before we were too old. So, in 2021, I was able to travel to Panama City, Panama, to receive Mesenchymal Stem Cell (MSC) Therapy at the Stem Cell Institute. This was expensive, but oh so beneficial. Since this first stem cell treatment, I began driving again, my dizziness that I had for four years disappeared, and my hand tremors improved! I started an Instagram page to share some of what I have learned @sofiawalkingwithms. I returned to Panama for more MSC therapy in 2022. I again received 132 million stem cells that revved up my healing!

Back in 2013, and then again in 2016, I tested high for Lyme disease. The diagnosis was always unclear whether I had it, so in 2019, I took a saliva and urine test that was positive for Lyme disease. My chiropractic neurologist ordered the urine test through DNA Connexions, and the saliva test through MacTech Imaging. Again, the results came back very high for Lyme disease. The lab technician called my doctor because mine was the highest load of spirochete they had ever seen. My chiropractic neurologist had me do a nebulizer treatment for Lyme. These factors, along with MS, Epstein Barr Virus, H. pylori, and my MTHFR gene, prevented me from improving, even though these treatments can be effective for others.

Prior to getting mesenchymal stem cells, I worked to detoxify my body and clear out heavy metals to clear the path for the stem cells. The first time, my acupuncturist recommended Chinese herbs, and the second time, I tried Extracorporeal Blood Ozonation and Oxygenation therapy (EBOO) to clear any obstacles for my stem cells. I found a healthcare provider in Pittsboro, NC, at Restorative IV Therapies, PLLC. They offer great nutritional IVs, as well as great healing advice. This treatment was actually very beneficial in removing biofilms, such as toxins, heavy metals, molds, and spirochete, from Lyme disease. A good amount of my energy returned after the EBOO treatments.

As strange as it sounds, I have become somewhat thankful for the education this disease, and its natural healing, has taught me. I am now able to share so much with my family and friends. Changing my diet has helped immensely. I try to cook at home as much as I can. It's important to make it fun, so my mom, sister, and I like to share recipes of what we have experimented with. I recommend eating dairy and gluten-free, as it is much better for your body. Now that I am doing better, my husband and I eat some gluten on occasion, especially sourdough bread because it has a lower glycemic value. I've learned that white cheese is better for you than yellow, so we have a little bit of dairy, but not much. When we do eat out, we try to eat healthily, even though it's more expensive. It pays off in the long run. Here is a recipe for my dairy-free parmesan cheese: almost 1 cup of cashews, 2/3 tsp sea salt, 1/4 tsp garlic powder, 3 tbsp nutritional yeast - mix all ingredients in food processor.

In January of 2023, I received stem cells and exosomes through an epidural in the U.S.! I was a little bit nervous because not many people have tried this—it is very new. I had great success. I just recently started walking without a cane! I am walking, driving, and feeling great. I began taking tap dancing lessons, which really helps with my brain-to-body coordination, and my drop foot.

Throughout my journey, I've gone to church and Bible Study Fellowship. I also continue to see a great chiropractor and a wonderful acupuncturist. I stay close to God, as He has seen me through and given me, "Peace beyond all understanding". I incorporate various practices into my routine for my health and well-being. These include prayer, yoga, exercising with a stationary bike, red-light therapy (Vie light), grounding, using some EMF protection, and little-to-no dairy or gluten. I also take daily supplements, based on my 23andMe gene test, use liposomal vitamins, such as C and Glutathione, occasionally use melatonin, and CBD oil almost nightly. In addition, I receive massage therapy, engage in physical therapy through tap dancing, take Epsom salt and baking soda baths, and incorporate liver into my diet. I prioritize cooking healthy, mostly organic meals with lots of vegetables, celery juice, and use all-natural cleaning and bathing products. I have gained a lot of viable information from the research by Dr. Jack Kruse, neurosurgeon, who strongly suggests sunlight, red-light therapy, and DHA fish oil for everyone with MS. I highly recommend reading some of his work. Other helpful reads include *Breath* by James Nestor and *The Brain Fog Fix* by Dr. Mike Dow, which I listened to through Audible. I also recommend following @themsgym on Instagram, who is a great resource with helpful neuro-based exercises.

I have experienced and learned so much. If I had to do it all over, I would 100% do the natural treatments. My hope in writing this is to encourage you. Don't panic. Start by making sure you are not anxious. Then, start praying, exercising, and sleeping well. The next step is to focus on diet and supplements.

It's been ten years since I was diagnosed with multiple sclerosis, and I'm so thankful for all the help, healing, and advice I have received. I have felt pulled in many different directions of healing. In an ever-changing world with a wide range of natural therapies, there are so many to focus on. We can't do it all. Remember not to get bogged down! You will become familiar with what works for your body better than anyone else. Listen to advice and pray for clear direction but know that you are in control of what paths you choose.

"Be joyful in hope, patient in affliction, faithful in prayer." Romans 12:12

25

Story by
ANDREA

Diagnosed in 2000
Currently 62 years old
Lives in Los Angeles, United States
Instagram: @graygator1

Hello, my name is Andrea, and I was diagnosed with multiple sclerosis (MS) in 2000 at the age of thirty-nine. Prior to my diagnosis, I lived a pretty simple life in the Santa Ynez Valley in California with my husband and three children. I had always been very healthy. The only big thing that seemed off prior to being diagnosed was an episode ten years earlier where I lost temperature sensation in my right leg. It did seem odd, so I asked my doctor at the time about it. He wasn't concerned, so I did not give it much thought, and it eventually resolved itself. I know it wasn't postpartum because I was way beyond that.

In the ten years that followed, I did have random things happen, like a strange tingling on the back of my neck that came and went, and an annoying itchy spot that moved from my wrist to my forearm. At the time, I did not think much of them, but once I was diagnosed, it occurred to me that those symptoms may have also been the beginnings of my MS.

Since my diagnosis, my life has changed in many ways. I can honestly say it has all been for the best, as the changes I made have led me to a healthier lifestyle. This is the story of my journey. It has been a long, winding mix of many different modalities, but none of the conventional types. In this story, I am only focusing on the different therapies, not the supplements I've taken—that could be a whole book on its own, as I have tried many different combinations.

It began with a case of optic neuritis completely out of the blue. I'd had a debilitating headache for about a week. As the week progressed, I started losing vision in my right eye. This was very scary for me, mostly because a friend of mine had just been diagnosed with a brain tumor, and her symptoms were identical to mine. Thankfully, her tumor was benign. Three trips to the emergency room, plus two different optometrists, and no one had any idea what was wrong with me. Desperate for answers, I made an appointment with an ophthalmologist. I told him what I had been experiencing, and he said without hesitation, "Oh, you have multiple sclerosis". Yep, it was a shock, but I was happy that someone finally had some idea of what might be wrong.

My general practitioner sent me to a neurologist who promptly scheduled me for magnetic resonance imaging (MRI). The MRI came back conclusive for MS. Based on the size, color, and location of lesions on the scan, he did not feel that any other testing was necessary. The first person I told was my husband at the time. My kids were eleven, thirteen, and fifteen. My immediate family was totally supportive of my decision to go at it alternatively and felt confident I was on the right path because they weren't comfortable with the pharmaceuticals either. But my mom was totally freaked out.

Still reeling from the news, I went home and immediately dove into researching what it all meant. I don't recall ever being scared about it. I think I was living in a bit of ignorant bliss, convincing myself that everything would be fine. I kept telling myself that people do not die from MS; they die from complications due to MS, and I was going to do my best to avoid the complications. At my follow-up appointment with the neurologist, he told me that he wanted me to begin treatment with Betaseron, which I believe was one of the newest drugs on the market for MS at the time. Again, I did my research. What I found was that this particular drug was a once a week injectable. I could expect to have two days of flu-like symptoms after the injection, and it would provide me with a 30% reduction in my symptoms. I did not feel that a 30% reduction in my symptoms was worth losing two days of every week for the rest of my life, plus I was not comfortable with using a drug that was so new that no one knew what the long-term implications of it were. I had to find another way.

When I went back to the neurologist and told him my concerns, he scoffed at me, and said, "You are a very foolish girl. You obviously don't understand the implications of this disease. I guarantee in six months you will be crawling back in here, begging for this drug!" Wow, I thought my diagnosis was a shock, but the arrogance of this man was astounding. Still, I was not deterred!

The next six months were full of stressors that could have kicked my MS up a notch. I turned forty, my dog died unexpectedly, and my grandmother passed away. I went back to the neurologist for my follow-up, but I was not crawling, nor was I begging him for the medication. I walked in, told him what had happened over the past six months, reminded him what he had said to me, and told him I still did not want the drugs. He actually apologized to me and said that based on the results, he did not think I should do anything different. He said that I should just keep doing the alternative things, like the supplements and dietary changes, I'd been doing since he saw me six months earlier because I didn't crawl back in begging for the pharmaceutical drugs like he'd predicted I would. This, by the way, was the last time I ever saw a neurologist. I have chosen to judge how my disease is doing based on how I am feeling and functioning. Some might say this is irresponsible, but the mind is a powerful drug. I felt that having someone tell me I have new lesions could send me spiraling and ultimately be more destructive to my wellbeing. In fact, I tried to go to MS support meetings, but it was so much doom and gloom that I just couldn't do it. That was so far from where I was at.

I was still unsure exactly how to proceed, so I returned to my general practitioner. He told me to give him a few days to do some research. What he proposed for me immediately was to begin a regimen of a therapeutic dose of both vitamin D3 (as cholecalciferol) and B12 (as methyl cobalamin), and to remove gluten and dairy from my diet, with the exception of butter and full-fat yogurt. I've taken 5,000IUs of vitamin D3 and vitamin B12 since the day I was diagnosed. I have my D3 levels checked every six months, and all the doctors I've seen like my number to be about seventy-nine.

Even though I said I wasn't going to tell you about my supplements, I mention these two because I feel that they are fundamentally important to where I am today. Many of the things I have tried for my MS have come and gone, but these two supplements have continued without fail to this day.

Resources for managing MS alternatively were few and far between in 2000, but one of the books I found helpful was Roy Swank's *The MS Diet Book*. This book was last updated in 1985, so it was severely outdated, but I read it and incorporated his diet suggestions into my daily routine. Today, the only thing I remember about it is that I removed red meat from my diet for one year. It took almost a year for my optic neuritis to heal, and my vision in my right eye returned to about 75% of what it originally was. A side note to my optic neuritis is that I walked away from that experience with a newfound appreciation for my vision... you don't know what you have until it's gone, right? The many months that I couldn't see out of my right eye impacted my life tremendously in ways I could not have imagined. Driving was next to impossible due to the loss of depth perception, and many simple tasks had become difficult because I could not see things the same way I was accustomed to.

As my MS journey continued along the winding road of alternative therapies, one generally led me to the next. I wasn't always sure whether the alternative therapy of the day was what kept me walking on my own two feet. I felt pretty good with no new symptoms, but I still struggled with crushing fatigue. It often felt like my legs and eyeballs were stuck in concrete. I had some serious brain fog and occasional trouble with my right leg.

My general practitioner was continually researching alternative modalities for me, which I greatly appreciated. About a year into my diagnosis, he found a clinic about five hours north of me that offered a promising treatment. This clinic offered Live Blood Analysis, something I had not heard of but was excited to learn more about. Now is probably a great time to mention that many of the modalities I tried fall into the quackery category, according to conventional medicine. I don't feel that anything I've done was quackery, but if you run it by a conventional doctor, or google it, they will tell you it is; I guess it all depends on who you ask. I always evaluated whatever modality I considered trying before jumping into it. Not everything worked, and maybe some were quackery, but who knows, maybe it did help because here I sit almost twenty-three years later with nary a symptom. Now, back to Live Blood Analysis. When I was a child, I remember going to the doctor. Every time, the doctor would take a drop of blood and look at it under a microscope before he would make any recommendations about treatments. I hadn't thought about this until I went in for my first Live Blood Analysis, so having this done regarding my MS made perfect sense to me.

Live Blood Analysis looks at a blood sample, magnified thousands of times, under a dark field microscope, looking for irregularities in the blood. Through this process, it was determined that I had something known as mycoplasmas in my blood, which are believed to be responsible for fatigue-producing diseases. The treatment recommended for this was an olive leaf supplement called d-Lenolate. If you google it, one supplement will come up. This is the one I took, as well as many of the MS patients they treated. I took one capsule every two hours for about one year and let me tell you—life goes by fast when you're taking a pill every two hours! But it was worth it, as it made a significant improvement in my fatigue. Not only did I feel the improvement, but I also saw it in my blood analysis as the mycoplasma diminished. The clinic is no longer open; both doctors that ran it have retired. There may be other places that do it, but I can't speak to the legitimacy of them.

A few years later, I was introduced to another interesting modality called Bee Venom Therapy (BVT). Sounds horrible, doesn't it? I read about it in an article my doctor gave me from a publication called *Self-Healing*, and it suggested calling the American Apitherapy Society for more information. From there, I did a bunch of research and interviews until I found a doctor that I was comfortable working with. I was hoping to reverse my optic neuritis and remain healthy and as free from MS symptoms as possible. It was an interesting process. First, I had to get an EpiPen (that I never had to use, thankfully). He was adamant about that for good reason. There was a manual with everything I needed to know before beginning BVT: how to hold the bee to only get stung where it was intended, where to administer the stings, how often, and how long to leave the stingers in. I was armed with information, so I needed to get my bees! I was surprised when they arrived in a little wooden box about the size of an index card via the postal service. I placed the box outside and opened it up. I had a mini hive of bees. Obviously not a real hive, so I had to feed them honey every day.

The therapy consisted of intentionally stinging myself six-to-eight times, several times a week, in a specific location. There was a routine to follow, and the locations were specifically chosen for their benefits—no two the same. My husband did the dirty work of grabbing the bee by its wings and carefully placing it on me, enticing it to sting me in the appropriate location. It wasn't bad the first few times, but I noticed as time went on, I wasn't feeling better anymore. In fact, I often felt worse. It almost felt like I had the flu after I did a session of stings. I reached out to the doctor about this, and he suspended the therapy. He felt that my body was not able to metabolize the venom, causing it to linger in my body, making me feel sick. He was worried about a potentially dangerous allergic reaction. I don't regret trying this therapy because I did see significant improvements in the lingering effects of my optic neuritis, but I was not sad when it was over! I don't remember exactly how long I did this therapy for because it was twenty-two years ago. All I remember is I did about fifty stings.

The next few years were a rollercoaster ride, feeling great some days and feeling like I was going to die from fatigue other days. When I started eating gluten and dairy-free, my body had some detoxing to do, so I didn't feel the results right away. It was hard to do because I still had so much to learn about eating gluten-free. It wasn't mainstream then, and finding alternatives was a challenge.

I had a laundry list of aches and tingles that came and went around different parts of my body; nothing that impacted my daily living, just annoyances that never seemed to go away. So clearly, I needed to dig deeper. I cannot remember where, but I learned about mercury fillings, and how detrimental they can be to our health. I don't know for a fact if the mercury fillings contributed to my MS, but my general practitioner, who helped me years later, agreed it was probably a trigger. I also learned that you cannot just have them removed. There is a very specific method that needs to be followed so as not to make problems worse. It took me a while, but I finally found a dentist about 120 miles from me, who was familiar with the process. I had six mercury fillings that needed to be replaced. He advised me that they should not all be done at the same time. First, he removed three fillings on one side of my mouth, waited three days, then removed the remaining three on the other side. I followed this with a series of supplements that the dentist recommended to assist in removing any remaining mercury.

Within a week of removal, I noticed that I was losing less hair in the shower, and my eyelashes were much fuller. I cannot say scientifically whether the fillings were responsible for my hair loss and thin eyelashes, but I was happy to see both improving!

As luck would have it, my general practitioner met a doctor who specializes in endocrinology and practiced medicine in a way he thought I'd appreciate. This was before functional medicine doctors had become mainstream. She did not officially identify that way, but her approach to health and wellbeing was exactly that—and I loved her!

She did a series of hormone testing through blood work, testing things I did not even realize were hormones. My results came back, and everything was out of whack. Next began the daunting task of trial and error to find the right doses and combinations that would balance things out. We started with the thyroid. She preferred using desiccated pig thyroid, also known as bioidentical. It's a prescription. I have used two different brands: Armor, and the one I currently use, ERFA. I started on one half grain and worked my way up, then back down to find the optimal dose, and settled in at two-and-a-half grains—which is where I remain today. I did try some of the synthetic versions of thyroid medications over the years, but they never balanced things out as well as the desiccated thyroid. Nowadays, I check my thyroid level every six months.

I also learned from her that estrogen is essential for the re-myelination of the myelin sheath that covers a nerve, so balancing my estrogen and progesterone was next on the list. This was another arduous process. It took a lot of patience—as it took several years and some trial and error to arrive at the right type and dosage. I varied the dosage over the course of the month to mimic my natural cycle until I went through menopause. Now, I do static dosing all month. Originally, I tried the bioidentical type of hormones, but ultimately had better results with Prometrium and the Vivelle Dot (hormone medications), both of which I still use today.

The next few years passed uneventfully. I remained gluten and dairy-free. I felt pretty good most of the time, but there were still days where the fatigue was oppressive, memory fog and cognitive function waxed and waned, and I still had a lot of random tingling in my hands and leg that would come and go. By now, I had put together a network of other like-minded people. One friend had heard about something called chronic inflammatory response syndrome (CIRS), and a doctor who had come up with a protocol for mitigating it. His name is Dr. Richie Shoemaker. Dr Shoemaker, a leader in patient care, research, and education, pioneered the field of biotoxin-related illness. Biotoxin-related illness occurs in certain susceptible people who are exposed to mold or have a tick-borne illness, including Lyme disease; are exposed to Dnoflagellates, like Pfiesteria; or come in contact with blue green algae, like Cylindrospermopsis, Microcystis, or Ciguatera. The people he found to be susceptible are individuals who have a specific HLA haplotype, inherited from both parents. He estimates that 24% of the population has this specific HLA haplotype. Genetically susceptible people have a problem with the production of protective antibodies that typically remove these biotoxins and mycotoxins, causing CIRS. I am not a doctor or a scientist, so this is as far as my understanding of the genetic process goes.

Knowing that inflammation is a key component in MS flares, I was very interested in this protocol. In 2016, I set out to find a doctor who practiced the Shoemaker protocol and found a woman in Montana who I was very comfortable with. The first thing she had me do was test my home for the presence of mold, using an ERMI test. Fortunately, my current home did not test positive for mold anywhere. Next, I did genetic testing for the presence of this HLA haplotype, and it came back that I do carry this genetic defect. Armed with this information, I began my treatment.

The symptoms of CIRS are as varied as MS symptoms, many of them being the same. Dr. Shoemaker found that most people with CIRS have at least six to eight of them at a time. Personally, I had at least half of them, rotating around my body all the time: fatigue, weakness, aches, headache, light sensitivity, decreased assimilation of new knowledge, memory impairment, decreased word finding, difficulty concentrating, joint pain, A.M. stiffness, cramps, unusual skin sensitivity, tingling, shortness of breath, sinus congestion, cough, excessive thirst, confusion, appetite swings, difficulty regulating body temperature, increased urinary frequency, red eyes, blurred vision, night sweats, mood swings, ice pick pain, abdominal pain, diarrhea, numbness, tearing of eyes, disorientation, metallic taste, static shocks, and vertigo.

The treatment plan is a twelve-step process that is very detailed. Moving from one step to the next is dependent on completion of the previous step. It was daunting, and I sometimes felt like I was never going to get to the next step. But I would remind myself of why I was doing it in the first place and refocus on the task at hand. There were medications I had to take, and I did Visual Contrast Screening (VCS) regularly. This is a test that measures your ability to see details at low contrast levels. It is considered a valuable diagnostic tool to measure the impact of neurotoxins on brain function. It was very interesting to see how my vision changed, often improving, from test to test along the way. It took about a year to make it to the final step in the protocol. The final step was a nasal spray called vasoactive intestinal polypeptide (VIP), a neuro-immune modulator that restores immune regulation. While using this spray, I was required to take my blood pressure and heart rate twice a day at the same time of day. This final step took me about two months to complete. It felt like I was never going to get through the process, but I did. Over that year and a half, I watched all the lingering, annoying symptoms either resolve all together or diminish to a place where they were no longer an annoyance. My brain fog greatly improved. I could not have imagined feeling so good when I started the process. I almost felt like my pre-MS self, and I was thrilled! As I look back, I think this process was probably the most transformative step in my health journey. You can find more information about the Shoemaker Protocol at https://www.survivingmold.com/docs/12_STEP_SHOEMAKER_PROTOCOL_FOR_CIRS.PDF

The next turn on my alternative therapy journey came the day my facial lady told me her story about a car accident she was in a few years earlier. She struggled with a lot of pain as a result but found great relief with something called cryotherapy. Cryotherapy is where the body is exposed to freezing temperatures between -120° and -180°F for about three minutes. Extreme cold exposure reduces inflammation, aids in muscle recovery, and reduces pain. I had to try it!

I started using cryotherapy about three years ago and felt a tremendous reduction in the arthritis pain in my lower back. I was hooked! Besides the improvement in my arthritis pain, I noticed an increase in my energy level, which was very exciting. I would leave my cryotherapy sessions feeling exhilarated with a spring in my step. I still do cryotherapy one-to-two times a week, as my schedule allows. I have recently added the infra-red sauna to my routine before cryotherapy. Saunas support detoxification and can be helpful in healing when used together with cryotherapy. I have only been doing the sauna for a couple of weeks now, so I cannot say definitively whether I notice any improvement from this combination. But thirty minutes in the sauna definitely contributes to my sense of relaxation, which is never a bad thing!

Exercise has always played an important role in my healing journey. We all know that staying active is important, but for those of us with MS, it is critical! I have always belonged to a gym and done heavy weight training and Body Pump for many years. During the COVID lockdown, I continued my workouts at home, and added walking three miles a day to my routine. When things opened back up, I did not feel like returning to my old gym. I felt like it was time to try something new. That something new was Reformer Pilates. Pilates seemed like the perfect option at this stage of my life because it is a mix of strength training, balance, and stretching—all very necessary not only as I age, but as I age with MS. I have been doing Pilates four times a week for over a year now, and I know it was the right decision. When I was younger, I was very flexible, but I did not realize until I started Pilates how much of that flexibility I had lost, whether it be to age or MS. Over the past year, I have seen my flexibility improve, and most exciting of all, my balance has improved overall—but markedly on my right side, the side affected by MS. Pilates has also been a good addition because it is a very calming form of exercise; it is a great way to reset in the middle of the craziness of life!

The most recent step in my journey was to do a DNA test through the DNA Company (www.thednacompany.com). This is not a DNA test like Ancestry or 23 and Me—this test is all about my genes and how they affect my physical health, mental health, sleep, and many other areas, and how to optimize all of that through supplements, food, and the lifestyle choices that I make. It was interesting to see that many of the traits that make me who I am are actually a result of my DNA. It also confirmed that my MS is real and not just another illness that presents as MS, which in a weird way felt good to know, as it confirmed that I had not been chasing the wrong diagnosis for over twenty-two years. Based on the recommendations of the report, I have updated my supplements and included the recommended foods as often as possible. Saunas and cold therapy were two recommendations that I was already doing, but now I know that there are some genetically beneficial reasons for it. It is something I will continue to incorporate as often as possible.

My diet has been pretty consistent since I started gluten and dairy-free. I was religious about not cheating for the first ten years and rarely ate out because it was so difficult. Like I said earlier, it wasn't mainstream, and a lot of people didn't understand when I told them I was gluten-free. Now, I occasionally have a treat, like a good slice of sourdough bread or a sweet treat like a donut (my weakness). I do eat out, but I try to remain mindful of my choices. I mostly eat organic, whole foods. If I eat meat at home, I choose grass-fed. Dairy is challenging because I love it, but I rarely cheat because it gives me a cough and horrible congestion. I found out from my DNA test that I am lactose intolerant, so dairy hits me hard.

I recently had my six-month checkup with my doctor, and she talked to me about some other modalities that I may want to try down the road, depending on what is happening with my MS in the future. This reminded me that the story that you just read is where I am at today, but I'm not done. This journey is lifelong. My health is a work-in-progress, and I will never stop researching and trying new things to stay ahead of the curve with regards to my MS.

I want to thank Agota for writing this book. Not only for the benefits it will provide others, but also because it gave me an opportunity to walk back through my journey. I had forgotten how difficult it was in the beginning, but I always knew that there was a way through. Almost twenty-three years later, I am so glad I made the choice to do it without the pharmaceuticals. I feel amazing today, almost forgetting that MS is part of my life. But I cannot get complacent. If I get lazy and do not take my supplements or eat whatever comes my way, I feel the little signs that remind me MS is a disease that does not go away. An amazing woman I met through the internet, when I was first on my journey to manage my MS alternatively, named Betty Iams, used to say, "I have MS, it does not have me." That is an adage that has stuck with me! I believe that I am in control, based on the choices I make. Anyone newly diagnosed, don't panic, don't let yourself be pressured into doing something you aren't comfortable with, do your own research, and don't make decisions out of fear—and most importantly, trust your gut! If you would like to reach out to me, you can find me on Instagram @graygator1. I would love to hear from you!

26

Story by

MERYL FAITH HUTT

Diagnosed in 1999
Currently 62 years old
Lives in Birmingham, United kingdom
Email: merylfaith@hotmail.com

"Multiple sclerosis (MS)? THE wheelchair multiple sclerosis?" I asked the neurologist. Even amidst the shock and devastation, I'll never forget that moment or his response.

"That depends on you."

It wasn't the answer I wanted. I was looking for reassurance and to be told everything would be okay, but it was exactly what I needed to hear. It started me on the path to where I am now—sixty-two years old and enjoying an active retirement.

So, how did I find myself—a thirty-eight-year-old mother of two—in the Neurology Department, receiving an MS diagnosis that day? It's a story all too familiar for many others. It started years before with symptoms that I didn't even realize were symptoms; symptoms we brush off as working mothers. We put things down to the strain of busy lives. I experienced dizziness, tiredness, numbness, or heaviness in my limbs. At first, the symptoms were episodic, and as they wore off, I carried on with life. Some were hard to ignore though. One night, when I was thirty-three, I was kept awake with what felt like an electrical current running through my body; little electric shocks, pins and needles in my fingers, and a burning sensation across my knees. Even though it was hard to ignore, I managed. I got out of bed the next morning and continued with daily life.

The following year, I landed my dream job as a Teaching Assistant, working with children with Special Educational Needs. I found I needed reading glasses and noticed problems with my hearing, especially within the busy classroom. Following a hearing test, I was told the problems were due to blocked sinuses and rhinitis.

Then, something happened that I firmly believe sped up my MS symptoms. The school I was working at was offering the Hepatitis vaccine to staff, and as a family member had recently died of the disease, I decided to have it. After that vaccine, my lower back pain worsened, and I started to have monthly migraines which made me vomit and faint. Then, one afternoon, a child fell over on the playground. I ran to help, but my leg gave way underneath me. With these new and worsening symptoms, I was sent by my doctor for an X-ray, and I was diagnosed with osteoarthritis. I wasn't worried though. My elderly mother had osteoarthritis, and it just seemed inevitable that I would, too. Naively, I started taking cod liver oil and believed that would do the trick. Needless to say, it didn't!

At that time, I ate standard British food. I have always loved trying new recipes, but back then, I cooked with butter and lard. Plus, I didn't eat as many vegetables or fish as I do now. However, it wasn't until the following summer, when my husband and children started to notice my disability, that I became concerned. Anytime we were out walking our dog, they noticed my "floppy leg" and the sound it would make as it hit the floor. At this point, my leg seemed to have a life of its own. It felt hollow as if all the muscle had disappeared. It started to affect my mood, too. We were an active family, but as my husband and children (eight and eleven at that time) climbed Mount Snowdon while on holiday, I was forced to wait in the car alone, unable to even start the ascent. My arm was also starting to bother me. Sometimes it would shake, and at other times, I'd suddenly drop things.

It was my mother who finally convinced me to return to the doctor as my symptoms were nothing like what she experienced with osteoarthritis. I was thirty-eight years old when I was sent for magnetic resonance imaging (MRI), which had to be rescheduled due to a broken machine (while I was in it), and then another two months before I was called in to receive my results.

That brings us back to being sat in the neurologist's office, asking whether my diagnosis would lead to a wheelchair. At that moment, it felt like my life was over. I immediately thought of my husband and children. Would I live to see my children grow up? Would my husband be forced to become my carer? What would our life look like moving forward? I had a lot of thinking time those next few days, as I immediately began three days of intravenous steroids. I had never taken more than one paracetamol, so I was reluctant. I told him that I didn't want it, but he said this is what I had to do, so I went along. Who was I to question a neurologist with years of experience? While they did seem to help initially, it was just days before the effects wore off, and at that moment, I decided to change my lifestyle. As a result, I never took another medication for my multiple sclerosis again.

The following year at my annual appointment, he wanted me to have steroids, but I refused as I couldn't see any difference. Every year when I attended my annual review, he would ask if I'd had any more relapses, and if I would like steroids or a trial of any new medication they had. I always refused, especially after my health had improved over the previous nine months, and I gained strength in my leg and arm. After ten years, my neurologist retired. I then had a much younger neurologist who was more interested in my diet and exercise, and he spoke about needing to research it further. About nine years ago, he told me I didn't need to come anymore as I hadn't had any relapses. My MS had remained benign/mild.

After I was diagnosed, the first step I took upon the advice of my husband was reducing my hours at work. Working in the mornings allowed me to rest in the afternoons. He also took on much more of the housework, and by now, my children were older, and they helped, too.

Next, I decided to start researching multiple sclerosis, so I might better understand my disability and be more informed in order to advocate for myself. The only problem was this was 1999. The internet was not what it is now, or at least it wasn't for me. I couldn't just pick up my phone and have a wealth of information at my fingertips. There was no social media to find others like me. The only book I could find about MS was depressing. A subscription to *MS Matters Magazine* didn't improve my spirits either. All the stories were of severely disabled MS sufferers.

There was not a hint of positivity or optimism to be found. The only seemingly happy people in the magazine were those raising money for charity by running marathons, and they did not have MS. I decided not to continue reading; all they did was add to my fears.

Six weeks after my diagnosis, we were booked to go on an all-inclusive holiday to a five-star resort in Crete. At the time, I was unsure about going as I felt self-confidence and my physical abilities slipping away. I decided, for my children's sake, I had to push myself to go. It was the best thing I could have done. The whole family was able to truly relax and unwind in the sunshine.

On returning home, I decided to focus on losing weight. Over the previous couple of years, I began piling on the pounds as I was not active. I started a low-fat diet, incorporating some of the Mediterranean recipes I'd enjoyed on holiday, and I cut back on sugar. I read about the benefits of the Mediterranean diet, so I started using olive oil, more vegetables/fruit in every meal, and ate more fish, nuts, and yogurt. Plus, I was cooking more from scratch. In a short span of time, my digestion improved, and I lost twenty-eight pounds. I felt much better! Gym visits left me feeling depressed, so when my niece mentioned a yoga class at the local Adult Education Centre, I decided to give that a try instead. It turned out to be the best decision I could have made. My yoga instructor, Ed, had experience working with clients with MS and knew exactly how to support me. I loved the classes. At last, I had found an exercise I could do that was beneficial. I attended classes for ten years until the class time conflicted with my work schedule. Yoga is still very much part of my life as I attend classes when I can and practice regularly at home. I firmly believe the combination of yoga, healthy diet, weight loss, and reducing my busy schedule allowed me to gain strength back in my body. My leg even stopped flopping! I started walking further, dancing all night at parties, and most of all, my fatigue improved. I also feel that my brain/ nervous system improved. When my strength improved, my limbs didn't feel hollow anymore. It felt like the transmitters had been cleaned out. Ten years ago, I joined a bowls team, and I enjoy playing four times a week. I play competitively in different leagues against men and women. One year, I was captain of the Warwick and Worcester team, and I managed eleven men!

As my strength returned, so did my confidence. I finally felt able to enjoy life without fear. I decided to travel more, visiting New York, Florida, the Deep South, and cruising the Mediterranean and beyond.

One thing I hadn't done up until about eight years ago was disclose my multiple sclerosis to anyone beyond family and close friends. I didn't want their sympathy or comments on what I could or couldn't do. One day a friend said to me, "People need to see that MS doesn't have to be life in a wheelchair." I thought back to that first appointment when I received my diagnosis and decided she was right. Many friends and colleagues were shocked as I had no noticeable symptoms.

Sharing my diagnosis with others not only opened their eyes to MS but also opened doors to new opportunities for me. A little over a year ago, a month or so into my retirement, a friend I'd met at work contacted me to let me know that our local MS Society was offering "Keep Fit", yoga classes, reflexology, and massage sessions. I now attend weekly, and I love it. I not only benefit from the exercise and relaxing massages but also the sense of community.

When I was working, I kept fit from bowling, walking the dog, and attending a yoga class once a week. After retiring last year, I started stretching every morning and doing some yoga poses, such as cat-cow, warrior, tree, sphinx, bridge, triangle, and to finish, child's pose. Alternatively, I will do a routine from YouTube. Currently, I attend yoga or an exercise class at an MS session at St. Giles in Sutton Coldfield. Afterwards, we have a chat or lunch together. The MS society in Sutton Coldfield offers reflexology/massage, plus exercise and yoga sessions. Hinna, my massage therapist (@relaxwellbeing), has been amazing this year for relieving tense muscles and giving me total relaxation.

Changing my diet has been vital in the improvement of my health. For breakfast, I'll have either a green smoothie (kale, avocado, spinach, oat milk, blueberries, banana, and a teaspoon of peanut butter) or yogurt with berries, almonds, and walnuts. I would love to eat more fruit, but my body won't allow it, so I only eat up to three fruits a day. During the winter months, I eat porridge with cinnamon and fruit. For lunch, I'll have a salad (typically Greek), homemade soup, hummus, or falafel. My favorite lunch is feta cheese with a drizzle of extra virgin oil and rosemary with red onions, cucumber, and tomatoes. If I'm hungry, I might have some granary bread, too. For my evening meal, I may have salmon or sea bass with spices and different vegetables. I love gnocchi with roasted vegetables, topped with crumbled feta, or cooked legumes with vegetable dishes. I love prawn linguine, crab, or pesto pasta. When it's cold out, I love cooking rustic vegetable stew, Mediterranean vegetable and chickpea stew, or butter beans stew. Alternatively, I enjoy chili and trying out new recipes. If I go to a restaurant, I enjoy eating meze with friends or fish. Very occasionally, I will have a filet steak. Now and again, I have some chocolate or a slice of cake!

When I was first diagnosed, every book or magazine spoke of getting used to a sedentary lifestyle—to take up knitting or jigsaws puzzles! This depressed me as I was so young and had small children. I suppose that spurred me on. Now, when I put my feet up, I love reading or doing crosswords, and my favorite codebreakers!

The reason I wanted to share my story is because I want others to know that life doesn't end with an MS diagnosis. I am sixty-two years old. I'm fairly fit. I enjoy walking and dancing with my husband, playing with my young grandson, weekly exercise classes, crown green bowls matches, and holidays with friends and family. Don't put life on hold because you have MS. My advice is to start with lifestyle changes. I have always been a positive person, but now that I'm retired and healthy, I enjoy every day.

27

Story by

CONOR KERLEY

Diagnosed in 2003

Currently 35 years old

Lives in Dundalk, Ireland

Instagram: @conorkerley.nutrition

Twitter: @conorkerley

Facebook: www.facebook.com/conorkerleyhealth

LinkedIn: www.linkedin.com/in/drconorkerley

It all started with a dead leg. It was a few days after Christmas in 2002. I was fifteen years old, a straight-A student in school, and a good athlete. Our school basketball team had just been beaten in the semifinals of the school tournament. Earlier that year, I got a very bad bang on my left knee, which eventually led to a large piece of cartilage becoming dislodged and essentially floating around my knee area, not attached to anything. When I told my Mam, she laughed and thought I had been drinking alcohol! But then I showed her that I could move this piece of cartilage from one side of my kneecap to the other. This required surgery to remove it, and the surgeon even let me keep the piece of cartilage in a jar. It has shrunk a lot, but I still have it! The reason I bring this story up is that for Christmas in 2002, all I wanted was to build my leg muscles without having to do too much running or jumping, which could affect my knee. So, my parents bought me a step machine. What normal fifteen-year-old wants a step machine for Christmas? Me! So, on the 27th of December, while my parents and sisters were chilling out with

Christmas sandwiches and chocolates in front of the TV, I decided to do 10,000 steps on my new step machine. The next morning, I woke up, and my left leg was dead. I could walk but not normally. I attributed this to the 10,000 steps and thought to myself how out of shape I had become.

We usually have a gathering at my parents' house a few days after Christmas. I was helping to get the house ready, carrying bottles around, but I kept dropping them. Since it was my left arm now, I knew it wasn't a dead leg from stepping too much! Over the next few days, neither my arm nor leg got better; in fact—they got worse. On New Year's Day, I went to the local hospital, which is very small. After conducting some tests, they immediately sent me to the nearest emergency room, which was in Dublin. Since the emergency rooms tend to get very busy on New Year's Eve, with drunken or injured people, I was admitted to the hospital immediately. They sent for a wheelchair, but I thought to myself, "If I can walk, I'm not that sick."

At the stroke of midnight on New Years Eve, I was receiving a computed tomography (CT) scan. I was then admitted to a brain surgery ward and spent most of the day sleeping. I have never felt sheer exhaustion like these few days. I would wake to see that friends or family had visited, and I hadn't even heard them. After many more tests, I was moved out of the brain surgery ward and into a brain injury ward.

The brain injury ward was empty as it was the holiday season. The entire ward had opened just for me. Then, a junior doctor came along to retrieve some spinal fluid from me. Easy, I thought...until he showed up with a massive syringe and spent forty-five minutes trying to retrieve the spinal fluid. That led to forty-five minutes of a massive syringe being poked into my lower back—repeatedly. I was later informed that nothing showed up on my lumbar puncture (spinal tap). Still, a forty-five-minute time span I won't be forgetting soon!

The hospital I was in is a university teaching hospital. Almost every day, someone would come around to assess me or ask me to be assessed in front of junior doctors or medical students. On one particular occasion, I remember I kept laughing. I knew I was ill; I knew this was a serious situation and that nothing funny had happened, but I laughed. This happened on several different occasions. Later, I realized that this uncontrollable and unexpected laughter affects roughly 10% of people with MS and is known as the pseudobulbar affect. This can also manifest as crying.

One question I was often asked by various doctors was regarding family history. My Mam is from a large, traditional Irish family—she is one of thirteen children! One of her sisters, now sadly passed away, had MS. Other than this one aunt, there was little other family history regarding health issues. Since the doctors always asked about family history, and because only one out of my sixteen aunts and uncles had MS, I didn't think I had it. Anyway, after more and more tests, including magnetic resonance imaging (MRI), daily blood tests, and two weeks of intravenous (IV) steroids, I eventually returned home.

On the way home, we met my uncle for lunch. I remember my Mam cutting up my food. I could use my right hand but not my left; eating was one of many things that was difficult. In fact, I pretty much had to learn how to walk again and how to tie my shoelaces.

There were no answers. What had happened to me and why? I just remember the overwhelming feeling of relief after getting out of the hospital. Although I slept a lot in the hospital and had visitors every day, it was very boring and lonely. The plan was intensive physiotherapy to get my arm and leg working again. Initially, I had physio pretty much every day, which gradually decreased to every second day, and then to once or twice per week. I was getting more energy and growing stronger all the time. But I was still napping a lot every day. There was no way I would be able to return to school yet.

A few months later (around March 2003), I started to feel tingling and numbness on the left side of my face. I was reviewed by the medical team who prescribed epilepsy medications. But still—no official diagnosis.

I eventually went back to school, at first for up to two half days per week, and then more and more. That June, I sat for the official Irish state exams after missing almost six months of school. It was around this time that I had a routine hospital clinic appointment for updates on what had happened to me and why. The doctor, whom we had never met before, had a very poor manner. Abruptly and casually, he mentioned that I might have multiple sclerosis, completely out of the blue. This frightened me as I didn't know much about MS, except the still common depiction of people with advanced disability. This wasn't an official diagnosis, so life went on afterward.

Every day I spent time exercising and getting stronger. I was keen to regain full control and power of my left arm and leg. One Saturday morning in August 2003, I was in our garage, exercising on my mini trampoline (again, to save my knee!). As I was jumping up and down, I kept veering to one side, even as I was conscious of this and tried to stop it from happening. A little concerned, I went into the house, and my godmother, an ex-nurse who happened to be visiting, said that we should get it checked out. On a Saturday, most local doctors (known as GPs in Ireland, similar to Primary Care Physicians) are closed, so we went to a locum GP, again—someone we'd never met before.

This locum doctor heard my history and sent me to the local hospital where I was admitted while waiting for a bed to open in the larger hospital in Dublin. This was certainly my third MS attack in eight months, but we still didn't know what was going on. Back then, there was no social media or smartphones. In fact, we didn't really use the internet at home. There was no such thing as "googling" my symptoms. The way I describe my first MS attack is the loss of 90% function of my left side. However, this third MS attack was more like losing 10% function, but this time on the right side. I was relatively functional, so I remember in the hospital there was a quiet staircase near my ward, and I used to run up and down, while holding the banister. This was partly due to boredom—no smartphones, Facebook, or TV streaming! But also, partially due to wanting to maintain my strength and fitness. But the main reason for wanting to run those hospital stairs every day was that I told myself, "If you can move and run stairs, you can't be that sick."

Testing facilities in this small regional hospital were limited, so I was moved to the larger Dublin hospital after about a week of IV steroids. I was admitted to the same brain injury ward as the first time I got sick. This alone gave me chills. However, I was much more functional this time. This hospital has a long driveway connecting to a main road. I used to walk up and down this driveway five times each morning. I remember once the doctors came around to assess me, but I was out walking! I got in trouble with the nurses, but I still remember my mantra: "If you can move like this, you can't be that sick."

I was scheduled for another MRI scan but thankfully no repeat lumbar puncture after the first one! A few days after the MRI scan, my parents and I were asked to meet with the entire medical team, including junior and senior doctors, as well as nurses. It was here that a single sentence changed my life:

"Conor, you have multiple sclerosis."
My Mam burst into tears and left the room. I'm not a parent, so I can't empathize with her. But I can only imagine how it feels to hear your child being told that they have a serious, incurable condition—especially

at the young age of fifteen. In addition, my older sister was born a twin, and my twin brother, Dara, passed away a month after birth. So, my parents had lost a son and now their only living son was being diagnosed with MS. In many ways, that day must have been harder for them than for me.

Strangely, my immediate reaction was relief—we had an answer, a diagnosis. We could come up with a plan and move forward. No more mystery. Except MS is very mysterious, but I didn't know that then. My second reaction was, "When can I leave the hospital!?" As I say, I was quite functional, having lost about 10% of function, but I could still walk unaided. One of my overriding memories of being in the hospital is boredom. There was nothing to do! I was the youngest in the ward by about fifty years. Although the other patients and I chatted, the days were long and boring. My third reaction was, "Will I be able to play sports?" This was one of my first questions for the medical team, and I remember them looking at me like I had two heads! I'm sure they were thinking, "We've just told this young fella he has MS, and he's worried about playing sports!?"

Thankfully, I was released! I was allowed to leave the hospital, but not before a serious discussion with the medical team about my treatment options, which were only presented as medications. No mention of exercise, nutrition, supplements, stress—medication only. Back in 2003, there were only three medication options, all injectable: two different types of interferon and Copaxone. The effectiveness of these three medications was very similar, so it was up to me to decide which I prefer. This would depend on how often I wanted to inject, the size of needle, side effects, etc. I went home to think about it, excited to be leaving the hospital. I later opted to go with one of the interferon medications.

As a young boy, the fact that school was about to start was just as significant for me. I was able to attend school, but I had to take a lot of time off for different medical appointments. The first relapse required almost an entire rebuild of strength and function, while the third relapse required more fine tuning. Both were difficult and frustrating!

At first, life went on, and I didn't really talk to anybody about MS. My friends were young, and there was (and still is) a perception that MS means life in a wheelchair. Not exactly a fun schoolyard conversation. I initially made some efforts to attend local MS meetups, but these were mostly attended by people fifty plus years older than me and with visible disability. So, I stopped going to these types of events. I was also advised against reading too much about MS as there was (and still is) a lot of misinformation. So, I avoided MS talk mostly, and life went on. But my medication, the interferon injections, were causing nasty side effects, from bruising and soreness at the infection sites to cold-like symptoms and sleepless nights—not ideal while trying to attend school, study, play sports, and chase girls!

The medication side effects were constant and made me feel miserable. I knew that being miserable was not healthy. It was at this point that I decided to start reading about MS—every piece of information I could find. I started in the local library–not with Google but using real books– and I read everything around me. The information was not consistent, and it was more than a little confusing. Nevertheless, healthy eating seemed important, as did moving my body every day, controlling stress, and sleeping well. I decided I was going to stop taking the medications due to the severe side effects, but only while changing my entire lifestyle simultaneously. At the next clinic appointment, I told the doctors that I was stopping the medications. They essentially told me that I was being foolish. My parents did not agree with my decision but said they would support me.

Leaving the clinic room that day, I felt free but also nervous. I already had a diagnosis, and my severe medication side effects were about to stop. But would I get sick again? I told myself to keep moving and educating myself. This sounds great, but initially it was an absolute disaster. I look back now at the information I was reading and believing, and I understand that a lot of it was rubbish. Some of it was dangerous information. Nevertheless, I was on a mission to live a healthier life.

I still had three years of school left before I would be able to go to university. Since my dream of being the first Irish guy to play in the NBA seemed doomed (jokes! I was good, but not that good), I decided to focus my energies on getting healthy. Nutrition seemed pretty important; I was always vaguely interested in nutrition but mostly from a sports point of view, not necessarily health. This was twenty years ago at the time of writing this. Thankfully, things have gone from strength to strength since then; I have been symptom-free, relapse-free, and medication-free.

My simple advice for anyone newly diagnosed is to connect with other MSers (in person and/or online). There are so many groups available, enabling anyone to connect anywhere in the world with similar issues, thoughts, questions and ideas. Ask questions to your medical team, including neurologists, pharmacists, physiotherapists, occupational therapists, dietitians, etc.

Educate yourself but be careful of the source. It has never been easier to access information than it is right now. However, finding trustworthy and reliable information is harder than ever! Be careful who and what you believe. A lot of social media influencers are not qualified on what they speak about. In addition, be careful because sometimes people talk about new research performed on animals (like mice or rats) and assume the effect is the same in humans! Engage with your local healthcare team(s), as well as national MS Societies and trusted key healthcare professionals.

Move! As you can tell, if you've read the first part of my piece in this wonderful book, I am a big fan of movement. You don't have to be a bodybuilder or marathon runner but try to move your body on a consistent, daily basis. Start where you are, be sensible, and find something you enjoy and will commit to. This could be a walk with a friend, swimming, gardening, or playing with the grandchildren, for example.

All diseases are complicated. MS seems to be one of the most complicated! However, there are certain things which seem important to help manage MS, based on my own opinion, experience, and most importantly, the scientific evidence.

I think nutrition is so important yet underappreciated and underused when it comes to health in general and certain conditions, including MS. As I mentioned previously, after I was diagnosed, I read a lot regarding nutrition and MS, but it was very conflicting and confusing. I became more and more interested in nutrition as a means to get healthy and stay healthy. My solution was to formally study human nutrition and dietetics at the oldest and most prestigious university in Ireland, Trinity College, Dublin. Following graduation, I completed my doctorate studies through the School of Medicine at University College Dublin in conjunction with two Dublin hospitals. For nutrition research, which I designed and conducted myself, I won multiple national and international awards.

But when it comes to MS, there is conflicting research and school of thought regarding nutrition. On one hand, there is the plant-based, low saturated fat approach. On the other hand, there is the low carbohydrate, paleolithic/ketogenic approach. These approaches are quite different! My chapter is not intended to focus on nutrition and the complexities of nutrition research. However, there is some consistency. For example, all plans recommend lots of vegetables. So, as I always say to my patients, adding more vegetables is a great place to start! Other antioxidant-rich foods, which are heavily recommended based on research studies conducted among those with MS as well as other neurological and autoimmune diseases, include nuts, seeds, and fruits, especially berries. Omega-3 rich foods, such as flaxseed (also called linseeds), walnuts, and oily fish, such as salmon, sardines, and mackerel, as well as certain fortified foods and omega-3 supplements, are also recommended. Some research supports small amounts of eggs and poultry products, but this is not consistent. On the other hand, foods which are not recommended based on research studies include processed meats, excess alcohol, refined cereals (such as white bread), high amounts of salt and sugar, fried foods, and trans-fats (e.g., processed salad dressing).

A fascinating area of research regarding health and disease, including MS specifically, is the gut microbiome. A really important nutrient for overall health and overall gut health is fiber.
And Kerley's golden rule of fiber is that it is only found in unrefined plant foods. This is a really useful guide when you are eating or shopping. Is there any fiber in milk? No, because it's not an unrefined plant food. Is there any fiber in white bread? Very minimal because although white bread is from plants, it is heavily refined. Is there any fiber in flaxseeds? Yes, because they are unrefined plant food. So, fiber-rich foods include legumes like chickpeas, lentils, kidney beans; nuts like walnuts; seeds like flaxseed; as well as wholegrains like oats, fruits, and vegetables. These foods form the basis of very healthy diets, including my own. Some research suggests that dairy products can be problematic for those with MS. I use mostly fortified soy alternatives, which are a great source of protein, as well as calcium, vitamin B12, and much more!

Here's a rough outline of my daily routine: As I've said throughout my chapter in this great book, movement is key for everyone, including those with MS. Initially, this was just my own thought as a stubborn, athletic boy, but modern science really does back up the therapeutic benefits of movement for MS (and other conditions). In the past, people with MS were encouraged to rest and not exercise. However, research conducted among those with MS and other neurological and autoimmune conditions has reported that movement and physical activity is good for muscle strength, bone strength, balance, coordination, brain function, and mental health, including mood, and much more! Research also demonstrates that exercise is actually beneficial for decreasing fatigue! I walk every single day outside in nature. I live on the third floor of a building and use the stairs down but also up multiple times per day. Using the stairs is a simple way to ensure that amount of movement throughout the day. I go to the gym most days and do a combination of strength activities with free weights and machines, aerobic training such as a spin class, as well as some yoga. I am terrible at yoga, but I know I really need to work on my flexibility (note that my poor flexibility has probably been from sports injuries, not MS). I play sports when I can, usually football (soccer) and basketball, but I love the chance to play pretty much any sport.

For anyone—with or without MS—it is important to try to move daily but start where you are and seek professional advice and assistance if needed. For some, a short walk may be a good starting point. For others, some gentle exercise while seated might be most appropriate. Brand new research from 2023 demonstrates that perhaps the most important thing when it comes to the benefits of movement is consistency. In other words, don't worry about the finer details, just try to move every day, or even better, several times a day! I am not a bodybuilder or an Olympian, but I do move every single day.

I do not currently take any medication for MS—or for any reason. In fact, I have not taken medication since late 2003. However, this may not be appropriate for everyone. Work with your medical team, especially your neurologist and GP (Primary Care Physician) to formulate a good plan, tailored specifically to you. And remember, this plan may change, but make sure you are part of the conversation to formulate a treatment plan for yourself, and make sure you have input into the treatment decision.

I used to work in a clinical respiratory department at a Dublin hospital, which included a sleep laboratory. My time here emphasized the importance of sleep and healthy sleep habits. Similar to other aspects of lifestyle, I think the benefits of good sleep are underappreciated and underused. Sleep is so important for us all, especially those of us with MS. I know when I don't sleep well, it affects my energy, my mood, my ability to concentrate, my food cravings, my appetite, and much more. I try to go to bed and get up at roughly the same time of day everyday— even during the weekends. I try to avoid eating late at night. I have also started to wear a night mask in bed, which helps me sleep better. In addition, when we are exposed to darkness, our bodies make the hormone melatonin. But ideally, when we say exposed to darkness, we mean not being able to see past our own nose. This is not always practical with city living, etc., so a night mask works great to help your natural melatonin production. Modern research has demonstrated that melatonin levels can be lower in those with MS and that increasing melatonin can decrease inflammation, even resulting in improved brain and physical function.

Regarding supplements, the most focused research has been on vitamin D. However, when we look at the research on vitamin D and MS, it is largely disappointing. For example, scientific reviews of original research studies published in 2022 and 2023 reported: "No significant therapeutic effect on MS, according to the disability scores and relapses during research," and "Vitamin D supplements (high or low dose) have no significant effect on relapse rate and disability during treatment in MS patients."

At the same time, vitamin D is important as some studies have reported seeing benefits in MS patients, but the overall picture is not as promising. I suggest you consider taking a sensible dose of vitamin D, for example 2,000IU (50mcg) daily with food, but do not expect vitamin D alone to work miracles. I do take vitamin D in the winter here in Ireland, but I opt for some sensible sun exposure when available during the Irish summer over supplements. In fact, there is some fascinating research suggesting that sensible sun exposure, without ever burning, has lots of other benefits besides vitamin D, including helping to regulate sleep cycles, improve mood, and provide benefits for blood vessels and blood flow.

But how do we know the sun is strong enough for us to produce vitamin D? Just look at your shadow and follow Kerley's rule: you want your shadow to be the same size or shorter than you for vitamin D production. When the sun is high in the sky, your shadow is short, and you can produce vitamin D. But when the sun is low in the sky, you will have a long shadow, and you can't produce vitamin D. Use Kerley's rule for any location in the world, any time of day, any time of year. Remember to never burn!

MS has also changed my attitude towards life. Health is so important, and I don't think most people realize this until we get sick. I certainly didn't think too much of my health as a fifteen-year-old…until I got very sick. I am not a health freak or overly strict with how I live my life, but I am healthy and have good, consistent habits. I would recommend that anyone with MS build healthy habits into their life, including movement, good sleep, stress reduction, and delicious, nutritious foods. You don't have to change everything all at once, but healthy habits really do help! As I say to my patients, stack the odds in your favor. Imagine you can place a bet with ten chips, and the bet is for a long, healthy life. There are some chips which might be healthy sleep habits, daily movement, stress reduction, daily vegetables, walnuts, flaxseeds, vitamin D supplement and/or sensible sun, stress, pizza, and excess alcohol. If you bet on all these chips, which are healthy except the pizza and excess alcohol, you have seven healthy chips versus three unhealthy chips (stress, pizza, and excess alcohol). Now, imagine that you can add in healthy or unhealthy chips to make the bet a longer, healthier life.

Personally, I don't listen to a lot of podcasts. Not because they're not good or I don't like them, it's just not a habit I have. However, there is a nice podcast from an expert neurologist in the UK that includes Dr. Agne Straukiene. The podcast is called *Bee Well with MS* by Dr. Straukiene. She is an MS expert, but she is very open-minded and speaks about all aspects of MS and potential therapies to help the disease, not just medications. In addition to Dr. Straukiene, some other prominent neurologists with multiple sclerosis expertise I followed include Dr. Aaron Boster (USA), Dr. Barry Singer (USA), Dr. Brandon Beaber (USA), and Professor Gavin Giovannoni (UK). I recommend following these experts for tips and updates.

When it comes to diet and diet books for MS, and as I mentioned above, there is conflicting research and schools of thought regarding nutrition. I am quite familiar with the Overcoming MS (OMS) program, designed by Professor George Jelinek in Australia. The OMS program includes advice on nutrition, movement, vitamin D/sun, stress reduction/mindfulness, with an option of adding medication. OMS has a great website and several books available. Their resources are very useful with recipes, meal plans, and an online community, as well as some offline communities. There is also the Wahls Protocol®, developed by Dr. Terry Wahls in Iowa, USA. The Wahls Protocol® is essentially a modified paleolithic diet with lots of meat, fish, vegetables, and fruit where dairy, eggs, grains, legumes, sugar, and some vegetables called nightshades are excluded. I recommend anyone with MS who is interested in nutrition to check out OMS and the Protocol®. I personally follow my own nutritional program based on my own reading and understanding of the research. This just so happens to be much closer to the OMS program than the Wahls Protocol®. But we shouldn't get overly bogged down. Anyone can start by simply adding more vegetables, fruits, nuts, and seeds, which everyone agrees is good for overall health.

I mentioned above that vitamin D is the most researched supplement for MS and gets the most attention, but evidence around vitamin D and MS is actually disappointing. During my own reading and research, I discovered that some natural compounds had much more powerful effects in research studies among those with MS than vitamin D. In fact, research with these plant-based compounds among those with MS demonstrated it. The effects included: less fatigue, less new MS lesions, less brain destruction, less disability, modification of the immune system, less oxidative stress and increased antioxidant activity, less inflammation, less fatigue, depression, and pain. I have formulated a unique and research-based nutrition product called "Nervous System Phix", which contains these compounds in the amounts demonstrated to be effective.

As a clinician, researcher, and patient, I try to keep up with all the new information about MS but also other conditions. This takes a lot of time! Some organizations I follow include Shift.MS and MS Lyfe, as well as MS News Today and MS Translate. There are obviously lots of different MS organizations around the world, but these are some that I find useful.

I am a fan of hip hop music. I found out a New York artist called Masta Ace was diagnosed with MS. He released a song call "Fight Song" where he says: "My spine's tinglin', my visions off and my fingers numb; he lookin' for a vicious fight, I'ma bring him one." In this sentence, he's referring to MS, so Masta Ace is saying he will fight MS. Later, he goes on to say: "You might slow me a little bit, but you won't stop me; you might stand in my pathway, but you won't block me." I love this song because of the clear defiance from Masta Ace. I try to live my life to defy MS, too!

A very brief summary of this short chapter and my attitude to MS and life: be defiant. Live healthy but enjoy life, especially exercise with friends and family. Connect with other MSers. Move it or lose it! If anyone reads my chapter in this book and would like to engage with me, ask any questions, or simply just connect, please do. I have included my contact details and social media links.

A final note: I've had MS well over half of my life. It changed my life in many ways—some bad but mostly for good. I think of how my attitude changed, all the great people I've met, and experiences I've had because of MS. MS used to be in my thoughts all day, every day; what I could and couldn't do. However, having had MS for over twenty years, I am delighted to say that MS no longer consumes me and my thoughts. I still think about MS but not every day. Just like Masta Ace, I choose to bring the fight to MS—in what I do and don't do, in how I think, and how I act. In this fight against MS, I am winning and long may it continue. I hope some of the words in this book can help even just one person in their fight, too.

28

Story by
PARMJIT (PAM) KAUR

Diagnosed in 2008
Currently 39 years old
Lives in Las Vegas, United States
Instagram: @stemcells_n_dumbbells
Facebook: Parmjit Kaur (Jersey)

Growing up in a strict, low-income, Indian household, I was consumed by duty; duty to my parents to be a model child, duty to my siblings to be their protector and set a good example, and duty to myself to get good grades and, eventually, earn a livable wage. While all that can be overwhelming for any one person, it can be that much more difficult for a child, particularly a highly sensitive one, which I absolutely was.

As if the stress of life at home wasn't enough, I was being bullied regularly at school. I loved school, but the thought of being confronted by my bullies put me in a constant state of fear and panic. I rarely, if ever, felt safe. I rarely felt secure. Rather, I often cried myself to sleep, praying for an escape from my reality.

Slowly, the escalating pressure and my constant state of fear began to take its toll on me…and on my health. You see, in those days (I grew up in the 80s and 90s), I hadn't heard anyone speak much about stress, mental health, and its sometimes-accompanying effects. I didn't know, nor understand, that the clinical depression I was eventually diagnosed with, and the regular stress, was introducing disease into my body. I first learned that lesson at only eighteen years old...

I was preparing for my first work trip to Las Vegas when I broke out with a painful, blistering rash on the right side of my chest and back. I writhed in agony as the blisters broke and stuck to my clothing. I fought a high fever, desperately wanting to see a doctor, but knowing I couldn't because I didn't have health insurance.

Eventually, the pain became so unbearable that I found myself in the Emergency Room (ER) at Trinitas Hospital in Elizabeth, New Jersey (NJ), where I was diagnosed with "Shingles". It wasn't until later in life, however, that I learned that Shingles usually presents in people who are in their fifties, or later in life. Shingles presenting before the age of forty is rare...

Rare. Rare. Rare. That word ruminated in my mind...over and over again. I couldn't quite understand how something that is said to be rare could've happened to me, an otherwise healthy, young female. But I soon learned that being an anomaly would be the running theme of my life.

One quiet evening, I sat with my brother and best friend, enjoying dinner at one of our favorite diners (NJ is well-known for having the most diners out of any state!) We sat with tears streaming down our faces from laughing entirely too hard, as we usually did, at the silliest of jokes that only made sense to us, when my friend asked, "What's wrong with your face?"

I assumed she was pointing at how red my face tends to get when I laugh too hard. It's something we've done since we were little girls—tease one another.

"HA-HA. You're so funny," I said, rolling my eyes.

"No, really!" She exclaimed. "You're talking, but only half of your mouth is moving!"

"Wait, what? You have to be joking," I responded.

I had to see this, so I walked over to a mirror and smiled. Sure enough, the right side of my face was motionless—almost frozen.

Soon after, I made another reluctant appointment to see a local doctor, who would eventually become my Primary Care Physician (PCP). I was astounded by yet another health event occurring so early in my life.

Upon entering his office, he knew almost immediately what I was dealing with. He looked at me with sympathy as he spoke my diagnosis, "Bell's Palsy". As for me, I wasn't quite sure how to react, as it had been the first time I'd heard of this condition.

My doctor put me on a treatment plan that included taking an oral medication called Prednisone, a corticosteroid. And while the medication was effective in eventually healing me and restoring muscle function to my face, it was not without side effects, most notably the effects on my joints. As I attempted to stand or move my arms, I felt as though my limbs were going to give way, and the severe pain would throw me into a sobbing frenzy. I communicated these side effects to my physician and vowed, in that moment, to never—no matter how challenging the health event—put my body through that again.

While Bell's Palsy was fortunately behind me, I needed to know more. I began looking into the age range that Bell's Palsy is typically diagnosed with, the likelihood of recurrence, and more. Once again, as was the case with Shingles, I was shocked to learn that Bell's Palsy most commonly affects those over sixty-five years.

Remember my life's theme: Anomaly.

Years passed. While I hadn't forgotten about my diagnosis (the mounting medical bills were a constant reminder of that harsh time), life forged on. I was in my early twenties and had landed a job with a mortgage company. I was thrilled, but my joy was short-lived. Around that time, I once again began experiencing unfamiliar symptoms.

My right hand and arm often became numb, and I regularly felt as though I was being poked with pins and needles. Perhaps, I should have been concerned, but I chalked it up to the way I usually slept, with my right arm beneath me. Soon after, I also began having trouble running up the stairs, but it wasn't until I had trouble opening the door to my office one day that I knew something was very wrong.

I remember naively wondering if Bell's Palsy had returned, not realizing that Bell's Palsy only affects the face. Once again, I made an appointment to see my PCP, who then recommended that I get a computed tomography (CT) scan.

I think I lived in a dream world at that time. I thought I was invincible. It was this innocence that led me to believe that the CT scan would be fruitless and that the results would show that my unusual symptoms were nothing more than a fluke. I truly believed this…that is until I walked into work one day, and my then-manager, who happened to be a friend of my PCP's, told me news that I would never forget.

"Pam, you need to call your doctor back. He got your CT scan results, and he thinks you might have a brain tumor."

Today, I know what a big HIPAA violation it was for my doctor to share my personal health information with someone other than me without my consent, but at that time, I could barely think. I was in shock. I was devastated. I called my doctor's office back and was told by one of his nurses that I needed to be seen ASAP. I made an appointment for the very same day. I called my fiancé at the time, choking back tears. I couldn't breathe and felt my chest tighten as I thought about the news I'd just received that I would soon share with him.

"Jaan (Punjabi translation for 'life'), what happened? Are you okay?" he asked, full of concern.

"The test results came back," I finally said, amid sobs that I could no longer control. He knew I'd had a CT scan prior. "Babe, the doctor thinks I might have a brain tumor. I don't want to die. Please, I don't want to die."

And with that, we both cried. He'd previously lost a friend to a brain tumor, and my news brought back memories that he'd never thought he'd have to relive. Next, I called my best friend, Melody, and still sobbing, shared the news with her, too. She cried.

"Don't you worry, Pam. You are going to be okay!" She comforted me. "I am going to go to the doctor with you." And she did.

She sat next to me and held my hand as the doctor pushed an image of a brain towards me, circling an area in which the CT scan had uncovered an unusual mass. "We will need to pursue further testing, Ms. Kaur, and I'm referring you to see a neurologist at the local hospital for follow-up."

He was extremely sympathetic as he said the next few words, but they hit me like a ton of bricks. "Unfortunately, I suspect that you may have a brain tumor."

I'd now heard that diagnosis for the second time in one day. I think I may have blacked out momentarily because my ears started ringing, and I don't remember what else he may have said.

I called the hospital to make an appointment with a neurologist; however, the earliest appointment available was a month out. I couldn't believe it. Here I was on the brink of death, or at least that's what I thought, and I was told it would be a month before someone would see me. So, I impatiently waited, each minute feeling like an eternity.

When it was finally time for my visit, a neurologist examined me, listening to my health history and making notes before ordering magnetic resonance imaging (MRI) of the brain. I felt claustrophobic and afraid as I laid in the noisy MRI machine. I no longer lived in a fantasy world. I no longer felt invincible. From that moment on, each test would bring with it an onslaught of panic and impending dread.

A couple of weeks had passed before my next appointment with the neurologist to review the results of the MRI. I showed up to my appointment, and he examined me, once again, asking a slew of questions. I sat on his examination table, the fresh paper beneath me, crunching every time I moved.

"Ms. Kaur," he said, "I have good news. The MRI results don't indicate you have a brain tumor."

I could hardly contain my joy and let out a long sigh of relief. Again, my excitement would be momentary.

"Rather," he said, "I believe you've had two silent strokes. We'll need to order more tests to rule out other possibilities." And with that, he ordered a series of tests, including an MRI of the spine, an electrocardiogram (EKG), and bloodwork. I was bewildered. It was 2008. I was twenty-four. How could this have happened?

More weeks passed, and it was time to visit him again to receive the results of the new tests. This time, another close friend, Kara, came to the neurologist with me. I felt more confident having her there because one, she'd always known how to make me laugh, and two, she'd worked in the medical field. I sat in front of the neurologist, with Kara to the right of me.

"Ms. Kaur," the neurologist said, looking me in the eyes, "We will have to do one final test to say with 100% certainty, but we are confident in our conclusion that you have multiple sclerosis (MS)."

I didn't have much of a reaction. I didn't know what MS was. But I glanced over at Kara and noticed her mouth was agape.

"Okay. What's that, and how do I get rid of it? My twenty-fifth birthday is coming up, Doc, and I don't want to be sick on my milestone birthday," I said, smiling. I'd thought MS was probably like a cold or maybe the flu—that I could just take medication for a few days, and it'd be gone. Oh, how innocent I was.

"Unfortunately, there is no cure for MS," he explained. It is a chronic autoimmune disease, and it will be important to manage it through disease-modifying therapy via injections."

"Oh. I'd prefer not to do injections," I said, not understanding that it was the only option available at that time.

He smiled at me; his face filled with compassion. "Currently, disease-modifying therapies are only available via injection or infusion."

I went home that day and began learning everything and anything I could about the disease, much of it alarming. I'd also learned that at that time, the highest incidences of MS were in Scotland, and that just so happened to be where I was born. A terrifying coincidence, perhaps.

The neurologist referred me to a different doctor in the same hospital, but one who specialized in treating patients with MS. This second neurologist ordered one last test, commonly called a lumbar puncture, or a spinal tap, to rule out a diagnosis of Lyme disease, which has symptoms similar to MS. During this procedure, a long needle was inserted between my vertebrae to remove a sample of my cerebrospinal fluid. It was pretty harmless, but the doctor instructed me to drink coffee if I found myself with a headache anyway. While that initial day went by like a breeze, the next day was like something out of a fiction novel. I woke up with an excruciating migraine that would only slightly lessen if I laid down. If I made the mistake of sitting or standing up, I would vomit profusely. It felt as though my brain was slamming against my skull.

I called the hospital, hoping for a solution, but instead was told, in so many words, to wait it out—that the pain would decrease over time, and

I had to be patient; that this was normal. It did not decrease. It was not normal. This went on for a couple of days, days that I spent curled up on a sofa, crying, feeling like I'd made the worst mistake of my life by agreeing to the spinal tap.

Melody and Kara would come over to try and cheer me up, but their sincere efforts were unfortunately futile. I couldn't bring myself to smile. I couldn't bring myself to laugh. I couldn't even bring myself to speak with my friends. They quickly saw the pain expressed on my face and described me as having become a shell of myself. I was becoming desperate, so I had my brother, the middle child, drive me to the ER. It was full, and I sat in the waiting room in tears, begging someone to see me.

Finally, after much pleading, I was seen by an ER doctor who inspected the site where the spinal fluid was removed and conducted another series of tests.

"I can't believe you were told to wait the headache out," he said, shaking his head after reading the test results. "You have a cerebrospinal fluid leak. This is very serious."

He immediately ordered an Epidural Blood Patch, a treatment that involved taking a sample of my blood and then injecting it into the spinal canal where the fluid was leaking. Although relief wasn't immediate, after the treatment and a short hospital stay, the horrific pain in my head went away. I then revisited the neurologist who'd ordered the test to hear the results.

"Ms. Kaur, your test results have confirmed that you have multiple sclerosis," she told me. "And we suspect you've had it for quite some time."

While I thought I'd be stunned, I was more so relieved—relieved to finally have an accurate diagnosis and relieved to have an answer to the mystery symptoms I'd been experiencing for years. While I wasn't thrilled about my diagnosis, I'd come to terms with the fact that I, Parmjit Kaur, at twenty-four years old, had MS, and my life was forever changed.

The first MS medication I started was Rebif, an injectable taken three times a week. From the first moment I injected myself, I felt happy and proud for having done it by myself. However, that feeling quickly dissipated as I began to experience the side effects of the medication, side effects that I hadn't been warned about, nor prepared for. Side effects that included flu-like symptoms, hair loss, and perhaps the worst of them all—suicidal thoughts.

In addition to the horrid side effects, my balance, along with the strength in my right hand, was getting worse. I was beginning to fall and drop things more often. My once beautiful handwriting began looking like that of a toddler's, and climbing stairs was becoming impossible unless there was a railing available to grab hold of.

I began missing work and cancelling plans. Every day I mentally devised a plan as to how I'd end my life; my quality of life was rapidly waning. I wanted to live…but not like this. Never like this.

One night, I grabbed the same bottle of aspirin that had provided me momentary relief from my fever-like Rebif symptoms all those days that I'd injected myself, and drove to an abandoned parking lot. I sat, contemplating life and death. Sadly, the choice for me was obvious; and with that, I began swallowing pills by the handful. I laid my head back… and then, the phone rang.

I answered, crying. It was the youngest of the family, my fourteen-year-old baby brother. He'd known I was upset when I'd left the house and wanted to know where I was.

"I'm somewhere. And I'm probably not coming home," I said, trying to remain elusive.

"What did you do? Did you take those pills?" He asked. It turned out he'd seen me grab them. All I could muster amid tears was, "I'm sorry."

"NO!" He said. "Pam, drive yourself to the hospital RIGHT NOW!"

I heard the anguish in his voice. Suddenly, the reality of what I was doing hit me…I was abandoning my brother, the brother I'd raised like a son.

Perhaps, my answering the phone was a cry for help. Perhaps, I didn't really want to give up. Whatever the case, that evening I drove myself to the ER where I was admitted and made to drink liquid charcoal to remove the self-induced poison.

Following my suicide attempt, I decided I needed to try a new medication. This time, my neurologist suggested Copaxone. After almost a year on it, my doctor ordered an MRI to see how effective the medication had been in slowing down the progression of the MS. Sadly, it had been ineffective, and the disease was still progressing, evidenced by frequent relapses. That news, coupled with several injection-site reactions, including the hollowing of my skin, was a clear indicator that we needed to go back to the drawing board. Except this time, I didn't agree with my neurologist's new direction: Tysabri, an intravenous infusion.

You see, Tysabri increases the risk of Progressive Multifocal Leukoencephalopathy (PML), a viral infection of the brain that usually leads to death or severe disability. That risk further increases if a patient has been infected by the common John Cunningham Virus (JCV), which a recent blood test had confirmed I'd tested positive for. My neurologist knew this, yet he was adamant that this was the best choice for me, and with that, my trust in my doctor began to wane. With limited options and feeling reluctant to experience the severe side effects that came with most MS medications, I decided to pursue a different route, one that didn't include medication.

I began looking into diets that would aid in healing, including the Wahls Protocol®, a modified paleolithic diet that focuses on eliminating grains, eggs, dairy products, etc., and a heavy emphasis on vegetables, fruits, meats, and fish. I also began working out more, particularly weightlifting, working hard to strengthen my legs. I was often heard saying that MS tried to take my legs, so I was building them up to take them back.

This approach worked well for me for a few years, but MS was relentless; unfortunately, the relapses continued. With each relapse, I lost a bit more function. I went from wearing four-inch heels to no heels at all, from wearing wedges to flats, from riding a bike and running to being unable to do either, and from walking up or down flights of stairs unaided to being forced to hold a railing when available. I was also falling more often, usually in public. Along with countless bruises, I was becoming a frequent flyer at the hospital. I even broke my ankle at my ten-year high school reunion. What was supposed to be a wonderful evening spent with friends turned into a night in the Emergency Room, surrounded by healthcare professionals.

I was shattered. With each month that passed, I found myself losing abilities that I once took for granted.

Then, a friend messaged me, telling me about Hematopoietic Stem Cell Transplantation (HSCT) for MS, a chemotherapy-based treatment for MS that aims to "reset" the immune system by eradicating the T and B cells in your body that have essentially gone rogue, and then using your own stem cells to regrow it. T and B cells are types of lymphocytes (white blood cells involved in the immune response). However, I'd read about snake oil salesmen, touting different methods that claimed to effectively treat MS, and I was wary of yet another treatment that would supposedly heal me. While I should've paid heed to my friend's recommendation, I put it out of my mind.

That is, until another patient I'd met through Facebook's MS community and become close to, messaged me upon reading of my many struggles with the disease. She urged me to consider HSCT, sharing that she'd had the successful treatment herself. She had been part of Dr. Allan Burk's clinical trial at Chicago's Northwestern University Memorial Hospital. Dr. Burke is one of the leading doctors in developing the HSCT approach for MS and other autoimmune diseases.

However, I was afraid. Although HSCT is over 80% effective in stopping the progression of MS for patients that have Remitting-Relapsing MS (RRMS), which is the version of MS that I had, I didn't want to put my body through chemotherapy. I also very wrongly equated femininity with long hair and the ability to bear children, both things that would be at risk if I went through chemo. So, I put-off having HSCT for two years. By then, not only had the clinical trial ended, but my prognosis was that I would soon have to use a wheelchair. While I still could've pursued HSCT at Northwestern, HSCT wasn't an FDA-approved treatment for MS. Only a handful of insurance providers covered it. Another option was paying for the treatment myself, but at an overwhelming cost of $100,000+, there was no way I could've afforded it. But with the MS rapidly progressing and not wanting to be trouble to my already burdened family, I knew HSCT was quite possibly the last chance at maintaining my independence.

My decision was made. I was going to figure out a way to get HSCT, and I was going to share this news with my neurologist, who I half expected to be supportive. Oh, how wrong I was.

I shared the news with him, and without so much as batting an eye, he told me I was taking a big risk, and I would probably die from the "experimental treatment". The distrust I began feeling toward my doctor only increased because I realized that he was trying to instill fear in me. Despite what he'd said, HSCT was not experimental; rather, it had been performed on cancer patients since the 1950s. While there is absolutely risk with all treatments, HSCT was less risky than the alternative MS drugs. But I didn't share all that with him. It wasn't my job to educate my physician about the best course of treatment. Instead, I asked him a question that he couldn't answer: "If you had multiple sclerosis, or any illness, wouldn't you also explore all credible treatment options?"

I began searching for additional locations that offered HSCT for MS and came across a forum for HSCT in Puebla, Mexico at a place called Clinica Ruiz. To my pleasant surprise, Clinica Ruiz was run by Dr. Guillermo J. Ruiz-Arguellas, an internist, hematologist, and one of the top twenty-five alumni out of Mayo Clinic. I read several positive reviews from patients from all over the world who'd been treated at Clinica Ruiz. That information, coupled with the treatment in Mexico being a fraction of what it would be in the U.S. ($54,500 to be exact), helped me decide that Clinica Ruiz was where I wanted to be treated. So, I rushed to apply. The application process was pretty straight forward. Within two weeks, I was approved. I was elated!

With my application approved, I needed to raise money for the treatment. While the cost of HSCT was significantly lower in Mexico, I still didn't have that kind of money sitting around but that, too, proved to be a monumental hurdle. I started a GoFundMe page, but unfortunately, I only raised about $7,000 of the $54,500 that I still needed, and my treatment date was quickly approaching. With my fingers crossed, I applied for a personal loan and anxiously waited to hear back.

I will never forget the day I received my loan application results; they temporarily crushed my spirit. I read the results and felt like I needed a drink of water to wash away the knot in my throat. I walked into my kitchen where my father and stepmother had been sitting around chatting. They knew I'd applied for a loan and were just as eager as I was to hear the news.

"Did you hear back about the loan?" My stepmother asked me. I took a big gulp.
"I did…My loan was denied," I said, fighting back tears.

At that moment, my youngest brother walked into the kitchen, reading my solemn face. "What's wrong?" He asked. I've always had trouble hiding my emotions from him.

"My loan application was denied," I said…and with that, I began to sob. My brother hugged me, and he, too, cried along with me. He knew that without HSCT, there was a good possibility that I'd continue to get worse. My father, seeing how distraught my brother and I were, made a grand gesture that would forever help to change my life. He offered to take out a loan against his existing life-insurance policy, so I could pay for my upcoming treatment. I can't put into words just how happy I was. And with that, I moved forward. In November 2016, I, along with twenty-five other patients, underwent a successful stem cell transplant in Puebla.

Even though HSCT was only meant to stop the progression of MS, almost immediately I noticed other improvements, starting with my balance. I no longer needed a railing to climb stairs. As the years passed, some of my lost abilities began returning. With this newfound strength, I also wanted to inspire other patients to continue pursuing their dreams, despite their disability. So, I set a new goal, and in 2018, I participated and placed in my very first bodybuilding competition.

Today, in 2023, I consider MS, for the most part, to be a distant memory. I'm running again, I can ride a bike again, I can wear heels again, and so much more! HSCT was a Godsend, and it truly gave me both a second chance and a new life, which I will never take for granted.

I've been asked if I am afraid about MS returning in the future. Truth be told, that's not something I've given much thought to as I've been very confident in HSCT's long-term effects. However, I recognize that to avoid introducing disease back into my body, I need to be in an environment conducive to healing. So, after getting HSCT, I moved out of my parents' home and away from the stress that came along with it.

These days I'm definitely much more cognizant of what I'm putting in my body. That is not to say that I always eat "healthily", but I do more often than not. I eat a balanced diet, paying attention to the ratio of carbs, protein, and fats in each meal. I've also taken advantage of supplementation and try to consume organic food whenever possible. My mindset and belief that HSCT treatment would work for me definitely contributed to its success! I'm a big believer in the power of the mind, of speaking things into existence, and of a positive mental attitude.

29

Story by

KADESHA ROSS

Diagnosed in 2012
Currently 24 years old
Lives in Winnipeg Manitoba, Canada
Instagram: @kadesha_ross

Most nine-year-olds start getting into sports and social life at school. I, however, was entering a world of blindness and paralysis. Oh, and don't forget the tingling sensation throughout my extremities. Although it was so long ago, I'll never forget my first multiple sclerosis (MS) episode. It was 2009, and I'd started experiencing vision problems in my left eye. I instantly thought it was from a laser tag incident. Why else would a healthy and active young girl's eye start to lose vision?

Allow me to rewind a bit. My name is Kadesha Ross, and I was born as a healthy baby on March 5, 1999, in Canada, Winnipeg Manitoba with zero pregnancy or birth complications. My father is from Jamaica, and my mother is from Canada. There is no known history of multiple sclerosis within my family. I was a happy, healthy child who loved gymnastics and anything artistic. I was quite the social butterfly with tons of energy, until one summer evening.

Everything that I once was began changing. My energy levels started diminishing, my athletic and social life became harder to maintain, and my artistic creativity took so much effort. I was no longer the Kadesha everybody knew. The change started after a friend's birthday party where we played laser tag. At one point in the game, one of the lasers from a friend's gun caught my eye. I felt fine, but it wasn't too long after that I noticed the vision in my left eye was weakening. I didn't think much of it. Assuming the vision problem came from the laser, I kept it to myself. The next day, it progressed so badly to the point where I had zero vision in my left eye. That really freaked me out. At first, I was hesitant to tell anyone because I was so scared of what would happen next. I truly didn't know how to share this news. Also, who would ever believe me when I told them I couldn't see out of my left eye? After a day or two, focusing during school became difficult. My right eye started hurting, as well, along with my head. With zero sign of improvement, I knew it wasn't going to get better on its own. I had to let my family know.

Initially, my brother thought I was pretending, and my mom thought I just wanted a pair of glasses since a lot of my classmates and friends had them. This made me refrain from expressing how bad it truly bothered me. After two more nights of zero complaints to my family, I felt the need to express that I still couldn't see out of my left eye. My mom finally took me to see an optometrist, where they said everything looked fine, throwing a pair of glasses on my face. Obviously, I still couldn't see. However, at the age of nine, I wasn't sure how to express this to my family, let alone, an optometrist. Time passed by, and my vision slowly started returning. Honestly, everyone, including me, sort of forgot about it.

For roughly a year and a half, everything seemed fine. I was healthy and thriving in my sports and hobbies again. Until one day in fourth grade, I started feeling a tingly sensation on my left side. It was predominantly in my left hand. I knew something was off when someone accidentally shut my locker door on my hand, and I didn't feel a thing. I still went about my day until last recess, the tingling and numbness started traveling all over my body. I knew I had to let someone know because it did not feel comfortable or normal whatsoever. I called home for my mom to come pick me up from school, and I'll never forget the look she had when she walked through the front door. She could see in my droopy face that something wasn't right. She calmly packed me in the car and headed straight to the children's emergency room. They ran a bunch of tests, beginning with bloodwork and computed tomography (CT) scans, becoming progressively more intrusive with the magnetic resonance imaging (MRIs), spinal tap, and so many others. After all these tests and hours of waiting, the doctors admitted me into the hospital, trying to find additional answers. At this time, they hadn't mentioned MS. They wanted to test for a variety of disorders of the central nervous system first.

A day or two went by, and we received news from the doctors that I may have had a stroke. A child having a stroke was unheard of and highly uncommon, so they wanted to do a few more tests. After a few days of prednisone, the doctors came back and announced that they thought I had something called acute disseminated encephalomyelitis (ADEM). This was a best-case scenario, as ADEM could be treated. With some treatments such as prednisone and tons of physiotherapy, I started to feel a bit better and was so happy to see positive results. I was finally able to brush my own teeth, feed myself, and walk, along with more daily mundane things. However, I knew I still didn't feel like myself. I was sent home after almost a month in the hospital with a misdiagnosis (one that I was unaware of until later). I slowly started regaining feeling and control back on my left side, but I knew I had many limitations that were not there before.

For my whole life, gymnastics had been a huge part of my identity. But around this time, gymnastics class seemed to be very hard. Even beyond physical and motor skills, I felt drained, mentally and cognitively. I had to put a lot of effort forward just to keep a conversation going. I'm not going to lie, even walking was something I would have to focus on deeply for it to work. My hand-eye coordination was terrible. The tingling sensation progressed, with pins and needles lingering on and off.

The cherry on top was a bad case of H1N1. Yep, I was one of the unlucky patients to be affected by the influenza A virus during the flu season in 2009, making me even more sick. Around this time in my life, I also started experiencing blood difficulties. My platelet counts would drop to an alarming level. It appeared that every other week I would be covered in bruises, along with something called petechiae. I was also suffering from internal bleeding. I remember one day, the internal bleeding in my stomach and digestive track was so bad that it produced tons of blood in my vomit, raising alarm in myself and others. Once again, I was sent to the children's emergency room where they treated me with transfusions and more prednisone.

Almost a year goes by of me trying to get my life back. After several tests and treatments at the Hematology Laboratory located at CancerCare Manitoba, I was diagnosed with an autoimmune disorder called immune thrombocytopenia (ITP). ITP is a blood platelet disorder that causes abnormal bleeding and bruising due to low platelet count levels. Platelets are small blood cells that stick together where blood vessels are damaged. When you don't have enough platelets, blood cannot properly clot to stop bleeding. ITP is an autoimmune disease caused by dysfunction in the immune system which attacks blood platelets with antibodies. If that wasn't enough for my now twelve-year-old self, I also had an MRI appointment with the neurologist. The results showed that I indeed have multiple sclerosis. Finally, I was properly diagnosed with Relapsing-Remitting Multiple Sclerosis (RRMS) in early March of 2012.

At the age of twelve, I didn't know what that meant, but I could see tears filling up my grandma and mother's eyes. That couldn't mean anything good. I just remember feeling so scared that my life was over before it had even begun. I was a 12-year-old kid, trying to figure out what two autoimmune disorders looked like. For me, it meant daily injections, lots of hospital visits, and extreme fatigue, as well as brain fog almost constantly. It also meant missing out on activities with friends and having many limitations. Pins and needles would sometimes be a pest but eventually felt like the norm. I felt trapped, stuck, and hopeless.

After a year or so of living with multiple sclerosis and feeling alone, I'd heard of something called a multiple sclerosis camp. A place where kids and teens like me, who were all diagnosed with MS, could get together for one week at a camp named Easter Seals, located in Ontario. MS camp was a place where the outcasts didn't feel like outcasts anymore. The daily problems we all suffered from (feeling fatigued, brain fog, or tingling) weren't a surprise to the people surrounding you, making us feel not so alone. I could talk to my peers about MS problems that my friends back home wouldn't understand. The average ages in the camp were twelve to twenty years old, as well as some peer support workers who were twenty-one years old and up. There was no disparity between boys and girls. Each day was filled with new information and insight regarding MS, giving me more of an understanding that MS looks very different for each person. When I watched videos about MS, it was always older people who were very immobile. Also, going to my appointments made me feel like the youngest person in the world to be diagnosed. At my appointment, I would have to fill out a questionnaire. However, the questions were for people much older than twelve. For instance, when it asked about how my MS was affecting my driving or work life, I never really knew how to answer. But at MS camp, I quickly learned that people of all ages were diagnosed. This is where I finally felt understood and didn't feel so alone. Multiple sclerosis camp is where I found my hope again.

The camp offered many activities, such as kayaking, arts and crafts, yoga, and much more. I found a passion for yoga. My MS symptoms were undetectable after each session, leaving me feeling tremendously relaxed. That wasn't the only spark that ignited through MS camp. I also felt a drive within me to share my MS story through a positive lens, inspiring hope in others who were diagnosed with multiple sclerosis. Although camp was filled with so many positive aspects, when it was time for the injections, I got very overwhelmed and just wanted my mom to be there to calm me down. I had never been this far away from my family, especially for this long. When my home sickness kicked in, I remember phoning home and crying for my mom to send an airplane to rescue me. Obviously, this couldn't happen. She encouraged me to try and enjoy the rest of what camp had to offer.

My MS peers consoled me, letting me express how much I disliked my injections. They told me that there were other medication options out there, ones that had never been mentioned to me by my neurologist. I was currently on Copaxone. These daily injections made me develop a phobia of needles. It was a daily battle for me and my mother during injection time. The needle itself hurt, but the aftermath left me with a burning sensation at the injection site. I could not live with the constant anxiety and fear surrounding my daily Copaxone dose, so I mentioned to my doctor another treatment named Tysabri that was shared with me by my peers from MS camp. This treatment could be given intravenously which put my mind at ease. However, I did not qualify due to the risk of getting progressive multifocal leukoencephalopathy (PML), a rare viral infection of the brain. After many complaints to my doctor, she allowed me to switch to weekly Avonex injections that I took for roughly six months. By then, my injection phobia and anxiety had returned. I also developed mild depression as a side effect. Luckily (and unluckily), I had two autoimmune disorders, which meant there were more options for medication. Why not kill two birds with one stone?

I started a medication called Rituximab (Rituxan and MabThera). It works by turning off a part of the immune system that doesn't work properly in autoimmune diseases. Although it wasn't guaranteed to help MS, my neurologist agreed it was worth a shot. If I remember correctly, I was taking Rituximab once a week for about five months. Then, I stopped responding to the treatment. I had to go in for a splenectomy in hopes it would help my blood disorder. After my splenectomy, I was placed on prednisone for about two years, which my neurologist had reason to believe would also help treat my MS. After the prednisone, I tried the Rituximab, once again, and it worked. So, I decided to stick with it. At this point, I was sick and tired of treatments.

In the midst of despair, I decided to attend MS camp once more as it was the final year that the program would be run through the Easter Seals camp. This time around, I was seventeen and able to enjoy the experience on a whole new level, allowing me to really connect with those around me and learn more about my disease. Although we shared the same autoimmune disorder, everyone around me was so individually unique, as well as their multiple sclerosis stories and experiences. One individual stood out to me the most. Jessica was diagnosed in April of 2007. Jessica was a bit older than me and seemed to be thriving. This gave me hope when it came to chasing my dreams and experimenting with different ways of life to help MS.

Jessica was very athletic. She experienced MS episodes that would limit her; however, she would always find a way to embrace her athletic abilities. I remember one day she invited me for a morning jog. Due to my ignorance, I thought it would just be a slow and short adventure. My whole life I was taught that individuals with multiple sclerosis are always limited when it comes to athleticism and energy. Jessica proved me wrong. Halfway through, I had to turn around. Walking alone on my way back, I realized that even with MS, you can almost always find a way if you stick to what works for you and listen to your body. At the time, Jessica was on a medication called Lemtrada and was living a vegan/ plant-based lifestyle. A yearning for a more natural lifestyle was ignited within me. Using what the earth has to offer by experimenting with different diets and activities that cater to you individually as a source to stay healthy can truly make a huge difference in your life.

When I returned home from camp, my old mindset on medication and life changed as a whole. I dove into research to see if I could live a healthy life with multiple sclerosis without medication. I continued to explore my love for yoga and started taking classes. I also practiced at home whenever I could. Apart from yoga, I love to walk. I found that these two activities alone made a difference in my mood and energy levels. Even if some days I had to turn it down a notch due to my MS, I always came out of it feeling better than before I started. Finding some sort of physical activity, in my perspective, is truly beneficial in sustaining physical health with or without MS. Apart from physical activity, I knew my diet had to change. I still ate desserts or indulged in the occasional burger and fries. But I tried to be mindful and pick whole foods and plant-based products whenever possible. I spoke with individuals already living this lifestyle and gained insight from them. I like to mix and match when it comes to my diet. I enjoy finding creative dishes on the app TikTok.

Being aware of what I'm putting into my body and reading up on certain diets for inflammation has helped me a lot. After getting my physical health and diet in check, I still felt like I was missing something. One of the biggest aids in my multiple sclerosis journey overall has been mindfulness practices and discovering spirituality.

Simply practicing mindfulness is amazing and beneficial for anyone, but it especially helped me with the everyday stresses of living with an autoimmune disorder. My whole view on life began shifting when I really started getting into spiritual practices. These practices consisted of meditation, manifestation, yoga, and working with the energy pools in my body. During my meditations, I would picture the lesions located on my spinal cord and brain being healed by a bright gold light. I was twenty years old when I started this specific practice. For manifesting, I would envision health and healing. During yoga, I could feel the healing taking place in my body. As for working with the energies in my body, I followed a guide to healing the seven chakras.

Emoha from *Emoha.com* says, "The seven chakras of the body are understood to be spinning discs of energy that should be open, aligned, and balanced for they have the vital task of absorbing our vital energy (prana) and redistributing it. For a balanced individual, these seven chakras deliver an adequate amount of energy to the mind, body, and soul."

Through my spiritual practices, I became grateful for the life I have. I no longer asked, "why me?" When I looked back at all my medical issues, I viewed them as lessons that have taught me to be a grateful, empathetic, compassionate, caring, strong, and wise human being. I finally accepted all the things that happened to me and looked at them with a different set of eyes.

I was able to help others just like me shift their perspectives to be more positive towards multiple sclerosis through the MS Society Peer Support Program. During this time, I also went to school to receive my Community Support Worker diploma and became a yoga instructor. Everything MS-wise seemed okay. I finally felt like I had control of my own life. I wasn't only living, I was thriving. I was doing things that many people warned me my complications would make impossible. I even had a baby in 2022! Many people told me my MS would get worse after giving birth, but it didn't. Apart from morning sickness the first trimester and hormonal changes, I experienced no symptoms at all during pregnancy.

Before having a child and falling pregnant, my daily routine typically started with me getting up early and going for a sunrise walk or jog. If I didn't have the energy for that, I would do a bit of yoga, followed by some meditating and journaling, or maybe read a book with some tea or coffee. Once I finished working for the day, I would return home for quality time with my family, then rest as I did tarot cards, energy cleansing, or painting. Now that I have a baby, the daily routine simply consists of taking care of the baby. Other than that, I like to make sure I have time throughout the week to do yoga or some sort of physical activity. The baby and I go on lots of walks together. The advice I would give to someone with MS wanting to start a family would be the exact same advice I would give to someone without MS. Yes, there may be limitations, but every family has some form of limitation. Creating something beautiful takes a village. Be sure to have a good support system, and if not, find resources that provide them.

I'm not quite sure if it's symptoms of being a new mom or MS, but sometimes I do get fatigued throughout the day. It's nothing a quick nap or coffee won't fix. Every so often, I tend to get vision abnormalities in my left eye, followed by a severe migraine. Tylenol, a dark room, and plenty of rest help when this happens. It's rare that these episodes occur. I see my neurologist and receive an MRI once a year. If there are any concerns, I can call my neurologist to make an appointment, but there hasn't been any need for that. I'm currently off all medications. The last medication used to specifically treat my MS was Avonex. Now, I take only vitamin D supplements.

I'm living proof that through a healthy lifestyle, you can treat your multiple sclerosis. However, that's only my perspective. In some cases, medication is needed. But I also believe that along with medication, a healthy lifestyle will make a huge difference.
The amount of physical activity or movement you do helps you to stay mobile and pain-free. Being mindful of what you put into your body helps a lot with energy and mood. It also helps with inflammation and cognitive levels. Lastly, and the most important for me, are my mindfulness/spirituality practices. Having my mood, attitude, and stress levels in check have helped me breathe and worry less about things out of my control.

If you focus on the negatives, your life will manifest what you constantly think about. So, why not focus on the positives? Train your mind to think positively about life, your experiences, and your future. I hope my story can inspire others or be relatable to those that read it. The divine light in me honors the divine light in you. Namaste.

Emoha, The 7 Chakras Demystified - Align Mind, Body & Spirit, Emoha.com, 2022, https://emoha.com/blogs/busy/7-chakras-meaning-in-human-body

30

Story by
MELODY WINSBORROW

Diagnosed in 2013
Currently 24 years old
Lives in United States
Instagram: @autoimmune.wellnesswarriors
www.autoimmunewellnesswarriors.com

My story isn't like most...Ten years ago, I was diagnosed with multiple sclerosis (MS) at fifteen years old. When I was in high school, I was an athlete and loved playing softball. One day, after a rough three-hour practice (these long practices were typical for me), I tried to pick up my fork to eat some of my favorite pancakes. Suddenly, I felt a jolt shoot through my body; I dropped my fork as my opposite leg started shaking. I didn't know what was going on—I was so stunned that tears came to my eyes (which was very unlike me).

I felt like I was going crazy before my diagnosis! My norm consisted of vision loss, muscle weakness, spurts of trouble with walking, vertigo, pins and needles, MS hugs, migraines, brain fog, fatigue, knives in my back, and so on. On top of everything, I was exhausted all the time.

I ended up in the hospital once due to severe chest pain and a feeling of breathlessness. My doctors attributed these symptoms to possible anxiety, and they also linked my daily joint pains to sports injuries, suggesting that physical therapy would solve the issue. They concluded that my symptoms were normal growing pains and sports injuries that needed some physical therapy, just like any other teenage athlete. This whole experience felt insane to me because I knew I was happy, and I knew it wasn't just a simple sports injury. Also, the "growing pains" were out of the question since I hadn't grown an inch since the fifth grade.

I am so grateful that my mom kept PUSHING the physicians to find more answers for me. After two years of doctors' visits, my neurologist diagnosed me with multiple sclerosis. It felt amazing to finally have an answer! The relief quickly ended when he told us that if I didn't go straight on medication, then I would end up in a wheelchair! I was devastated. The life I was planning—all my dreams—went out the window then and there. When he presented my options, I knew that there was no way needles or pills would be my answer. My mom and I felt something deep inside of us telling us to continue looking for alternative answers. I said no to the medication, and it was the best decision I made.

My mom, my angel, dove into research for me. She found Dr. Wahls—my biggest inspiration. Even though she had "limitations" to her diet, she was alive and truly healthy, which seemed like a blessing. The Wahls Protocol® answered so many questions and, at the same time, saved and changed my life. After complete focus, determination, and patience, I was able to feel like me again!

When I went off to college three years after my diagnosis, I thought I could be more lenient with my diet. Since I felt so many symptoms completely disappear for so long, there was a part of me that thought I was healing from my MS and that it would be just fine if I had a little sugar and dairy here and there. It was hard seeing all my friends living their lives fearlessly and not joining in with them.

A couple years after starting those "small cheats", I had to remind myself that even though I felt better, I wasn't "healed" from the disease. All those traces of food from cheating (sugar, dairy, etc.) hit me so much harder when a big stressor came into my life; it felt like a ton of bricks. I went partially blind, I couldn't walk far, brain fog returned, and I lost use of my hands for months. Throughout the entire process, one thing remained clear: I had healed myself through dieting before, and I knew I could do it again! Positivity with my MS didn't come easy. I learned one lesson though: no matter how far I have fallen, I can always come back.

Since regaining my health through nutrition and lifestyle habits, I knew it was my mission to guide and teach other warriors to do the same. In 2019, I became a holistic practitioner. I then became a Nutritional Therapist and a Wahls Practitioner, and then, in 2020, I began working with clients. I wanted to let them know, "I'm here with you. I stand with you because I was you. Here is a way to gain hope and get power back!" In a lot of ways, I am grateful for my diagnosis! Without it, I would have never found my purpose—helping autoimmune warriors take their lives back.

Being diagnosed with MS at the young age of fifteen made giving up my favorite comfort foods difficult, like ice cream and pizza; but once I understood "why", it became so much easier. And once I started feeling better, I knew this was what I had to do. I wasn't blindly heading into this; there is science behind it.

When I began my wellness journey, I wanted to eliminate all the common autoimmune trigger foods to get rid of excessive inflammation in my body. I first removed gluten, dairy, and eggs. The first two, gluten and dairy elimination, are absolutely critical. Gluten and dairy have similar molecular structures, and they turn into morphine-like compounds in the brain, stimulating opioid receptors. So, if these foods are extremely hard for you to eliminate, it's because your body is addicted to them.

Let's look at gluten first. Gluten is everywhere in our modern society. Modern-day gluten is NOT made of the same ingredients that our grandparents ate. Our bodies are unfamiliar with this new form of gluten that can dissolve into our meals, shampoo, and even toothpaste. Our bodies do not know what to do with this new "gluten" strain.

Gluten has three main detrimental effects that cause chaos in the body. Firstly, it is the primary culprit of leaky gut, as it weakens the gut barrier. I love the following analogy by Dr. Myers: "Think of your gut lining as a drawbridge. Teeny tiny boats (micronutrients in food) that are meant to travel back and forth are able to go under the bridge without a problem. However, when gluten releases zonulin, it causes the drawbridge to go up and allow bigger boats (large proteins) to cross over that aren't meant to travel through. In the case of your gut, its microbes, toxins, proteins, and partially digested food particles passing under the drawbridge and escaping into your bloodstream." When you eat a piece of gluten, it travels to your stomach, eventually arriving at your small intestine. This triggers the release of zonulin. Zonulin is a chemical that signals the intestinal wall to open, creating a "leaky gut". A leaky gut allows proteins, foods, and toxins throughout the body that contribute to our inflammation.

Secondly, when the body detects a foreign invader, its natural response is inflammation. It's trying to eliminate anything it sees as dangerous. As a result of being overworked and overstimulated, chronic inflammation occurs. Our bodies are constantly working to protect us, fighting off viruses, gluten, and other foreign substances that may have penetrated a compromised gut barrier.

Your stressed immune system is less able to attack pathogens and invaders with precision. Instead, it begins indiscriminately, sending wave after wave of attacks, eventually hitting your body's own tissues, which leads us to the third reason of why eliminating foods, such as gluten and dairy, is so critical. Leaky gut is a main factor in the manifestation of autoimmune disease. When gluten molecules slip through the leaky gut, the body wants to fight it off. This is when the PROBLEM arises. This phenomenon is called molecular mimicry because its identity can be mistaken for its similar structure. The immune system is memorizing these structures, and it will not be able to tell the difference between these "foreign invaders". The body is trying its best to keep us safe, but when it's overworked, antibodies do not function perfectly. It eventually starts accidentally attacking us. This is why we need to help our bodies out. We want to make sure that the drawbridge is shut, so the foreign invaders don't pass through because it will cause the body to constantly overwork and create persistent inflammation.

Just like gluten, dairy has a similar molecular structure and the same inflammatory response throughout the body. The casein in dairy creates gut issues and worsens autoimmune diseases. Eggs are also a potential risk factor. They can allow proteins (usually lysozyme from the egg white) to cross the gut barrier where they don't belong and contribute to molecular mimicry. A lot of people with autoimmunity will notice that eggs are triggers for them, but it's not the case for everyone. To test if you are sensitive to eggs, cut them from your diet completely for at least sixty days and slowly reintroduce to see if they are a trigger for you.

When a client of mine goes gluten or dairy-free, I'm always asked if substitutes, such as dairy-free ice cream or gluten-free bread, are compliant. The answer is yes, they can be. This is how I started my wellness journey, too. It made the transition accessible for me. No one is expecting you to be perfect. These foods are so hard to give up! But I will ask that you read the labels. Make sure there are no refined sugars, gums, or oils. This will only create other problems in your body. Stay mindful of how these foods make you feel. If they cause symptoms, it's a good idea to stop immediately. Keeping a food journal to track your food sensitivities provides valuable insights into your body and helps you better understand the impact of your diet.

If you're starting your own wellness journey, there are a few things you need to know before officially diving in. I wish I had this knowledge when I completely changed my entire diet and lifestyle regimen.

Before embarking on your wellness journey, it's important to remember that you may initially experience temporary discomfort, as your body undergoes the detoxification process. However, this is a natural part of the healing journey, and it will pave the way for better health. I want to remind you that this process is temporary, and the length of time and intensity varies from person to person. This process is also known as the "carb flu", so if you start experiencing headaches, increased fatigue, brain fog, and/or flu-like symptoms, just know this is all natural, especially if you are significantly decreasing your carb intake and are not used to eating lots of fiber and nutrients daily.

With the rapid changes in diet (increasing fibers and fats while decreasing carbohydrates), it is normal to experience temporal gastrointestinal issues (loose stools, bloating, constipation, belching, etc.) within the first few days or weeks. Your gut microbiome is adapting and becoming healthier by producing more acids to absorb, digest, and assimilate nutrients properly. Again, these symptoms will be temporary. Keep in mind that your body is starting to cleanse itself. These increased symptoms are normal at the beginning; this does not mean that the process is not working for you. It means it's just starting. Remember each person is different. These symptoms can last anywhere between a few days or over a month. Stay strong and keep going; it's worth getting over the first part of this hill.

During this time, drink lots of water to stay hydrated and help your body flush out toxins. Water is crucial—not something to skip out on! Fill your body with complex carbs from fruits and root vegetables. This will also help you manage cravings at the beginning and help fill that sweet tooth while staying compliant to the journey.

Another trick I have also found helpful is taking activated charcoal during the withdrawal period. Activated charcoal binds to toxins or substances in the body to remove it faster and decrease inflammation. Start with one per day. I recommend not going over three per day. Only take activated charcoal for two weeks at the most since it is known to cause constipation if taken for prolonged periods of time.

Starting this journey is definitely tough. Remember, giving yourself grace during this healing and wellness process is critical. You may have a few slip-ups, especially at the beginning. Just because you had a cookie does not mean you messed up the whole process, and you should just give up. NO! Not at all! I do not want you to give up. Making mistakes just means you're human. This is called a journey for a reason, not a destination. Forgive yourself, get back up, and start over.

Healing isn't linear; it is going to have many twists and turns. There are going to be times when you're getting better so quickly, you'll think you finally figured it out. Then, out of nowhere, symptoms will rear their ugly heads, and you'll feel like you're going backwards again. Don't get discouraged. Sometimes we must get worse to get better. We have to be extremely mindful and tune in to what's working for our bodies and what's not. It's all part of the journey! When riding this rollercoaster, it helps to reach out to a fellow warrior who is on a wellness journey for encouragement and support. More often than not, you'll find fellow warrior friends who are going through extremely similar things. You don't need to go through any of this alone!

The foundation of my daily routine for managing life with MS begins with the food I eat. I aim to eat six-to-nine cups of veggies daily, along with fermented foods (apple cider vinegar, bone broth, sauerkraut, or yogurt). I make sure my macronutrients (proteins, fats, and carbs) are balanced. I completely eliminated gluten, dairy, refined sugar, and refined oils. I do light exercise every day, like walks, Pilates, yoga, or stretching. Hydration is key! Also, a good night's sleep (six-to-eight hours every night) is a must for me to feel great all day.

Warrior, if you're looking to take a holistic approach to managing your autoimmunity, it's 100% worth it! What we feed our bodies, what we tell our minds, and what our daily habits are (such as sleep and hydration) all play a role in our vitality. Aim to give your body the tools (nutrients) it needs each day. Find a support team to help you. Stay determined, patient, and consistent. Focus on progress, not perfection. I know it's tough, but I promise you'll be thanking yourself in the long run. You got this!

31

Story by
LIEZA

Diagnosed in 2016
Currently 32 years old
Lives in Christchurch, New Zealand

My story is one of resilience, perseverance, and unwavering optimism. Despite facing challenges and setbacks, I never lost sight of my goals and refused to give up. I moved to New Zealand (NZ) from Belgium when I was twelve years old. I'd always loved horses. In NZ, I started competitive horse riding. I loved competing! Eventing (which is what I focused on), consisted of three phases: dressage, show jumping, and cross-country. In the cross-country phase, you have to go fast over jumps for three-to-four minutes. I think I experienced my first multiple sclerosis (MS) symptom (blurred vision) when I was seventeen years old, during the cross-country phase of a horse-riding event. I knew that I had to jump between the red and white flags. Luckily, my horse and I had a strong bond, so he would just jump. I didn't experience blurred vision every time, so I assumed it was just adrenaline from competing.

When I was twenty-two years old, I gave up horse riding as it was too time-consuming, and I needed to focus on my university degree—a Bachelor of Science majoring in Physics. To "relax" from the stress of university, I took up running. I loved putting on my running shoes and hitting the road. I'd run everywhere. If I felt sad, I'd run. If I felt happy, I'd run. I ran to think about things. I ran to forget about things. Running gave me so much freedom and happiness. Some of my fondest memories are running with my dad on the beach and in the hills of our hometown.

I didn't want to just run; I wanted to be great. I trained six days per week, religiously following a schedule I put together. My dream was to qualify to run the Boston Marathon one day. On trail runs, I'd often trip over tree roots. My dad and I would laugh about how clumsy I was. Little did I know, this was a sign of what was to come. I competed in three full marathons and numerous half-marathons, road races, and trail runs.

When running, I sometimes experienced strange things that I couldn't quite understand. I was not able to completely focus my eyes, and my balance was not as good as usual. I'd slur my words a little afterward, and my feet would sometimes feel heavy—I felt like I was stomping my feet on the ground. These strange symptoms would come and go. I thought maybe my blood sugar was low, so I ate sugary foods during my runs, but that didn't help.

In June 2016, my sister and I decided to run a half-marathon together, aiming for a sub one hour and thirty-minute time. I was doing a lot of treadmill running leading up to it as I was close to submitting my master's degree. By the time I could train, it was dark outside. When I was driving home from the gym, I'd have to cover one eye to properly judge the distance between my car and the car in front of me.

The first three kilometers (km) of the half-marathon were good; then my legs started feeling heavy, and I stomped my feet down on the ground. I kept going but was rapidly giving up on my desired time. At eighteen km, I had blurred vision and could no longer run in a straight line. My sister had to hold my hand. I was stopped by a race marshal and given some soft candies. I was told to rest and wait for the ambulance to arrive. She suspected I may have diabetes.

I got sick of waiting and asked if I could continue. I only had three km left and wanted to finish. She said that I could continue if I walked. I walked for a bit and then decided to run. My legs started feeling heavy, and my vision went weird again. So, I walked the remainder of the course but ran through the finish line, with my sister by my side.

I didn't run again because I feared a repeat of what had happened. I underwent a myriad of tests; none of which provided an answer. Four frustrating months later, my parents paid for a private neurologist appointment. I explained my experiences to him, and he mentioned something called Uthoff's phenomenon, but no real explanation. He got me into the public health system and ordered magnetic resonance imaging (MRI). No words of MS had been mentioned at this stage, though the neurologist probably had his suspicions.

While I was waiting for the results from my head and neck MRI, I completed my master's degree, and my sister and I traveled around Peru for three weeks. I hiked Rainbow Mountain (5200 m altitude), Machu Picchu, and visited the Amazon Jungle. I didn't experience any strange symptoms during this time.

After my trip to Peru, I started my PhD in Medical Physics. In December 2016, I had an appointment with the neurologist to discuss my MRI results. In NZ, to obtain an MS diagnosis, lesions need to be detected on an MRI, and you must undergo a spinal tap/lumbar puncture. A few days before Christmas, I received my spinal tap. They accidentally punctured my spinal sac, and I spent the weeks around Christmas vomiting and having terrible migraines whenever I stood up. It was performed by a registrar, but I recommend seeing someone who has extensive knowledge regarding the procedure.

In January 2017, at the age of twenty-six, I was officially diagnosed with Primary-Progressive Multiple Sclerosis (PPMS). I remember sitting in the neurologist's office with my mum, not really knowing what this meant, but knowing it wasn't good.

A few months prior to my diagnosis, I began to study for my PhD in Medical Physics. Immediately after receiving my diagnosis, I thought to myself that I'd better get on with my life. I was symptom-free, other than not being able to walk or run quickly. I didn't want to know what could possibly happen; knowing the worst-case scenario is not helpful for me. Ignorance is bliss, right?

The only time I heard from my neurologist after my diagnosis was when she called me to ask if I was interested in participating in a drug trial. I researched the drug and decided no—it wasn't for me. I felt fine; I didn't need medication. I never heard from my neurologist again after that.

So, I continued living my life. Over the next three years, I traveled to China, India, Nepal, Sweden, and visited family in Lithuania and Belgium. I completed my PhD in three years. I had an active social life and met the love of my life. I had MS, and life was pretty good. I was proud of myself! Even with MS, I was living a life better than I could have imagined.

Fast forward a year and a half. In October 2019, I had the opportunity to live and work in Hong Kong for one year. I loved Hong Kong. My symptoms hadn't changed much since my diagnosis, and I felt very grateful. I couldn't run, so I found refuge in going to the gym for strength training six days a week, but the pandemic took that away from me. My walking deteriorated. Walking from my apartment in Hong Kong to the bus stop (about 500m) was a real struggle. Walking downhill was the worst. My legs would shake and feel like jelly. Walking was awful in the tropical Hong Kong climate, especially with a mask.

At this stage, I was alone. My boyfriend had come to live with me in Hong Kong for six months, but he went back to NZ as he couldn't find a job; Hong Kong is not cheap. I felt hopeless. I was in a foreign country alone, experiencing something that I'd never experienced before. I turned to MS support groups on Facebook for help and advice. I joined quite a few of them, but I felt like none were right for me, as the posts were often negative and quite depressing to read. I felt even more hopeless, like my life was going downhill from here. Then Facebook suggested a group called "Overcoming MS". I joined the group, not fully knowing what it was about—I just liked the name. The first few posts that I read were about people being positive and helpful! I was hooked.

Soon after, I met up with a member from the group, who had MS and also lived in Hong Kong, five minutes away from where I lived. She explained the seven-step Overcoming MS (OMS) recovery program to me. It consists of the following steps: Step one focuses on diet. Step two highlights the importance of vitamin D and sunlight exposure. Step three encourages regular exercise. Step four emphasizes the practice of meditation and mindfulness for stress management. Step five addresses the use of medication. Step six focuses on preventing family members from developing MS. Step seven emphasizes changing your life for life.

She had been following OMS since her diagnosis, and she managed to shrink some of her lesions. Shrink lesions?! How is that even possible? After meeting her, I followed the diet part of OMS 100%. I was taking 50,000IU of vitamin D orally—one capsule per month. Although I didn't feel changes immediately, I did notice that it helped my energy levels. Now, I try to aim for a vitamin D level in the range of 150-225 nmol/L (or 60-90 ng/mL), as per the OMS guidelines. I get my vitamin D levels tested about twice a year: once at the end of winter and once at the end of summer. I also made sure that I exposed myself to the sun as often as I could. I was doing resistance training in my apartment at home, taking two tablespoons of flaxseed oil a day, and my OMS friend had even convinced me to do yoga.

The amount of resistance training that I did was dependent on my symptoms and mobility level (this was also pre-baby). I used to work at a gym as a receptionist, so I had friends who were knowledgeable and helped me develop my own program. I mostly did strength training with two upper body and two lower body days per week. For my upper body, I trained chest, shoulders, back, biceps, and triceps. For my lower body, I trained my quads, glutes, hamstrings, and calves. My cardio was walking on the treadmill or using the rowing machine. I wasn't really seeing any big changes, but I believed in the science of OMS, and I knew that it would take a long time (years) to see and feel the difference.

My year in Hong Kong was up, and I declined the offer to extend my contract for the sake of my health. At this point, simple tasks were a struggle. Leaving the house was nearly impossible. Every move that I made was calculated. Is it worth it? Is it important? Will I benefit from using what little energy that I had?

I was so happy to get back to NZ, where the climate was cooler, to be reunited with my family and boyfriend, to not have to wear a mask all the time, and to have access to my gym again. I had to do two weeks of managed isolation in a government quarantine facility due to COVID, but that was okay; it was two weeks of rest. I'd managed to organize all my meals to be OMS-friendly, and I even ordered some flaxseed oil from the local health food store. The OMS diet is plant-based, but it also includes seafood, so I got a lot of salmon, rice, and steamed veggies. Life was pretty good.

I'd completed one week of managed isolation when I was reading in my room one morning, and the vision in my left eye started going blurry. A few minutes later, I couldn't see anything out of my left eye. I was experiencing, what I later found out to be, my first bout of optic neuritis. Optic neuritis is often associated with an MS relapse. I had another week stuck in my hotel room all alone! Who could I ask for help? I then remembered that I had a tattered old card in the back of my wallet that had the contact details of my MS nurse on it. I'm surprised and grateful that I remembered I had this.

I was given a five-day course of oral steroids for my eye (I'd had a phone appointment with a neurologist from my isolated hotel room), and I regained some of the vision back in my left eye within two weeks. At this stage, I was at home with my family and boyfriend in Christchurch. My eye recovered more every day, until my vision finally returned fully.

"Phew, I'm through the worst," I thought. But MS had other plans. Before the steroids, I could walk fairly normally. I couldn't walk for long, but what I could do appeared "normal" (except for walking downhill or downstairs). After the steroids, I couldn't walk straight, my balance was all over the place, my legs would shake and felt like jelly, and I had a limp. I'm not blaming the steroids; it was probably just my MS progressing. I felt awful, embarrassed to be seen, and not like myself. But, as I told you earlier, I'm very stubborn.

Nearly everything that I'd heard and read about MS told me that once you start getting worse, there is no way of going back to where you used to be. I kept following OMS and trusting the process in hopes that it would speed up my recovery. I upped my vitamin D dose three months after starting OMS, from my monthly 50,000IU to 10,000IU a day. I started supplementing with magnesium, and I started meditating daily.

I also went back to the gym. Using the knowledge that I'd gained on my own and from my personal trainer that I'd had in Hong Kong, I started training myself. Initially, I couldn't walk on the treadmill without holding the sides with both hands (since the treadmill felt narrow and required balance for me). Then, I gradually transitioned to holding on with one hand for one minute, and then the other hand for the following minute. Afterward, I progressed to using alternating fingers for support, followed by fifteen seconds of walking without holding onto anything. Now, I am proud to say that I can walk on the treadmill for five minutes without holding on to anything. That was in the space of about six months.

When I first came back from Hong Kong and was able to drive with my eye, I started working full-time at the medical imaging company that I had worked for prior to moving. Parking is bad where I worked, so I had to walk about one km to work and one km back every day. In the beginning (November 2020), that walk was so difficult. It felt like a walk, or hobble, of shame. My limp was so noticeable.

After I'd finished my job for the day, I'd make myself go to the gym (three times a week). Then, I'd come home and cook myself an OMS-friendly meal. At the end of the day, I was exhausted. "Was it all worth it?" I asked myself. Some of my family members thought that OMS was too restrictive, especially concerning the limited saturated fats. I also lost about ten kg when I first started, but then I got pregnant while following OMS, and that was that.

After a few months, my limp that occurred while walking to work in the morning disappeared. I transitioned back to walking like a "normal" person, at least for a few hours. A few months later, I noticed that my limp wouldn't start until the walk back to my car in the evening. Presently, my limp only shows up when I've done something "wrong".

Following my discovery of the strong link between gluten and inflammation, I have embraced a gluten-free lifestyle as part of the OMS diet. I also repeat a lot of the same foods to make it easier on myself as I can prepare in bulk. For breakfast, I have scrambled tofu, beans, potatoes, and spinach with two tablespoons of flaxseed oil drizzled on top. Or I eat rice flake cereal (like porridge) with cocoa powder, maple syrup, and banana with flaxseed oil drizzled over the top. For lunch, I have vegetable lasagna/pasta, vegetarian sushi with miso soup, salmon with vegetables and rice, or curry. I typically eat the same foods for dinner that I eat for lunch. My go-to snacks are bananas, toast, and rice cakes with tahini and honey.

In August 2022, I found out I was pregnant. My pregnancy was very good, and my MS was very well behaved. I'd heard this might happen; nine months of bliss. I was not completely symptom-free, but I had definitely improved!

On May 1, 2022, I gave birth to a beautiful baby girl. I probably didn't eat as much or as well as I should have (still 100% OMS compliant with my diet though). I definitely didn't get as much sleep as I needed. I didn't exercise or meditate regularly. My daughter was my number one priority. But I quickly learned that you can't pour from an empty cup. About three months after the birth of my daughter, my MS symptoms got worse. I think old symptoms were flaring up. Months of sleep deprivation and my crazy hormones were probably the cause. I was, and still do, exclusively breastfeed my daughter, who is nearly fourteen months. I decided I would do everything it took to get better for my daughter. She was my "why". I was still following the diet portion of OMS faithfully, I started meditating again daily, supplementing with vitamin D (I never stopped this), and I also became a paying member of the MSGym. The science behind the MSGym really resonated with me, and it made so much sense! I highly recommend you check it out, regardless of your abilities. There is a lot of free information, as well as paid membership options.

I don't currently take any MS medication. There is no medication funded for people with PPMS where I live, but even if Ocrelizumab/Ocrevus was available, I'm not sure if I'd take it. The main reason being that so little is known about MS, so how can they develop effective medication for it? I wish more research was focused on finding ways to better the lives of people living with MS today, rather than solely pursuing an elusive "cure". I prefer lifestyle changes as opposed to medication being the first thing that is offered. Lifestyle changes and medication can coexist. Why do some neurologists see them as being mutually exclusive? Can't you do both?

I don't undergo regular MRI's because I don't believe they are necessarily an accurate representation of MS progression. There are two reasons behind my skepticism. Firstly, so little is known about MS, and new research is constantly emerging. It raises questions about why individuals without detected lesions on an MRI scan still experience disease progression. Is there another underlying factor at play? Lesions alone may not provide the complete picture. Secondly, an MRI machine's ability to detect lesions could be limited by its resolution. This means that different scanners might yield varying results, further challenging their reliability as a diagnostic tool.

To prioritize my health, I engage in several activities that have been beneficial for me (in no particular order). I follow the OMS diet and take vitamin D3 supplements. I include two tablespoons of flaxseed oil in my daily breakfast routine. Getting good sleep, natural sunlight, meditating daily, and engaging in regular physical activity are also part of my health regimen. For meditation, I use apps like *Calm* and *Balance* for guided sessions. I practice breathing exercises for relaxation (non-sleep deep rest) and energy boosts (cyclic hyperventilation/Wim Hof techniques). These habits contribute to my overall well-being.

I've found cold baths to be very beneficial for my well-being, and I incorporate them into my routine whenever I find the time (three-to-four times a week), both in the morning and evening. I stay in for two-to-four minutes at a time. They help to improve my mood, energy levels, sleep quality, and mobility. I feel great whenever I take them. I recommend listening to Andrew Huberman's podcast, as it offers a lot of information about cold exposures. I've noticed that taking a cold bath before a hot shower helps me tolerate the heat better during and after the shower.

Am I grateful to have MS? Yes and no. No, because I wish I could still run on the beach and in the hills. But yes, for so many more reasons. Being diagnosed at a young age made me become a "yes" woman. I say yes to things without overthinking and sorting through all the possible outcomes. I deal with issues as they arise because 85% of what you worry about won't happen anyway, so it's just a waste of time and energy. Everyone has something "wrong" with them; MS is just my thing. I am not symptom-free. My gait is affected, and my left hand has unauthorized parties (among other symptoms). I can do 98% of what a "normal" person can do. Some things I can't do as fast as others, but I get there in my own time.

Life, regardless of whether you have MS or not, is full of ups and downs. I know that I will probably have another "down" period in my life, but I also know that I have tools to fight whatever comes my way. I will never give up; I will continue to learn and educate myself. I will live a life that I have decided, not a life MS has decided for me.

Through my continuous research on neuroplasticity and the power of the mind, I am convinced that the mind can heal the body. Things are looking up. I will leave you with a few things that I have learned on this crazy journey so far: never compare yourself to others, especially considering the unique effects of MS on each individual. While improvement with MS is very possible, there are no quick fixes. Stay consistent and persistent. Take care of your body with nourishing food and positive thoughts. Remember, your subconscious mind is always listening.

Having MS has made me even more determined and resilient. I want to prove people wrong. Pursuing a Ph.D. despite English being my second language and dealing with an MS diagnosis? No problem. Completing it within three years, while managing MS? Absolutely achievable. Residing and thriving in Hong Kong? Yes, indeed. Embracing the joy of motherhood? Certainly. As for running again, just watch me exceed all expectations.

32

Story by

JASMIN DUNCAN

Diagnosed in 2008
Currently 35 years old
Lives in Los Angeles, United States
Instagram: @j.kristophr

Welcome to my multiple sclerosis (MS) Journey. In this chapter, I share my journey of living with and healing from MS, from the onset of symptoms to finding a path of holistic healing. I aim to inspire and provide valuable insights for others facing similar challenges. I was diagnosed with toxic shock syndrome, caused by a Staph infection in 2007. After fighting for my life and coming out on the other side a year later, I was diagnosed with MS at the age of nineteen.

My journey started with intruding unfamiliarity. I noticed changes in my speech and an unexplained slurring of my words that would only happen for a few seconds at a time. Then, the tingling sensations in my fingers and toes followed, a strange numbness creeping up my legs and arms. Not the kind that comes from being in one position for too long, such as your foot being "asleep", but a more profound, bone-deep sensation. The kind that can't be cured by getting up and shaking it off. Overall, my coordination seemed a little off.

After a few days, I decided to see a doctor, who then referred me to a neurologist upon hearing about my condition. The neurologist ordered magnetic resonance imaging (MRI), a spinal tap, and even a visual test, which led to the diagnosis that would drastically redefine my existence: Multiple Sclerosis. I was blindsided. MS, a chronic disease that affects the Central Nervous System, was now a part of my reality.

My initial reaction was fear, so deep and overwhelming that it threatened to consume me. How could I lead a normal life? What about the rest of my life? What will that look like for me? Instantly, fear turned into hope after hearing that my grandmother also had MS; she was diagnosed in the early seventies. I spent my entire childhood with this superwoman, who lived her life to the fullest every single day, and I had no clue that she was living it with this vicious disease. She is now eighty-eight, and she remains unmedicated. Her fullness gave me hope. Still, her only beauty/ health secret is to rest and not worry about a thing.

At the time of my diagnosis, conventional medicine offered me a treatment called Rebif. I embarked on a year-long journey of self-administered injections, but the side effects took a toll on my well-being. Discontented with the impact on my quality of life, I explored alternative approaches. I decided to educate myself more about MS, learning about its potential progression, available treatments, and coping mechanisms. The more I learned, the more I came to accept my condition. This wasn't the end of my world, but the beginning of a new, challenging chapter.

I began by making lifestyle modifications. I desired a more natural approach, so I shared my decision with my doctor to discontinue Rebif. I would embrace a holistic approach to managing my condition, prioritizing a healthier diet, regular exercise, vitamin D supplementation, stress management, and plenty of rest. This lifestyle became my new mantra for navigating life with MS. However, my doctor expressed concerns and predicted a bleak future, stating that I would be in a wheelchair by the age of twenty-five. I refused to accept this prognosis and told him that I had too many fabulous shoes not to be able to walk in them again. I resolved to take charge of my health and explore natural healing methods.

Despite my skepticism, I maintained a positive mindset and believed in the healing potential. I refused to let MS define my life or dictate my future. I found motivation in envisioning a life filled with vitality, adventure, and the ability to wear my chosen shoes—progressive actions and advancements. With advancements in MS treatment, I started disease-modifying therapy (DMT). While committed to a natural path, I remained open to medical advancements and the possibility of oral medications. A year after I decided to discontinue Rebif, the FDA approved the first oral drug called Gilenya. Recognizing its potential benefits, I weighed the options. I resumed treatment to manage my MS symptoms—the treatment aimed to reduce the frequency and severity of relapses, slowing the progression of the disease. Despite how I felt about conventional treatment options, it was a placeholder to manage my condition.

Life changed when I became pregnant with my first child in 2015. That's when I stopped taking Gilenya, and since then, I haven't taken any prescription medications. As a mother-to-be, I had to prioritize the health of my unborn child while managing my MS symptoms. Through navigating pregnancy, I found a delicate balance that allowed me to embrace the joys of motherhood while maintaining my health. I learned to adapt my healthy habits to accommodate my new reality. I've also found that walking can be therapeutic. My journey isn't over. I am not just living with MS—I am thriving, and I am resilient.

Throughout my journey, I discovered the power of holistic healing approaches. I explored various lifestyle changes, including diet modifications. Managing MS started in my kitchen. I swapped processed foods for natural, whole foods, concentrating on lean proteins, fruits, vegetables, and whole grains. Regularly consuming fish rich in omega-3 fatty acids became a ritual. Cutting down on sugar was challenging, but my determination kept me on track. Moreover, I stayed well-hydrated with celery juice and supplemented my diet with essential vitamins, particularly vitamin D and turmeric. In addition, I eliminated all toxic chemicals from the beauty products I use and the cleaning supplies in my house.

Recognizing the intimate relationship between the mind and body, I delved into the power of the mind-body connection regarding healing. During my second pregnancy in 2020 and the subsequent years, I experienced a remarkable absence of MS symptoms. I attribute this improvement to being pregnant and combining factors, including an active lifestyle, mindful eating, and emotional well-being. I cultivated resilience, inner strength, and renewed hope through mindfulness practices, exercising, meditation, and positive affirmations. All of these were a cornerstone of my life with MS, which improved my strength, balance, and aided in stress management. On good days, I walk a minimum of 10k steps, taking care not to overexert myself. Exercising helps me feel more in control of my body, giving me a sense of accomplishment and uplifting my spirit.

Usually, my days start with a good morning stretch and meditation to set a positive tone. I then enjoy warm water with lemon, followed by celery juice. Taking my supplements is an essential part of maintaining my health and well-being. In the evening, we like to go for another walk. Before I go to bed, I do lymphatic drainage massage while putting my legs on the wall to reduce the day's inflammation. I don't follow a strict day-to-day routine; instead, I prioritize staying in tune with my body and listening to its needs. If it suggests going for a walk, I embrace it. However, what truly matters to me is finding stillness. I feel my best when I allow myself to be still, as it is during those moments that I know my nervous system is healing. My body requires a less rigid routine and more attentiveness to its signals.

It is important to note that every individual's journey with MS is unique, and what works for one person may not work for another. Connecting with your inner being and making informed decisions based on personal circumstances is essential. My collaborative chapter aims to share my experiences and insights. I hope my story makes your healing journey a little easier.

Dealing with MS is a balancing act. I found my rhythm by juggling herbal supplements, an active lifestyle, mindful eating, and stress management techniques, like acupuncture and an undying spirit. I have maintained moderate-to-zero MS symptoms in recent years. Today, as I reflect on my journey, I celebrate the triumphs and the lessons learned. Earlier this year, I went in for a well overdue checkup with my neurologist. I was curious about what my body looked like on the inside. It had been seven years since my last MRI. After the MRI showed no active lesions on my brain, I embraced the idea that natural healing is a lifelong process—but it is happening.

It goes beyond managing the symptoms of MS. Through resilience, determination, and a commitment to holistic well-being, I have surpassed expectations and continue to thrive. I take each day as it comes, celebrating small victories, learning from the setbacks, and forever remaining hopeful.

We all know that every day with MS brings new challenges but also new growth opportunities. Taking a holistic approach has given me the power to take charge of my health and live a fulfilling life beyond the limitations of MS. I am incredibly grateful to my tribe for their unwavering support and encouragement. Together, we have faced challenges, celebrated victories, and embraced the beauty of life.

33

Story by
MEGAN LEWELLYN
Diagnosed in 2007
Currently 52 years old
Lives in Sedro Woolley, Washington State, United States
Segway Into My New Life - Available on Amazon
Instagram: @bbhwithms and @campsunshine420
www.BBHwithMS.com

Although it was over sixteen years ago, and my damaged brain struggles at moments to function through the lingering fog caused by the pharmaceuticals and the disease's progression; even though I have years with few to no memories, I remember the day I was diagnosed like it was just last week. Granted, it helps that I wrote a book about it. But truthfully, it's hard to forget a life-changing moment like that. It becomes imbedded in your mind, playing on a constant loop: you have MS, you have MS, you have MS....

You fucking have MS.

Your life is instantly split in two: the "before diagnosis" and the after.

Shit gets redefined. Instantly, priorities shift. Your one driving hope is to stave off the progression of the disease...or slow it down. At least, that's how it was for me.

I was thirty-seven years old. Up until this moment in my life, the biggest medical procedures I'd been involved in was shooting children out of my vagina, and I'd done that with as little medicine as possible. I avoided pain pills after being struck by a vehicle as a pedestrian, waived offers for sleeping aids after going through a bank robbery, and shooed away even Tylenol after the aforementioned births because I really didn't like taking medicine. Something in the back of my mind told me to avoid it.

And yet, in the span of just a few short months, I went from defining myself as a "young, fit mother of three who had strong hippy tendencies" to "a patient dependent on chemicals and drugs to get through my life."

And I remained that way for ten years.

Having been born and raised in New Haven, Connecticut, home of the prestigious Yale University, and its acclaimed medical school, I was taught to trust doctors—to respect their expertise and knowledge in the field of health, the human body, and the ways to care for and heal it.

So, when I needed hope for my future after being faced with a major medical road hurdle, when I needed to know that I could continue to be the mom I wanted to be—out and about with my little people—and not confined to a life at home, I turned to doctors for answers. I looked to the people I thought were the experts on my condition, and I was led to believe my hope for that future lay within the world of pharmaceuticals.

I remember sitting on the couch the night after my diagnosis, watching a video my doctor had provided me with at my appointment earlier in the day. It was an advertisement for one of the drugs he thought I should consider starting. As I watched the actors on the screen smile and laugh, I made the decision. There, at that exact moment, on the battered, burnt orange leather couch, stained with the messes that come with a life of little kids and dogs. Watching that dumb promotional video, I decided that I would use pharmaceuticals to fight the monster that was living within my body. I would sign up for a lifetime of needles and pills, appointments and infusions, if it meant I could still be the mom I had always dreamed of being.

It worked for the people in the video, so hopefully, it could work for me.

It seemed foreign to me, the idea of being someone that was on medication. A sick person, reliant on pills or infusions to live.

To cope.

To survive.

Being a patient was not my best role. I hadn't been good at it during childbirth, and I wasn't sure how it was going to go over now. However, my thought process was that it may not be a cure, but the video people seemed happy and active. Someone was even skiing, so this must be the way to go.

Truthfully, there had been a bit of research done prior to this visit with the couch and the drug video. After my brain and thoracic magnetic resonance imaging (MRIs), while waiting for the results of my spinal tap from the Mayo Clinic, I had begun to suspect it was multiple sclerosis, and I investigated it.

I'd seen articles and blog posts as I'd delved into the world of the internet on the kids' computer while making dinner over the past few weeks. My parents called to say their neighbor in Martha's Vineyard was the former CFO of a major pharma company that was producing a drug that looked very promising in research and studies…

A woman from the local chapter of the National MS Society called to introduce herself and invite me to participate in the fundraising events they were planning—sponsored by pharmaceutical companies whose names were becoming familiar.

When people in my life heard about my possible diagnosis, they would send emails with articles from the *Boston Globe* or *The New York Times*. They sent anything promising and always about a new drug or research for a drug.

Pharmaceuticals kept popping up, over and over. What I kept hearing was that being on pharmaceuticals, or more specifically getting on pharmaceuticals as soon as possible, seemed to be everyone's number one way to fight the disease.

I was told the longer I waited, the worse it could get.

I didn't want to get worse.

I wanted to get better.

So, I didn't wait because I didn't want to fail my kids.

In hindsight, the decision I made seems moronically simple and lacking any true research. But at the time, I was juggling three kids under the age of ten, my marriage was a sham, and my condition seemed to be getting worse. Crazy shit was happening to my body, and I needed it to stop.

I'd peed myself at the playground earlier in the day—just after being given the diagnosis and picking the kids up from school. I was standing there talking, and then there was urine running down my legs…

I was in front of a group of other parents.

Thank goodness for forgiving woodchips and short, breezy sundresses worn in late fall.

My point being, I had just been told I was going to live with this disease for the rest of my life. I wanted to believe that the doctors would guide me in the right direction.

I needed to believe it.

For a decade, I was a diligent patient. I had MRIs, spinal taps, and follow up appointments.

I did the drugs.

I started by stabbing a needle in my thigh once a week. When that failed to cease the incessant lesions and the disease's progression, I drove myself to an infusion center every twenty-eight days for someone else to put the drugs in my body. As my mental and physical health waned, managing my disease and its ever-increasing side effects became a full-time occupation, despite my already packed schedule as a single working mom.

I threw myself into being a patient, and I was encouraged by everyone. They said I was strong for going through the procedures, brave for taking the medications, for sticking myself with a long-ass needle once a week. These words helped spur me on. They gave me strength to push forward, even though I encountered many setbacks.

I was made to believe that by taking them, even when they made me feel like shit, by enduring the infusions, even if they lead to bad reactions and god-awful side effects—I was fighting the best fight I could fight.

That's what I was led to believe. Those were my dark years.

In the end, I tried four different disease modifying therapies (DMTs) over the course of ten years. None of them agreed with me, and some did significant long-term damage. In addition to the medication I took to try and alter the course of my disease, there were drugs for all the other symptoms: the pain and the numbness; the spasticity and the agonizing muscle spasms. Drugs to help me sleep, and medications to lessen the ever-present fatigue.

By 2016, I was on a handful of prescriptions, and there had been discussion of implanting a pain pump in my hip. I was on methadone for the pain. Gabapentin for the spasms and spasticity. Ambien to help me sleep. Ampyra to help me walk. Amitriptyline, and then nortriptyline, for the depression.

And alcohol. Always alcohol.

Drinking became a really important tool in my wheelhouse.

Throughout the years of living with my disease and pharmaceuticals, I self-medicated with alcohol. When the pills didn't work, when the pain became too overwhelming and completely unmanageable, alcohol helped. I knew it was bad for me. I knew it was harming my body, but the pain was just too much, and the relief it provided was too tempting...

On top of all of that, I decided to return to smoking cigarettes. I was angry at my body for getting sick. I felt that overall, I had lived a relatively healthy life, and I was livid that things were failing me so early on.

I told myself I deserved them, and my disconnected mind and body said it was okay.

Needless to say, I didn't become one of the people in the video. I wasn't active, and I wasn't happy. One decade in, and I was a complete mess. Every fear I had of what my life with the disease would look like had come to fruition. I was seventy-five pounds overweight, divorced, unemployed, and unable to walk the dog around the block. And my memory had gone to shit.

I once prided myself on my ability to remember things—multiple things —for long periods of time. But the new version of me, the "me" that was saturated in pharmaceuticals, couldn't remember jack shit.

My life had become pathetic...

I lived on our couch, watching endless hours of television.

I hated myself.

I hated what my life had become.

I hated myself for allowing it to get that bad.

I hated myself for hating myself.

I had no motivation to do anything that would better my situation. The brain/body connection was severed. Contrary to how I had lived my previous thirty-six years, I became a victim, looking for someone else to fix my problems, rather than taking care of myself.

As I said, dark years.

Six years ago, I made the decision to come off all the pharmaceuticals and try naturally managing my disease and my health. I decided to stop all prescription medications to see if I could live life without them. The results have been absolutely life changing. I'm down to my fighting weight, I walk three plus miles a day, help with chores around our five-acre property, go for hikes when we can fit it in, and I remember things far better than my aging old man.

I have hope for my future, both physically and mentally, and there are no pharmaceuticals involved.

After years of giving shit up, I am currently on the kick of adding things back into my life.
I'm lifting weights. Walking. Hiking. Running. Granted, it's an ugly run, and I definitely peed my pants in the process, but I'm used to that these days. What's really important is—I ran!

And I'm driving!

This one is kind of huge! After not driving for over five years due to vision and focus issues, I've taken to the roads again, and it's going well.

I haven't hit anything or anyone. I've also gotten into a routine of doing some of the household errand running all by myself. Gaining back some level of independence is a big deal.

Next on my list, try skiing. I'm not particularly driven to become a full-blown skier again, like I am with driving, but I want to give it a shot to see if I can still manage a trip or two down the slopes. Just to say I can.

After spending ten years giving things up, saying goodbye to activities and experiences that I loved, I'm up for the challenge of figuring out how to do things again, despite my limitations. I am so grateful for all that past "me" did to get me here. I made getting healthy my full-time job, and I've got to say, I kind of feel like a promotion might be in order.

I spent eighteen months slowly tapering off all the prescriptions. One by one, I would slowly reduce my consumption levels until I was off all of it.

I then spent a few months living "raw"—not using any form of medicine (natural or unnatural) to clean out my system and get a sense of just how bad things were. The alarming discovery was the pain was the same, screaming and crashing through my body, just like it had been for as long as I can remember.

Truthfully, I had expected it to be worse. I buckled down, preparing myself mentally for what I thought was going to be unimaginable levels of pain. Given how bad it was while on all the drugs, I feared that coming off the prescriptions would leave me at an even more intolerable level (if that was possible), and a raging alcoholic. But it seems the medications that had once helped were no longer doing anything to assist me. Instead, they were harming me.

And so began my journey to what I now call "naturally managing my shit", and my kids call "my weed phase". I had the nurse practitioner at my doctor's office prescribe me a Medical Marijuana Card (referred to as an MMJ card), and I began doing research online. I discovered *Leafly.com* and began learning about things like strains and terpenes. I found a few bloggers who wrote about using cannabis as medicine, and I tried figuring out what exactly I was supposed to ask for at the local dispensary. I didn't know much about cannabis (or CBD) and walking in uninformed seemed like a recipe for disaster.

Anxiety that stems from living with an invisible disease, along with brain fog, makes any form of shopping extremely uncomfortable for me. Being in a strange place, not knowing what I want, and the looming fear of potentially getting stoned off my ass and having our five kids make fun of me for all of eternity, scared the living crap out of me. So, I dragged my feet. I put it off… Eventually, after weeks of agony, I packed myself into my Subaru wagon, drove to a pot shop, and made my first purchase of marijuana as my medicine.

Having grown up in the eighties with a brother who was "into the weed", I had been around it. I'd even puffed and inhaled on occasion (bathroom of a fraternity house in the 90s), but it wasn't something I enjoyed. After that incident at the frat house and a mean visit with paranoia that same night, it was honestly something I avoided. So, this was a huge step for me.

I began visiting dispensaries on a regular basis. I looked for people that had knowledge about cannabis being used for medicinal purposes. I called to speak with people at weed shops all over the country. I found people on the internet. I met people at cannabis conventions. I hung out with people who consumed weed, and I connected with people who grew it. Anyone knowledgeable and game for talking about medical marijuana became my new best friend.

As I began to understand my consumption levels (I consume a lot due to an enzyme deficiency, but that's a topic for an entire book—specifically a "healthy edibles" cookbook I am currently working on) and I learned of questionable practices when it came to organically grown weed, I realized growing my own would be necessary.

I flew to Colorado to attend a "grow expo", an event all about growing cannabis. Shortly after my return home, we were gifted with our first clone (a plant derived from cutting a piece off an existing plant), and our journey to growing my own medicine began.

I was off the pharma, and I had weed. But beyond the whole "I'm going to try pot" thing, I didn't have a clear direction. I didn't have a plan to get my health back on track, other than always trying to listen to myself and my instincts. I didn't have evidence that what I was doing would work, but I knew I had to try something different. I knew that I could not continue living the way I was living.

My years on pharma had not been kind, leaving many things to be fixed. I feared that fixing the damage caused by the pharmaceuticals and helping manage my chronic illness with all its craziness, would be asking too much of nature. But I had nowhere else to turn and nothing left to lose.

So, nature it was.

Once I had the drugs out of my system and had procured the weed, I slowly began chipping away at my health.

I started with exercise.

I started walking.

Rain or shine, hot or cold, I committed myself to walking every day. I would consume my cannabis, and I would walk. It started with one block. Every day, my goal was to walk farther than I had walked the day before—even if it was just one more driveway.

The elimination of pharmaceuticals, plus the addition of walking and weed in my life, wasn't an instant fix. I had major issues to tackle. I was still drinking alcohol, and sadly, I would arrive home from my walk and promptly light up a cigarette after smoking a joint. I hadn't yet amended my diet, hadn't learned about CBD, grounding, Epsom salt baths, or my beloved pot powder. At that point, I don't even think I had pulled my foam roller out or begun yoga, but I was moving again, and that was something.

And that little something, along with the small connection between my brain and body that the cannabis created, lit a spark in me. It made me feel like I could actually do this: get better and get my life back on track. That little spark and the weed reminded me of who I was beneath the toxins and chemicals. It made me want to retrieve that version of myself, dust her off, and get her back in shape.

Around this time, I took on a whole new attitude about my health, and my physical and mental well-being. My direction became clear once I began viewing myself and my health as an old, classic car I was restoring. As a young girl, I fell in love with a 1965 convertible mustang that an older boy in my hometown had purchased and was working to restore. It was a rusty mess and a slow process, hindered by his lack of money (caddying at the golf club could only earn a sixteen-year-old kid so much) and time (caddying was time-consuming). On top of his obligations with school and sports, time for working on the car was limited. But slowly, over the course of about two years, with a lot of love, a ton of elbow grease, and an unfaltering commitment to the project, that beat-up old car slowly became beautiful again. By the time graduation rolled around, she was purring like a kitten and shining like a bright star.

I realized that is what I had to do with my body and my brain—how I was going to fix things and manage my health going forward. Give them the love and attention they need to become bright and shiny.

I wanted to purr again.

Once I had that analogy firmly planted in my mind, my path became super clear. Only do things that will help in the restoration process. Never do things that will hinder my progress. I cleaned up my eating and began the long process of trying to heal my gut. My years of living on pharmaceuticals had wreaked havoc on my digestive system, and my gut biome suffered greatly. Unlike my previous efforts and endeavors, I did not look to others for advice, suggestions, or solutions. I didn't jump on anyone else's diet or protocol. Instead, I turned inward. I made friends with that little voice in my head, the one that so often makes suggestions, and I encouraged it to speak up.

I tried things. I paid attention to how my body felt, and I listened. I made decisions for my health based on my own feedback and experiences. For the first time since being diagnosed, I did what I thought was right for my body. Every change I made, every shift, every adjustment was made based on how I felt, how my body reacted, and how my brain responded. I stepped up my exercise by adding strength training and weights back into my life. I began working on my balance and strengthening my core to counter my numb legs and incessant vertigo.

I quit smoking cigarettes, I haven't had a sip of alcohol in three years, I avoid refined sugar, and I don't eat anything processed. With the "restoring an old car" analogy forever on a loop, I find it impossible to put these things in my body. If I ever slip and think it would be a good idea to eat something crappy or to have a drink, I think about my purring mustang. I would never put rocks, pebbles, or dirt in the gas tank and think that it wouldn't have negative repercussions on the way the car runs. So why would I put shit in my body and think that it will function properly?

When I look at it like that, it seems simple—logical.

Everything I do is an attempt to better myself and my health. What it came down to was I stopped bullshitting myself about my condition and the current state of things. I stopped telling myself it wasn't that bad, and I allowed myself to see it for how bad it really was.

And it was bad. I had gotten to a point where enjoyment of life wasn't possible. The pain and the mental disconnect were so severe that the path to healing was almost completely obscured. I forgot how to care for myself. I forgot to care about myself. And somewhere along the line, I had decided it was okay to do myself more harm.

I am eternally grateful for this new chapter of my life, and I am thankful for the relief I have found. As I mentioned, we now live on a five-acre piece of property, which has been the ideal setting for my healing. Being here, stashed away from the world during the months and years of the pandemic, spending time alone with myself, day in and day out, has allowed me to heal on levels that I didn't know were possible.

I still have my disease, and I still live with chronic pain, plus all the sensory and vision issues I had when I was on the pharmaceuticals, but everything is far more manageable now. I have genuine hope that they will continue to lessen over time. I've come to realize that if I continue on my journey of using mother nature and her powers to fix things, there really is no limit to how much I can heal.

As hippy dippy as it sounds, I have fully bought into the idea that naturally managing my health is a far better way to go. I've begun putting together my "healing team"—a group of professional people with likeminded views on how to manage one's health, who know me, know my story, and know my goals. So far, I have an amazing naturopathic doctor (Dr. Ed rocks), a phenomenal dentist (fun fact, pharma can cause massive tooth decay), a chiropractor, and a massage therapist who performs pure magic with her hands and smells delicious. I'm still looking for an acupuncturist and may find a few other fields of healing that I need to incorporate into the roster, but having flown solo for the past six years, it is nice having people in my corner again.

I haven't had an MRI since breaking-up with my neurologist in 2015, so I don't have "scientific evidence" that I am better, but I can assure you, I am. I'm better than I ever hoped I could be. I'm still working the kinks out of my routines and diet. As things heal and other issues arise, I make adjustments. From years of chronic constipation to a run-in with severe anemia (common with autoimmune diseases, and I've always been anemic) to my current visit with small intestinal bacterial overgrowth (SIBO), I shift foods and occasionally supplements, to help my body run as well as it can.

I'm slowly working more significant cardio back into my life (hello, hiking!) to increase my heart's strength and help my lungs begin to heal. Now that I have eliminated combusting cannabis almost entirely by using my infused oils, healthy edibles (weed gummy worms and cannabis-infused granola are my favorite) and pot powder (ground up decarboxylated weed I put in my morning smoothie), I figure it's time to give my lungs a bit of love.

Beyond not doing my lungs anymore harm, each of these methods allows me to use more of the plant, which is called full spectrum. It provides me with incredible pain relief and a level of mental clarity that I thought was gone from my life. It means I use all of the plant, wasting less of what we work so hard to grow.

The plan is to add some serious elevation to our future. As we hike, I will breathe in as deeply as I can to clean out all of the toxins. I'm healing shit left and right over here.

Basically, my Mustang looks bright and shiny. She's ready to purr.

When I started out on this journey, I didn't know whether managing my disease without pharmaceuticals was possible. I didn't know if I could manage my shit without pills and needles. But now that I do know, I can't help but share.

Because I wish I had known.

Honestly, if someone had told me back then that instead of heading to the infusion center to heal myself, I should head out for a hike, I don't know that I would have believed them.

If someone had said, "Clean up your diet, quit drinking, get a divorce, and get out in nature, then you will feel significantly better", I don't know if I would have listened. I know the ones around me (my family and friends) wouldn't have bought into the whole "naturally managing a disease" thing either.

Despite my lifelong aversion to medication, I waivered because this seemed different. Everyone was in support of pharmaceuticals, and I was led to believe that I needed them to survive. I sure as fuck wanted to survive. So really—what other choice did I have? Looking back at it in this light, it seems almost obvious that I would have gone down the path I did. But I still wish I had known.

My husband and I are in the process of opening a cannabis retreat and educational center, where others can come to learn about using plants as medicine and how to grow plants of their own. The goal for Camp Sunshine is to have cannabis-friendly events and classes (small, weed-friendly musical concerts, weed-infused yoga sessions, cooking with cannabis, or a beginner's class on growing weed). The plan is to have campsites, and eventually small cabins, on our property where visitors can come chill, heal, and learn in a quiet, safe place.

I am currently working on my cookbook, my husband I have begun a podcast (Weeding Through Life - available on Spotify) and I hope to resurrect regular contributions to the blog (bbhwithms.com) again soon. If you would like to know more about my diagnosis and my years on pharmaceuticals, I encourage you to read *Segway into My New Life: A Book About a Diagnosis*, available on Amazon. It's a raw look at what it was like, being the mom to three young children (ages five, seven, and nine) and being told I would have this new label for the rest of my life. In keeping with my general outlook on life, I approached this new hurdle with humor and optimism. From deciding what kind of underwear is appropriate for a spinal tap to learning how to shoot-up an orange—I spill the tea on what it was like to be diagnosed with MS. From the sheer terror of the unknown, to the tears of loneliness and the small triumphs of learning how to navigate life with my new found disabilities—you are along for the ride as I set out to redefine my life.

As for my more recent activities, I have voraciously documented my journey over the past six years on Instagram (@bbhwithms), much to my children's chagrin. From my very first visit to the pot shop, to buying Camp Sunshine and having our first ever events here at the property, to our own wedding in 2018—it's on "the gram". I encourage you to check it out.

There is also my blog, bbhwithms.com, which I began in 2013. It's a lifestyle blog (how I live life with my MS), and it has a ton of multiple sclerosis information within its walls. It has some gems like "My Naked 911 Call" and "Wearing Diapers in My Skinny Ass Jeans", and even a post about making a booty call after my marriage had dissolved. But, mixed in with the humor, dabbled amongst the many opportunities to laugh with me, are valuable life lessons on how to live with ease despite this crazy disease.

I took a healing hiatus and haven't written in a few years, but I have a goal of writing weekly again. Truthfully, I am hoping that writing this chapter for this wonderful book about naturally managing ones' multiple sclerosis will be the spark that I need to follow through with that goal. Between our continued journey to make Camp Sunshine all that I have dreamed about, growing lots of weed and hemp, my husband trying out retirement, and the constant antics that just seem to arise in our lives, I have plenty of words and life experiences to share.

Being diagnosed with an incurable disease has turned out to be one of the best things that has happened to me. It allowed me to clean up my act, purge the bullshit from my life, and live a genuinely happy life, despite my disease. My children (now twenty-five, twenty-three, and twenty-one) are amazing human beings—strong, smart, and funny, but most importantly, kind. They've learned empathy. 1 learned I'm strong. I learned to be creative in my pursuit of doing things despite my limitations and to let humor guide me through life. I have found an unwavering faith in myself and my path.

I am back in control, I know can get through anything, and it feels fucking fantastic.

34

Story by
GABRIEL

Diagnosed in 2018
Currently 33 years old
Lives in France
Spotify Podcast: Chronic Stories
Email: ghfrancon@proton.me

On June 18, 2018, I was diagnosed with multiple sclerosis (MS). The diagnosis hit me like a punch by Mike Tyson in his prime—only I was blindfolded and never saw it coming. The notion was so surreal that it all sounded like a terrible nightmare you can't wake up from. Your mind immediately jumps to an analysis of all the potential implications, which, frankly speaking, you can barely comprehend, considering the emotional rush you go through simultaneously.

I'd been told repeatedly during the first few days that I was one of, if not, THE strongest person some people knew, which ordinarily comes as a great compliment. This time though, it made me feel so powerless. I would discreetly tear up when someone said it to me. At the same time, you know deep down that you must demonstrate strength and character to lift the hearts of your loved ones. I am not saying that you need to lie about how you feel. Keeping a positive mindset is ultimately what you'll need to do if you want to tackle a disease that feeds off stress and sorrow. Aside from being deeply hurt psychologically, beyond your own self, you think of your loved ones and how this will impact them, too. The feelings you are forced to deal with are so powerful that it would take hours and countless characters for me to explain it all.

I've never cried so much in my life. I cried every single day for an entire week, hidden from view, most of the time alone in my room at my parents' house. "I never hurt a fly...I don't deserve this," I would tell myself.

When you realize that you're getting better at verbalizing it, you let your head fall within your hands and exclaim: "I cannot believe this is happening to me." The spiral of self-pity and despair can suck you in at the speed of light. I know it because I felt it nearby, but you must stay away from it.

That being said, the situation is inevitably sad and stressful. Finding the right balance of expressing your feelings, even alone in your room, while being optimistic is tough.

One of the hardest comments to hear at first is, "You know, people can live very well with it, nowadays!" To which you just want to answer, "How about we switch places, and you tell me how things are going five years from now? Nah!?" Knowing that we can have a normal life, contrary to what others may think, is not comforting at all. It didn't make me more willing to experience it whatsoever.

The lack of information at first is also something that is hard to deal with because you feel disoriented but don't know where to go from that point, what your journey will be made of, or if you have the necessary courage to succeed.

Handling the sadness of those who love you and understanding that you are not the only one affected is also important. Ignoring their pain is denying them the same right that you have to suffer. The news is so painful that you can easily become selfish, thinking this is only happening to you. But just as the death of someone affects an entire family, so does a bad diagnosis. Even though you must put yourself first, you somehow wish to watch over them, not worrying them more than needed.

They say, when it rains, it pours. This is exactly what happened to me. I lost my dad to cancer eight months following my diagnosis. Yeah...those eight months were tough, man. I had been so intensely sad over my diagnosis that, although crushed by my dad's death, I did not show any emotion. I had no tears left in the tank. It was like my diagnosis had pumped them all out. The urgency I was in to find the key to my health overshadowed the imminent death of my father, too. We already knew by July 2018 (I was diagnosed in June) that the doctor had run out of solutions for my dad, so I had to manage my feelings over my own health, as well as my parents' emotions.

My dad knew that he'd be soon gone—which is hard enough to fathom by itself—but on top of it, he had to accept the idea of leaving both my mom and me to deal with my MS. This is probably what haunted him the most over his last six months. I had to show resilience not only for me, but for him, too. He took his last short but loud breath on the night of February 26, 2019, as I was holding his already cold hand. You see, the body is quite amazing. As all his organs were shutting down, his body redirected his blood towards the heart to help it until the very last moment. This is a known mechanism and the reason why his hands were cold. I forgot to mention that I received my diagnosis on the same day I buried my fourteen-year-old dog in my backyard after we had to put him down…what a great fucking day that was. When it rains, it truly pours.

"I will turn this thing around," I told myself. I went from being devastated to being hopeful, taking matters into my own hands. I'd never researched as intensively and purposefully in my life more than when I was diagnosed. Neuroscience, microbiology, gastroenterology, micro-nutrition, epigenetics—you name it. I just couldn't get enough.

Considering the side effects of medications available to "MSers" and the corruption in the pharmaceutical industry that just wishes to bank on sick people (fifty thousand dollars a year, so two million dollars over forty years for people with MS), I understood that I was on my own. I rejected treatment, and I am happy I did. Although I do not take any medications, I would never point a finger at someone who does. We're in the same boat, after all.

I probably spent several hundreds of hours devouring books and various peer reviewed studies. The first book I read was *Overcoming Multiple Sclerosis* by George Jelinek. This book saved my life. Dr. Jelinek is an Australian emergency doctor (retired now, I believe) whose mom had multiple sclerosis and who was himself diagnosed later in his life. As a researcher, Dr. Jelinek also directed a medical publication, which allowed him to accelerate his research into ways for staying healthy with MS. Visit *overcomingms.org* for more information. His findings have helped hundreds, if not thousands, of people by now. I was floored when reading about one lady who followed his program. Her name is Linda Bloom, an Australian woman who was diagnosed at age twenty-eight like me, and whose latest MRIs do not show any lesions in her brain or spine—as if she never had the disease. In other words, she healed her multiple sclerosis through diet and lifestyle, refusing treatment. When I read about her, I decided that I, too, could do it. Then, I found out about Kristen, who cured her MS without treatment, using a different technique but still revolving around lifestyle. You can read about her in an interview on *medium.com* from 2013. (https://medium.com/cured-disease-naturally/the-woman-who-cured-multiple-sclerosis-11d2ebe47162).

Later, I stumbled upon Mathew Embry, who was diagnosed at nineteen and also chose lifestyle over meds. He is now in his forties and runs like a madman every morning. Not only is he in top health, but he is also in far better shape than the average man—a true inspiration. Mat and his father, Dr. Ashton Embry (Ph.D.), have founded a movement called MS Hope that you can explore via their website called *mshope.com*. As a movie director, Mat also made *Living Proof*—a great documentary about multiple sclerosis that I urge you to watch if you have not yet. It's available on Amazon Prime. It shows well-functioning alternatives to treatment, going at length to demonstrate the cynicism and corruption that surrounds the pharmaceutical industry.

There is also Dr. Terry Wahls, who built on Ashton Embry's work and experimented on herself, creating the Wahls Protocol®. Terry had severe symptoms that made her bedridden. She recovered so well that she can now ride a bike. I do not remember if she takes treatment, but what I do know is that it is her lifestyle and what she puts in her mouth that helped her recover—not the medication. I follow a lot of principles that she applies to her daily life.

There is plenty of hope, as you can see and read in this book. Once I found out about all these people, I felt relieved. They do not follow the same methods to heal their MS, but what they do is obviously working. I kept telling myself, "If they can do it, so can I!"

There is obviously a way for me to be healthy and even heal myself. My diagnosis was a red flag from my body, notifying me that something was not working, and we needed a change of course. The body's first and constant purpose is to be healthy. It is my job to provide it with what is needed, so it can perform its job properly.

When I was diagnosed, I was the healthiest person anyone could think of. I worked out five times a week and ate my veggies and protein. I respected the eight hours of sleep rule. I did not smoke or drink. I would rarely enjoy a cheat meal. I checked every single box the general consensus has to define a healthy, fit individual.

As we know, multiple sclerosis is a chronic disease whose way of treatment resides in its nature: chronicity. You must eat, sleep, and exercise chronically well if you wish to get ahead of the game—and even heal. Let me share a few thoughts on what MS is in my eyes and the current status quo of medicine. First things first, let's tackle the way I see multiple sclerosis working. This is how I explain it every time to people.

Picture Clara going along on her bicycle. She loves it! Until suddenly, she falls. You see what happens and rush to help her back up, assessing if she's hurt. Turns out, she cut herself deep on the knee and does not seem able to get back on her bike. Her knee is sore and bleeding, so she will need a couple of stitches and some time to recover. The cut will leave a mean scar—that's for sure. There are two scenarios possible here to help Clara. One is short-lived, while the other is much more promising:

1. You can apply an antiseptic, stitch her up, and put on a bandage before letting her go.
2. Or you can do all the above, plus investigate why she fell off her bike.

If you only conduct the first part, Clara will eventually get back on her bike. Surely enough, she'll fall again. Every time she falls, she will be left with yet another scar, until her body cannot take it anymore. Eventually, she'll never be able to ride her bicycle again. Multiple sclerosis is no different. If we do not figure out what is causing the body to express itself in such a way, what they call Relapse-Remitting Multiple Sclerosis (RRMS) will perpetually repeat itself until the left overs (the scars) of each relapse (or fall) leave you with too much damage to your nervous system for the body to cope.

I am voluntarily making it sound simple, but I am under no illusion that it is. What I am saying is that we must investigate and experiment on ourselves to put an end to that mechanism, so we do not fall from our bicycles ever again. My message to you is simple: You are not condemned to go downhill as many doctors politely insinuate. You can actually turn this around. You got this! Own your MS narrative. Multiple sclerosis does not define you. It is merely a part of who you are.

I realize as I am writing this that I would have a difficult time saying this to someone in a wheelchair. The scene of Mathew Embry in *Living Proof* where he goes to meet a fellow woman with MS who must use a walker, even after stem cell treatment, rushes to my mind. He manages to keep his emotions in as the interview proceeds but has to let go of them as soon as he leaves her home. That scene is powerful. Just a note here that Mathew recently shot *Living Proof 2*, which we hope will be available sometime in 2023. To you who have lost a lot of your independence and maybe most of your faith, whomever you might be, just know that I have deep love and empathy for you. I have those feelings because being in your position is my worst fear if I am being honest.

But even if I lose my battle because of X and Y, and indeed end up losing my autonomy, I must keep faith that what I practice daily can put anyone back on track. I must hold on to that thought, if only to keep sane. And because part of me strongly believes in it. Some fellow MSers have had incredible comebacks against all odds, like Terry Wahls, but she is not the only one. This book is proof. And as I often say, "If they've done it, there is absolutely no reason that you can't!"

Multiple sclerosis can be a pivotal moment in your life to discover true health, which is not only summed up by diet and exercise. Diet, sleep, and exercise are of course paramount, but nailing all three while living in a toxic environment will not be enough. Make sure that those who surround you support you in every possible way, and make sure that no one in your intimate circle causes you stress beyond reason.

When it comes to food, it might not always be so easy to eat out because you will not be able to have the same food as others—but that's fine! You know why? Because these foods and behaviors are probably what gave you MS in the first place and what powers the skyrocketing of all chronic illnesses in society. Do not let MS define who you are. You are not "that guy" or "that girl" with MS. No one is allowed to stick any label on you, period. You can be that incredible human being who is kicking ass at life —a leading example of resilience for your friends and family, who are in awe of all that you achieve and who almost forget that you have MS.

People would never guess I have multiple sclerosis. My relatives actually forget sometimes because I have not changed one bit. I even have to explain to people who don't know about the disease that it can be serious because, as they see me, they think it's a walk in the park—haha! I should probably clarify that this is not medical advice, and you should consult with your physician. But this isn't going to be a place for me to lie, so I'll be as nuanced about it as I most honestly can. It is my opinion that your health is your responsibility and yours only. Any doctor is an advisor, not a decision-maker. You make the decision for what treatment you take or do not take. No one should ever force you to do anything—treatment, MRIs, whatever. I do not receive any treatment, and honestly, never would for many reasons.

I believe that the probability for doctors to be wrong in their approach is as high as their certainty that going without treatment is bad for people with multiple sclerosis. In more blunt terms, taking a medication without changing your lifestyle has a very high probability that you will relapse again, and your doctor will prescribe you more and more potent drugs, "until there's nothing left on the shelf"—an expression from my dad who died from cancer.

Whether or not you decide to undergo treatment, changing your lifestyle represents the highest probability for you to stabilize and eventually heal. This is the part where I must tell the truth about what I think. I believe available treatments to date have a higher probability of endangering your health rather than helping it. I simply will not lie about it. There are many reasons why I think this. It intoxicates your body and worsens what we call the "toxic burden". The toxic burden refers to the accumulation of harmful chemicals, pollutants, and toxins in the body over time. Treatments force your body to work harder to detoxify when its energy could be spent on healing. Although they refer to them as immunomodulators, they really knock your immune system out, which is unnatural. Imagine being semi-consciously in a state of drunkenness forever. That's essentially how your immune system is probably feeling when undergoing treatment. Stopping treatment will put your health at risk because once you stop, your immune system will attempt to wake up by jump-starting itself. This will probably cause a massive inflammatory reaction. As we all know, inflammation equals a high likelihood of relapse. If by all accounts, doctors agree that MS is a snowflake disease, meaning that every case is different, then why standardize treatment as if we're all the same? It makes no sense to me. Some of the side effects of these treatments are horrendous. I almost considered trying Lemtrada because it's a once-in-a-lifetime treatment. But the main possible side effect is that you have a fifty-fifty chance of getting chronic thyroid disease. I mean, seriously. And guess what? I know two fantastic women who have taken it in the UK (where it is mostly used), and sure thing—one of them must take thyroid pills for the rest of her life. So, thank you, but no thank you.

With all that being said, I will repeat it again: I would never point a finger at anyone who takes medication. We are in the same boat. I wish to help, not to blame. I am just being my authentic self. The reason I am sharing my story in this book is to help as many people as possible, not to criticize you for your choices. I am not a doctor or a researcher. The points I've just made are my opinion, based on my personal research, analysis, and understanding of what living with a chronic disease entails. The golden rule is that you decide for yourself. And just like the quote by Bruce Lee says, "Absorb what is useful, discard what is useless, and add what is specifically your own."

What I learned from reading about these various people mentioned before who were handling their multiple sclerosis successfully but with different methods is that there isn't a one-size-fits-all remedy. I have changed many things in my lifestyle and am doing very well. I train five times a week and am still very strong, if not stronger, than three years ago. You must create your own recipe for your personal, unique success story. But there are some key elements that we cannot ignore, such as the absolute necessity to cut all dairy because it not only activates the disease, but it also sustains its process. That being said, Kristen (who was mentioned before) consumes goat dairy from time to time. That is a risk I am not willing to take, but hey, it is working for her, and she is doing very well! Mathew Embry eats chicken, along with Terry Wahls, who also eats ghee and game meat. They also both advise against gluten. George Jelinek cuts out all meat but allows for fish, egg whites, and gluten. His program is the one I decided to follow the most from day one. I, however, do not consume eggs anymore. I usually say that I am pesca-vegan.

Here are the daily practices I've adopted to live my life to the fullest. These are based on my experience and what I've seen working for other MSers who are doing fantastic, as well. Let's start with what they agree upon and build our way from there. They all agree that dairy is poison for people with MS. That means no butter, milk, cheese, cream, and nothing containing them. Vitamin D3, B12, and Omega-3s are crucial, along with antioxidants. Loading your plate with plenty of vegetables and fruits, especially greens, is vital. Also, eating homemade, organic food as much as possible will benefit you immensely. They suggest exercising as often as possible. I exercise five times a week.

Now, let's build up from that list and add whatever I found to be useful, taken from various people working in health research. I also consume zero dairy. If I mistakenly ingest it, I either drink a draining smoothie to rid my system of it, or I make myself vomit, then drink the smoothie. Sounds radical? So does being in a wheelchair. Fasting is one of the most powerful tools in your arsenal. I would suggest looking at the work of Professor David Sinclair from Harvard University. He dedicated his career to researching longevity, and he wrote a book called Lifespan.

There is a great podcast of him and Shaun Parish on The Knowledge Project. He speaks at length about the positive impacts of fasting.

I also eat mainly homemade food, not the food-like substances that make up 95% of most supermarkets. Industrial food is garbage. If you consume it, make sure to eat very well afterwards to make up for it. I wouldn't make a habit of eating industrial, premade food. All good things in life take time. Shortcuts never do you any good. I also eat more than eight vegetables a day. I usually make a salad consisting of lettuce, cilantro, carrots, cucumbers, and endives. I eat lentil dahl almost every day with green lentils, beluga lentils, onions, garlic, and avocado. Dahl rice is a dish that can be made with any type of lentil. I usually eat dahl with potatoes (sweet or not). For your salad, you could also add purple cabbage, peppers, or beets. I often have a daily smoothie to sustain my training. It consists of banana, blueberries, peanut butter, and vegan chocolate protein. So, I total between fourteen to seventeen veggies on average—sometimes even more. I have found that eating fermented foods full of probiotics helps to populate the gut with healthy bacteria that help ease digestion. Lastly, I take a freezing cold-water shower for one-to-three minutes upon waking. This has a tremendously positive impact on your health. Andrew Huberman covers it in his podcast. Cold showers can be used for either physical or mental purposes. What you need to remember is that both play to each other's advantage. Improving your overall physical health will promote mental health, and vice versa.

Although I am doing very well today, I felt like shit when I was diagnosed—just like anyone else. I built myself into what I am today. It took true grit and was not always easy. From the moment the diagnosis was confirmed, everything I did after that became a first—first drive being sick, first training, first shower, first plane ride, first breakfast, lunch, dinner, and so on. I knew that my life would never be the same. There is a "before" and an "after". I wouldn't go as far to say that it feels as if you suddenly acquired ten years' worth of wisdom, but you sure feel as if life, along with everything you enjoy in it, is far more precious than you ever could have realized before. The phone calls warning all of your family and close friends are awful because you have to experience the same feelings every single time, saying, "I'll be fine," although you have no idea if that's true. Saying to yourself, "I am sick" is the strangest thing I've experienced so far in my life. I can now confidently say that no one understands this unless they have lived through it themselves. It was the first time that I experienced what "heartbroken" truly means, but I refused this new reality that was forced upon me. And it has helped me grow in ways I never expected. Being diagnosed with multiple sclerosis sucks but having it doesn't have to.

35

Story by

TALIA

Diagnosed in 2016
Currently 37 years old
Lives in United States
Social media: ALFA by Talia
www.taliahalberor.com

When I was twenty-six years old, I moved from Israel to the U.S. and started fresh in all areas of my life. I was in a new relationship with a wonderful person who, over time, became my husband, and it seemed as if life couldn't get any better than it was.
I had a great partner, I lived in a beautiful house, I had a lot of freedom in so many ways, I didn't lack anything, and I had all the freedom to choose how I wanted to design my life. When I was twenty-nine and already married, even though to one's eye it still seemed as if I had it all, inside of me it felt like something was still missing. Saying that I was "unhappy" would be an understatement.

Around this time, I traveled to Israel, from there to China, and as soon as I landed back in Miami, I got sick. It felt like I initially caught a bad cold, but unlike any other cold, this one wasn't going away, and it was accompanied by an unexpected bad headache. The whole experience was quite unusual for me since I rarely suffered from headaches. As time went on, the headache worsened, and I experienced very low energy levels. I made an appointment to see a virtual doctor because I was too ill and fatigued to travel to the doctor's office. His answer was that it was a sinus infection. A few days later, I saw him again because I noticed a "cloud" starting to form over my left eye, and the pain around it worsened. He diagnosed it as a severe sinus infection and recommended over-the-counter medication from the pharmacy, reassuring me not to worry.

I followed his advice and didn't worry at first. But a few days later, a startling revelation struck me—I had lost my ability to see almost completely. It became apparent when I met my now ex-husband for lunch at a nearby restaurant. While walking through a store, I unexpectedly bumped into a wall, realizing that I didn't see it, even though it was right there in front of me.

That day, we went to see an optometrist, who referred me to another doctor. By the end of the day, we had seen four different doctors before we finally landed with a neurologist. He gave me steroids after just a couple of tests because he was concerned my vision wouldn't return. I had no clue what was going on, so I did everything they suggested.

The neurologist ordered magnetic resonance imaging (MRI), and the test results showed a clear lesion. I wasn't diagnosed then and there. Instead, he told me, "Because we already injected you, I can't tell you 100%, but we want you to know that it's most likely multiple sclerosis (MS)." He sent me to an MS specialist that immediately suggested I start medications. Since it was easier for me to believe it wasn't an official diagnosis, I carried on with my life and began feeling physically better once the relapse subsided.

As I reflect on that period of my life, I now recognize that if someone had assessed me, I would have received a definitive clinical depression diagnosis. The challenges I faced, both internally and externally, took a toll on any area of my life, and not very long after, my marriage came to an end, as well. After separating, I devoted considerable time to introspection and embarked on a profound journey of self-discovery. It became clear to me that despite having everything that many people desire, I felt an inner emptiness and unhappiness. The word "gratitude" kept echoing in my mind, as I longed to experience it but didn't know how.

I decided to attend a Tony Robbins event. It was a transformative experience that opened my eyes to numerous insights. The most significant realization was that I possess the capability to think, feel, and become more than what I had been, and that ultimately, I am responsible for my own growth. This journey of self-exploration led me to meet someone who suggested I enroll in a personal development course called Gratitude Trainings. The mere mention of the word "gratitude" resonated deeply with me, prompting me to eagerly sign up. The intensive four-day course proved to be one of the most enlightening experiences I'd ever had at that time. By the end of those four days, I felt an overwhelming sense that I could achieve, pursue, or embody anything I desired. This emotional and remarkable experience left a profound impact on me.

After participating in the program, my beliefs underwent a significant shift. I realized that I had the power to choose my path based on the life I truly desired, not just what I had been taught was right or wrong. Coming from Israel, a region plagued by ongoing conflict and suffering, I felt compelled to bring this transformative work back home. My aim was to bridge the divide between Palestinians and Israelis, helping them understand that love can replace fear and hatred. I firmly believe that by connecting with their inner power and making choices that align with their vision for a better life, peace could become a reality, leading to positive changes for many.

I immersed myself in the world of personal transformation, pursuing training to become a creator and facilitator of transformative programs. As a student of the International Coaching Federation (ICF), I developed my skills as a coach. Guided by my vision to bring about transformation in Israel, I also took on the role of a coach, helping individuals in their journey to transform specific areas of their lives.

Around that time, another flare began. This time, I was affected a lot worse, feeling a constant sense of numbness and tingling sensations. It started with my feet and traveled up my legs, but I did my best to ignore it. I began feeling tired, which gradually turned into daily fatigue, becoming a regular part of my life. It got so bad that sometimes I had to take a nap in the middle of lunch just so I could finish eating. When I drove, sometimes I'd have to pull over and rest because I didn't want to fall asleep at the wheel. I had tingling in many parts of my body, and my left hand felt very weak. When I found out what "brain-fog" was, I later connected it to my MS symptoms.

One morning, I noticed my left knee and ankle weren't functioning properly. The discomfort persisted and eventually worsened to the point where I could barely walk. I ended up in the emergency room, where the medical team suggested spinal surgery. As I shared my previous experience with "MS" and the vision loss, additional tests were conducted, revealing more lesions on my brain and spine. It became clear that optic neuritis was not a one-time occurrence but a progressing disease. This time, the doctor officially diagnosed me with multiple sclerosis and emphasized the importance of medication as the main treatment. They discussed the likelihood of needing a wheelchair in the future and advised me to prepare for the life-altering changes ahead.

I was told that medication was the only thing that could possibly slow down the progression of MS. When I arrived at the hospital to receive my first dose of the medication I chose, after being instructed by my doctor to do so, the nurse used extreme caution when administering the drug, which made me ask some questions. She warned me that even the slightest contact with any portion of this drug, which resembled a chemotherapy drug, could result in severe health consequences for other individuals or pets involved. I was very upset with the fact that no one had explained what I was about to put into my body. I researched and compared drugs online, but I didn't realize how extremely high the risk was. I remember the level of fear and confusion at that time. They say medications are the only route with MS, but those medications could majorly harm other parts of my body that would then require other medications to "help" with. This whole concept didn't make much sense to me.

I remember my doctor saying, "You know, MS medications can be tricky. We'll probably change your medication later on, so just go with what you want for now, and we'll adjust." It seemed as if he knew it might not be effective. At that time, I didn't fully understand his words, but soon I began experiencing the harsh side effects of the medication. My body was covered in rashes, and I suffered from stomach issues and headaches. I don't remember much from that period, except that my entire body was in constant discomfort and pain. What I remember very well is that there was a lot of fear involved in the process.

Eventually, I had to sell my business since I was the only one running it; I couldn't handle the daily tasks due to how I was doing. The amount of mistakes I was making due to what I later realized was brain fog affected the quality of my work. It was stressful, which I believe caused more symptoms in my body. This is when I noticed that every time MS took a turn, I was experiencing stress in my life.

This was a tough time in my life. I kept thinking about living without mobility, not fulfilling my dream of being an independent woman and a mother, not clear about my future...I knew I was in victim mode but didn't know how to escape it. Brain fog and fatigue made my journey very challenging. I felt like I was stuck in a never-ending cycle, until one day, I had a revelation. A voice from within whispered, "This doesn't have to be your life; there is a better life out there, waiting for you."

That small voice within me became the catalyst I needed to push myself forward toward my goals. It sparked a realization that I was in control of my own life and possessed the power to pursue anything I desired. I couldn't help but envision a future, filled with happiness, good health, and the opportunity to share my passion for coaching with others. However, I also recognized that clinging to a victim mentality and self-pity would only stop these aspirations from becoming a reality. I knew I wanted to travel and thought of how I could help others while staying in beautiful places. So, I spent most of my time studying, taking courses, reading books, and following the most influential teachers, leaders, and scientists—to regain control over my own decisions and reclaim autonomy, ensuring that I, not multiple sclerosis, was the one determining my path.

Little by little, my body started responding favorably due to my newfound optimism, the changes I was implementing in my life, and the way I was perceiving my reality. Gradually, I began to gain confidence that my dedicated efforts were paying off, ultimately resulting in full reversal of all the symptoms, weakness, and limitations I lived with, leading me to make the decision to discontinue the medication. I was very happy to put an end to the side effects and the unnecessary toxins the meds brought to my body. It was like magic; one after another, my symptoms were disappearing. The numbness and tingling vanished, spasms stopped, the effects of optic neuritis completely healed, and fatigue lifted. I regained strength and control in my hands and legs, allowing me to never use the cane again. Thankfully, my mind became clear and focused once more.

My diet had been fairly healthy before, but even more so since I started my healing journey. I pay attention to which foods nourish me. I make sure to eat foods that give my body the power to take care of itself, and I nourish both my mind and body on a daily basis. I understood that many people, upon receiving a chronic illness diagnosis, often focus on changing their diet in hopes of achieving significant results. However, despite their best efforts, they may still find themselves falling short of their desired outcomes. Through my studies, knowledge, and personal experience, I came to understand the profound impact mind transformation has on our health goals. I learned that our thoughts, emotions, perception of reality, and lifestyle choices can actually influence the expression of our genes. As I dove deeper into research, I began to realize what people with MS might be missing. Despite their dedication to a healthy diet, they often struggle to heal. I discovered that true healing becomes challenging when the body is constantly in survival mode, burdened by low-vibration emotions, fear, and chronic stress.

Around the same time that I had this realization, people with MS began appearing in my life (prior to my own diagnosis, I had never heard of MS). As they applied the insights and strategies I had developed for myself, remarkable changes took place, and they began experiencing notable shifts in their physical well-being. I realized none of this was coincidental—I don't believe in coincidences. I believe everything that appears in our reality has a purpose; everything is designed carefully and specifically for us by the universe and our higher selves, including chronic illness.

In my mind, I started to think that this was one of the reasons MS showed up in my life because I held knowledge and understanding that I could share with my community. Slowly, I was shifting my coaching practice to working only with people who were living with MS, and the results have been amazing. I now help men and women around the whole world through their healing journey from MS and other autoimmune diseases, and I am coaching health coaches to improve their skills and expand their ability to support people on their healing, and I feel better than ever, both in my mind and my body. I believe that love is the answer for healing, and the moment we truly fall in love with ourselves, with our lives, and with the present moment—true healing can be achieved.

These days, I don't feel like I'm just managing MS; I've gone beyond that. MS no longer manifests itself in any form. Through a complete transformation of my life, I no longer take actions to prevent MS from appearing. I've found a sense of freedom within myself that takes care of everything. I think differently, I process information differently, and my beliefs about myself have undergone a profound transformation. Not only have my beliefs about myself changed, but also my beliefs about human beings, the world, and reality. Meditation has become a regular practice for me, allowing me to focus inward rather than seeking external validation. As a result, I no longer feel vulnerable to others' actions or words. This heightened sense of responsibility brings me freedom and peace. When there is peace within, the body no longer engages in a war against itself.

I meditate regularly and maintain a very clean diet. I prioritize making choices that align with my personal values and the life I aspire to live. I have come to realize that I have a purpose on this planet, and in order to fulfill it, I must prioritize self-care. If I neglect my well-being, I may not be able to offer others what I am destined to share. As a result, I operate from a different perspective, a heightened level of responsibility that empowers me to prioritize self-care each day when I wake up.

Through my work with different individuals that were living with MS, I developed a program called "The Mind 2 Body Program". I felt it was missing from the MS landscape because this is specifically what I realized I needed on my healing journey, but it didn't exist. Each professional was offering a specific healing modality, and with autoimmune diseases, including MS, there can be multiple underlying causes, making it difficult to pinpoint the specific trigger for each individual. So, if somebody wants to truly heal, there is no other way but spending tens of thousands of dollars to acquire the necessary knowledge, like I did. Clearly, we all know that the body needs more than just dietary changes to facilitate healing. While adjusting one's diet is important, the disease can still progress during this time, potentially leading to feelings of discouragement and a sense of lagging behind others who seem to be recovering. This uncertainty can have a big impact on people's lives. My program tackles these concerns by including different approaches that help the body focus on healing and regain its natural healing abilities. It empowers individuals by tapping into the body's own wisdom and healing capacity.

It breaks my heart every time I meet someone who doesn't believe that they have the power to heal themselves because I see those "miracles" in my practice every day. It is all backed by science—none of it is miraculous, and it is so unfortunate that we live in a world where most of our doctors don't voluntarily share this information with us. These cases only seem miraculous because we're often told we can't do it, not because they are miraculous. I hope this message reaches those who want to empower themselves because we all have the capability, and we all deserve it.

Someone once asked me the question: How can I eat healthy when I travel so much?" It's easy! I take responsibility and plan ahead. I prefer to book an Airbnb versus a hotel because Airbnb provides me with a kitchen. I travel with my blender and other kitchen essentials, even if they add extra weight to my luggage. This way, I'm not dependent on the people I travel with or the restaurants they offer. As soon as I arrive, I visit the supermarket and buy the necessary ingredients that will serve me best. This level of responsibility to myself is essential, and I rely on it. I don't have any expectations from others to provide what I need. Smoothies make it easy for me to consume great food daily, no matter where I am. I often laugh that I make salad smoothies, mixing vegetables, leafy greens with some fruits for flavor, chia seeds, and water. I avoid processed food and animal products, focusing mainly on vegetables and fruits.

If you are reading this and are newly diagnosed, the most important message I have for you is to take a deep breath and understand that everything that happens in life is a course correction. It's a message we receive that is designed for us in a way that, if we end up tuning into and listening to it, it ends up working for our highest good—even though I know it doesn't feel this way necessarily. Once you realize that, you can allow yourself to process it and make decisions to overcome it. If you succumb to the fear that comes through what you read or hear, you're likely to make choices that keep you trapped. Even if a small part of you wants to heal, focus on the positive stories out there. Learn from those who achieved the results you want, and stay curious about why life, God, the universe, or whatever you believe in, has temporarily slowed you down. Then, take immediate action. You can reach out to me or someone you trust for support, and go for it. Don't waste time. Every moment counts in these circumstances.

Looking back, I can say that I unknowingly took immediate action, but it also took me three-to-four years to realize I could have changed my diet right away. I used to eat healthily because I cooked most of the time. Being from Israel, the food in the United States often tasted bland to me, so I preferred to make my own meals. Additionally, I liked knowing what ingredients were in my food, although my knowledge had its limits, and I wasn't aware of how bad any processed item in the states can be. I was not aware of many things. My diet consisted of a lot of eggs and chicken. Each morning, I would have bread before going to the gym, and when I returned, I would eat eggs for protein. I also made smoothies and ate vegetables because I always enjoyed them. Overall, my diet was a lot better than the common American diet, yet I wasn't aware of what my body actually needed. I had food sensitivities to many of the most healing vegetables at the time, so even though I thought I did great, my body was still lacking what I didn't know I needed at the time.

Prior to my diagnosis, I suffered from ongoing digestion problems throughout my entire adulthood, starting at the age of eighteen. It was tough. Unfortunately, I didn't recognize these symptoms as indications that something was not working properly in my body to such an extreme.

I should have paid attention to these signs and taken different action. However, I was repeatedly told by doctors that it was just irritable bowel syndrome (IBS) and that there is nothing that can be done. Additionally, I used to consume processed foods and alcohol to have fun. Thankfully, those habits are now in my past. I hardly drink anymore. Instead, I've learned to create happiness, joy, and energy from within myself. I teach exactly that—this is what true healing entails. It involves recognizing that we came into this world with a clean slate. But as we went through life, we absorbed beliefs about ourselves, some of which we realize, and some we don't. These beliefs end up being the designers of our lives, whether we like it or not. Healing involves peeling back those layers and reconnecting with your true, authentic self, without judgement.

Real happiness comes from within; seeking it in external things, like money or job titles, is temporary. What happens when those things disappear? Who are you without them? It's about being true to yourself from the inside, not relying on external factors. That's where the real work lies. And even with conditions like MS, when you stop fighting yourself, your body stops fighting you, too. That's why I always say that true, lasting healing can only happen from the inside out.

I love the concept of this book. Instead of sharing fear with each other, we get to share love, inspiration, and empowerment. My wish is that it reaches as many readers as possible. I always say that if even just one person receives a message that inspires them to take action and conquer this disease, then my purpose is fulfilled!

You have more power than you were led to believe, and you have everything it takes to successfully overcome this challenge called MS.

Sending you love, light and healing,
Talia

36

Story by
ALICE SYDOW

Diagnosed in 2007
Currently 48 years old
Lives in St. Louis, Missouri, United States
Social media: @styleyourglow369
www.styleyourglow.com

My journey with multiple sclerosis (MS) has been a lengthy one, navigating a course filled with medications resembling a passport's array of stamps. Instead of traveling to somewhere fabulous, I received a one-way ticket to Crazytown and Depressedville, with many stops at red lights on Anxiety Avenue. If you are reading this, perhaps you can relate. You see, I was never taught how to regulate or manage my emotions, and I was always a deeply sensitive girl. As I grew up, even during my grade school years, I found myself attuned to other people's emotions. I can recall being on the playground when bullies would tear down those who could not defend themselves. I would stick up for them and try to console the victims because I could feel what they were feeling. It hurts badly to feel others' emotions. When my own emotions became big, I didn't know how to regulate or process them. I would bury them inside my body. I never learned how to let them out, even though I wanted to SCREAM. Over time, those feelings and trapped emotions built up inside my body, which is what I attribute to the dis-ease that unfolded in my life. Alongside this, I encountered other factors like mercury fillings (mercury poisoning), residing in a dorm room during college that had been closed-down due to asbestos, six months after I had moved out, that resulted in losing my sense of smell (fungicides/toxins/asbestos), and picking up parasites during a trip to Paris when I was twenty-two.

Adding to the burden of the viral load in my body, I endured both verbal and physical abuse as a small child, unable to defend myself. I never learned coping skills for handling the shame and sadness brought on by these experiences. Seeking validation, I resorted to love, alcohol, sex, shopping, and more addictions, unable to build a strong foundation. My saving grace came with the diagnosis because it forced me to heal unresolved trauma that I never even knew I had. It wasn't until I was diagnosed with MS, numb from the waist down, bedridden, handed a cane, bankrupt, and broken that I had the time to process and look deep within. I finally found the freedom I had been searching for my entire life. Now, as I put the cane in the closet and begin to walk freely, I bring more balance to my life. Gone are the days of people pleasing, playing the nice girl, the good girl, the victim, and the girl with the disability/cane. The old story was about me reaching for a cane, or anything outside of myself, to help me cope with the pain. NOW, I tell a NEW story: a story of resilience, a story of compassion, a story of grace, a story of accomplishment—a story of FREEDOM.

My intention in sharing my story is to shed light on the workings of big pharma and how I felt trapped within that system. I found a way to break free and learned that healing IS POSSIBLE. Instead of accepting the notion of "impossible" or "incurable", words doctors often use which instill fear, I want to spread the message that healing is within reach. My aim is to inspire hope and show that there are alternative paths to wellness and empowerment. Audrey Hepburn once said, "The word itself spells 'I'm POSSIBLE'." In my discovery, words have power. When I began to look at the root cause of my health condition, I realized that it was my body out of alignment and flow that led to dis-ease. Suddenly, I found myself using a word I never thought would apply to me—disability. But then, I decided to take the "dis" out of the equation and get to the root of the problem. I discovered the ABILITY to find healing and balance.

It wasn't until I challenged and reversed all the programming I had been taught about the condition that I began to create a new story. I wanted to redefine not just the "dis-ease" portrayed by the western medical model as multiple sclerosis, but to tell a new story about my journey of healing.

Every day, I shift my mindset and am retraining my brain to live a life of freedom, ease, and grace.

However, before I share with you where I am now, I need to introduce you to a version of Alice who was diagnosed with a condition doctors call MS, and what I refer to as
"The body being out of flow and balance". We'll call her "Adderall Alice".

Let's begin, shall we?

We all know the story of Alice who goes down the rabbit hole. Like Alice, my own journey began as I traveled the world to far-flung destinations, having the time of my life as a Travel Director. I was constantly on the road with a travel company, working 320 days a year for five years, conducting corporate events and business meetings for Fortune 500 clients. At twenty-three, I was living the life at first class VIP events, such as the American Music Awards, the Super Bowl, the Kentucky Derby, the Indianapolis 500, and several other high-profile events. I was getting a taste of what life was like in the fast lane through VIP clubs, red carpets, and five-star resorts. I traveled to far destinations, such as South Africa, Buenos Aires, and the Greek Islands. It wasn't until I became burnt out and tired of traveling that I began to look for another opportunity.

Unfortunately, at that time, the job market was challenging as September 11th had happened the prior Fall, and no one was hiring. I ended up finding a job that paid twice my salary as a Business Analyst, which relocated me from St. Louis to Minneapolis earlier that year. I had majored in marketing in college and always wanted to be in sales, so I thought that even though I disliked math, I could transition into sales once I got my foot in the door. I had a beautiful, large office; yet I felt like a caged bird, analyzing sales data. A dark contrast from lying on a yacht in the Mediterranean, being sprayed with a water bottle by a hot Danish man in full uniform.

Despite being far from following my passion, my goal was to adopt a mindset of "getting a few years of experience, then transition". I disliked the job very much; however, the management and training were exceptional. I ended up excelling and received a promotion almost a year later to a Retail Sales Representative role. This time, I was wearing khaki pants while walking into accounts, like Walmart and PetSmart, selling pet food and schlepping fifty-pound bags of dog food as I stocked the shelves of major retailers. Again, I disliked the role, but I felt I needed the experience. You might be wondering how different it was to go from traveling the world, staying in luxurious hotels, like the Ritz-Carlton and the Four Seasons, in the exciting travel industry, to working in the pet food industry. Let me tell you, it was a stark contrast, and this is where the dis-ease in my body began to take shape.

One day, I was in a Walmart, looking at a shelf stocked with cat food (snooze), reading the pricing labels. I saw one price tag above another. I didn't realize what was going on, so I sloughed it off as just being overly tired. The following day, I was on my way to the airport during the week off for the Thanksgiving holiday to work an event in Scottsdale for a golf program. As I walked to the gate to catch the plane, the double vision started to resurface. I called the Lead of the program, and he suggested I go to a LensCrafters (an eyewear retailer) before going to the work room at the hotel.

After arriving at the mall, I managed to see the ophthalmologist, and he examined my eyes. Concerned about what he saw, he recommended immediate magnetic resonance imaging (MRI). Despite it being Thanksgiving week, I got the scans done. When the radiologist approached me afterward, they informed me that the staff had left but felt compelled to tell me that I might have a brain tumor. In utter shock, I went back to my hotel. I spoke with the team, and they suggested I fly home immediately to be with my family. It was a celebratory holiday, and all my family could focus on was the thought that I had to undergo brain surgery. I was twenty-nine years old; it was a very scary time.

I had to wait almost a week to see a neurologist. She said that my scan indicated a possibility of MS, but she couldn't officially diagnose it as it wasn't within the guidelines of the MS rule book at that time. I had no idea what MS was. Back then (circa 2005), doctors did not give an official diagnosis until the patient experienced a second flare-up or occurrence. The neurologist recommended that I undergo an evoked potential test and a spinal tap, which involves inserting a needle into the spine. I agreed to the evoked potential test but decided against the spinal tap because of my severe fear of needles. Little did I know that within a few years, I would be giving myself a shot every day for the duration of SEVEN YEARS! The doctor told me to wait until I had another flare-up, then she could officially diagnose me and prescribe the necessary medication. I went home and lived my life, trying not to focus on the unknowns of my future. The rules around this are different now. They suggest medication immediately following diagnosis.

The second flare-up didn't occur until two years later, after I had transitioned from the pet food industry to managing events for a company run by one of the largest liquor companies in the world. My job entailed hiring youthful looking models to serve liquor in bars, restaurants, and events. After my success in implementing great processes and improvements in that role, I received a promotion and was managing all the restaurant sales for the entire state of Minnesota. I had achieved my goal of making six figures, but life had a different plan for me.

I was now thirty-one. One day while I was working out at the gym, I noticed tingling on the bottom of my feet. I initially thought it was my Diesel tennis shoes, as I had purchased them in Italy, but unfortunately, I was wrong. Over the course of a few days, the numbness and tingling traveled up to my waist. I called my neurologist and was finally diagnosed with multiple sclerosis. I was devastated and felt like my life had shattered, convinced I was going to end up in a wheelchair because that is what I was initially told.

During this time, there was so much activity taking place, which only added to my mind-body-spirit dysregulation. When I look back on how I was living when numbness overtook my body, it dawned on me that perhaps I became numb because I was numb to life! This made sense to me because I was not in alignment with my true self. I was working a job I didn't love, ignoring the signs, chasing the dollar, and attempting to numb the pain by not dealing with the root cause of why dis-ease manifested in my life. I knew something was wrong, and I was not caring for myself like I should. I was completely disconnected from my body and my life.

The day I was given the news, the neurologist prescribed a medication to help with the condition, which to my dismay, was a shot I had to give myself everyday (Copaxone), a stimulant for fatigue (Ritalin, then Adderall), antidepressants, anti-anxiety medication, and sleep medication (Ambien). There were never any suggestions on holistic or more natural approaches, like mindfulness, mediation, yoga, supplements, homeopathic remedies, etc. I hope that today, more neurologists are aware of these tools that are readily available to help manage symptoms, emotions, and stress. But sadly, I think as a patient, YOU are responsible for being your own advocate. This is why so much fear lives within the autoimmune world because doctors are still saying that the body attacks itself. I understand why they say this, as the myelin sheath gets diminished; however, that narrative needs to be reframed. As an abuse survivor (mental and physical), I've carried a lot of shame around my body. So naturally, when the doctors told me it was my body's fault for attacking itself, it triggered self-hatred and anger because of the trauma I endured as a child.

Now, let's continue down the rabbit hole. Once I was diagnosed and in shock, I pretty much lived with the shame that there was something wrong with me and constantly put myself down in my head. I eventually (thank GOD) regained all feeling and function in my lower extremities after eight months of being bedridden. It is also important to note that at the time of the initial diagnosis, I was extremely depressed and shared with a not-so-close friend that my life would be better if I jumped off the balcony of my condo because I could not handle this diagnosis. She took me to outpatient therapy where I had to go daily for months. While I was there, they pumped me full of more drugs like Ambien and Zoloft, Abilify, etc. so I recall feeling strung out. I continued taking them, but in hindsight, I believe I was situationally depressed because of the multiple sclerosis diagnosis, and I might not have needed such heavy doses or combinations of medications. If more time was spent learning emotion regulation verses pumping my body with pharmaceuticals, I feel things would have been different.

As time passed, I started feeling better, and my friends invited me to go out and meet them. I remember choosing a beautiful dress in blue and green colors that brightened my skin tone. When I looked in the mirror, I thought to myself, "I look pretty; I don't look or feel sick." It amazed me how dressing up lifted my spirits after being bedridden. It made me realize that if I could feel this good by putting on a great outfit, I could potentially help others feel better, too.

Over the next week, I discovered the image consulting industry, and to my surprise, it turned out that being an image consultant was an actual career. Excited about this career, I immediately approached my mom and told her my plan to fly to NYC for certification in image line design and color. Off I went to pursue my newfound passion, and in doing so, I found my JOY. Corporate America was no longer my focus; instead, I was working for myself, doing what I loved. I was so excited to create a new life for myself that I did not put any focus or attention on my health condition. I did not speak about MS, and no one around me knew I had it. I hid behind the closed doors of shame, morning, and night, while administering my Copaxone shot, suffering silently on the inside. If that is not closeted shame, then I don't know what is, right, Brene Brown?

From my viewpoint, I acted like I did not have MS. I did not give it airtime in my mind. However, I was not working on the inner shame and anger; I was just stuffing it down, which is how I was taught to deal with emotions. It's no wonder I like to use the acronym "MS" for "Must Scream", as I was never taught how to let my emotions out and that it was okay to do so. According to Louise Hay's book "You Can Heal Your Life", she states, "MS indicates mental hardness, hard-heartedness, iron-will, inflexibility, and fear. She suggests a new thought pattern, "By choosing loving, joyous thoughts, I create a joyous and loving world. I am safe and free." I wish I had known this then as I would have written this down on notecards and hung them on my mirror. Instead, I took my daily shot and focused on what brought me joy—helping others feel good and showing them their own inner beauty. I thought I was doing the work, but I was scapegoating and bypassing.

Although I was teaching others how to love themselves, I was not in alignment with my truth. Deep down, I had not done the inner work of truly loving myself, accepting the diagnosis, and understanding why the diagnosis had shown up in the first place. Six months after I flew back from NYC with my certification, my career took off. I started doing live TV shows, made appearances on Twin Cities Live, worked with radio stations, and styled photo shoots for newspapers and magazines. Additionally, I began consulting with clients, helping them with wardrobe and color choices. I even appeared on the hit reality show produced by Rachel Zoe called *Resale Royalty*, which is currently on Amazon Prime.

It was a successful seven-year fashionable run, until it wasn't!

During those years, I was on Copaxone until Tecfidera came out. My neurologist suggested I try it because it was the first oral drug to hit the market. I had been on Tecfidera for a short time, and when I was heading to a closet edit appointment with a client, my phone died. I knew the general vicinity of where she lived, as I had been there before but made a wrong turn off the highway. I found myself in an industrial area and pulled over to an auto body shop to ask for directions in a sea of office buildings. I walked into an all-male body shop, dressed to impress. They were perplexed by my random appearance in their garage. I asked for directions to the Eden Prairie mall in Minnesota. I knew how to get to my client's house from the mall, so this was my rationale. They wrote directions down on a small piece of paper, and I went on my way. I could not find the mall, so I went back the way I came. This time, I asked them for a phone charger. They agreed to find a charger and disappeared in the back of the building. At the time, I recall standing in their waiting room, feeling nervous because I could not call my client to share that I was going to be late for our session. I feel this must have triggered the mania in my body, and it is likely they sensed something was off. When someone is manic, they may speak very fast and can exhibit illogical thinking. A few moments later, they returned, saying I had to come outside because they had called the police. The police officer put me in the back of a cop car as if I were a criminal. I asked them what was going on, but all they told me was that I had to stay in the back seat. Then, an ambulance arrived. They took me by my arms, put me on a gurney in the ambulance, and impounded my car. I had no choice, and none of my contacts were called. Throughout all of this, I was kept in the dark as to what was happening. Looking back, the least they could have done was allow me to call a friend and have them come pick me up, versus hauling me off to the hospital.

Once admitted, I recall being in a room with a man who proceeded to take my blood and check my vitals. Then, unexpectedly, two large men forced me into a wheelchair, pushing me down and restraining my arms. They didn't allow me to call anyone for help. I was a victim of the medical system in a cage of misfortune. I went from complete freedom at 9 am to feeling stuck in purgatory by 2 pm. Nobody was ever informed or notified about my situation.

Once I was forced and wheeled into the psyche ward, I was put on a forty-eight-hour hold. They would not let me take any of my Adderall, but they allowed all the other meds I was on. I pleaded with the male doctors that I needed to taper down off the Adderall, which, by then, I was on 60-70mg per day. I knew the side effects of going off Adderall cold turkey were intense and varied. I would need a small amount of it, or else my body would go into shock. Unfortunately, they didn't listen to me, my voice wasn't heard, and I was completely cut off from the meds. My body went into shock, as they cut me off the stimulant. I understand their reasoning, as they may have been considering a normal, able-bodied, healthy person, without a prior diagnosis of MS. However, I was not harming anyone, and they completely disregarded my diagnosis, my sensitive nervous system, and my pleas for them to taper me down from the medication, which is where the fault lies. Within forty-eight hours after the cutoff, my body began to break down, and I found myself grasping onto walls and losing my balance. In my opinion, being taken off the medication abruptly, and the stress of not being heard, threw my body out of balance, causing a flare-up. I went into the hospital fully mobile but came out needing a cane and handicapped.

My hope with this story is to shed light on the concerning treatment of patients in these hospitals. A protocol should have been in place for individuals with a history of being on antidepressants, having autoimmune disorders, and/or sensitive nervous systems. It's crucial to address this concern and adopt a more sensitive approach to tapering off medications.

In addition, since being admitted, I continued to urge the staff to let me see a neurologist. I explained that I was a successful business owner and had been diagnosed with multiple sclerosis, and my neurologist had prescribed the medication to help with fatigue. It took them a staggering NINE DAYS to finally allow a neurologist to come see me, but it was too late; the damage had already been done.

I strongly believe that if I had been able to call a friend or loved one, the unfolding events could have resulted in a completely different outcome. The way mental health is addressed in this country is completely broken and backwards. I hope my story sheds some light into the darkness of the entire mental health field. The crazy thing is that I wasn't even taking the Adderall for what it is prescribed for—I was taking it solely for energy to combat the fatigue due to a diagnosed medical condition. Stimulants are prescribed like candy to those suffering from fatigue in the autoimmune disease community. However, it only lasts for so long, then you need to bump up the dosage. For example, when I was first diagnosed, I was given 20mg. Over the course of seven years, my doctor had increased it to the point of 30mg two times per day, with a bump of 10mg in the afternoon when needed, and it fried my brain! Not to mention all the side effects from mixing this drug with antidepressants, Ambien, and a cocktail of other drugs I took solely due to the diagnosis. I tried to speak with a lawyer about medical malpractice/negligence, but I was suffering emotionally from such severe PTSD, depression, and shock, and I could barely walk. I recall the moment I had the strength to finally call an attorney, but I was advised against it. Hospitals have insurance, and the people admitted to psych wards are often in a distressed state, causing them to regularly lose their cases. I should have fought harder, but I was in shock, living alone in a city without family or support. By that time, I had lost my downtown high-rise condo, had to go on disability because I was unable to work, and found myself on welfare, living in government housing.

My life was spiraling, and I found myself going from Prada to PayLess.

Since I started using a cane while on Tecifdera, my neurologist suggested that I might be transitioning to Primary-Progressive MS (PPMS). They prescribed Tysabri, an infusion treatment. However, before starting it, I had to ensure I tested negative for the JC virus because, if positive, it could lead to progressive multifocal leukoencephalopathy (PML). She suggested that I go on the medication, even though my test returned back positive for the JC virus. I was in such a low place and disconnected from life and body, I followed her suggestions. After I started Tysabri, my gait became worse, and I would feel sick after each infusion. I repeatedly pleaded to discontinue the medication. It's important to emphasize that this was how my body reacted, and I understand that these medications can be helpful for others with the same condition. I'm just sharing my experience that they didn't work for me.

At that time, I sought second opinions on what my next move should be. I met with two different neurologists and asked if they would have taken me off Copaxone. Both of them pointed out that my MRI tests were stable, and they would have advised me to continue with that treatment. I was furious; this led me to question EVERYTHING! If I had tested positive for the JC virus, could I have other viruses in my system, like Epstein Barr? What if I had PML because it manifests as mental slowness, disorientation, and behavioral changes, which I experienced at the time of my MS diagnosis? What if MS could be caused by a virus? Maybe I had something other than MS? I was so confused! I went down the rabbit hole, as every good Alice does, and I began to uncover a lot of information. This all made sense when I read *The Medical Medium*. It explains how the root cause of MS is the Epstein Barr virus. More studies are coming out about Epstein Barr virus being the root of MS; however, my current neurologist says there are not enough studies to determine this.

About a year after I was released from the hospital, I was mailed the book *The Wahls Protocol* by Dr. Terry Wahls, and I saw how others were managing and thriving by changing their diet. Following her recommendation to visit a functional medicine doctor, my perspective started to shift around the diagnosis. So, thank you, Dr. Wahls, for the work you do. It gave me hope when I saw countless people's success stories about how they were changing their diet and coming off their medication. Also, her recommendation on removing heavy metals from your mouth made sense to me. I followed her protocol for three and a half years, and then plateaued. I had not yet delved into the trauma. Instead, I switched from the paleo diet bandwagon to the vegan bandwagon and decided to try following the Medical Medium. I stuck to this lifestyle for another three-and-a-half years, but unfortunately, I wasn't getting better with this approach either. Initially, it always started out great, but the positive results didn't last long. I felt good and would notice my body becoming more flexible, or I would have more energy here and there.

I then began to work with a specialist here in St. Louis and found results with his approach to prevention and healing. I conducted more tests, which found large amounts of mercury still in my body, so I did heavy metal chelations, along with many parasite cleanses. I have to say that western doctors, who are covered by health insurance, do not offer the same tests as functional medicine doctors. Reviewing the test results from the doctors who I have paid out-of-pocket to are remarkable. Learning about the amount of lead, arsenic, heavy metals, and toxins I had in my body, along with fungicides, pesticides, parasites, and bacteria, was helpful in connecting the dots and discovering what was causing the MS or dis-ease in my body. I feel when we detox and get the viral load down in our body, it helps the body to heal, repair, and renew. Taking action by doing things to support my body physically was very empowering, especially when I began to see a difference in my fatigue, brain fog, foot drop, hips, balance, bladder incontinence, focus, and overall flexibility.

At one of my vitamin C infusions, I was given *The LDN Book 3* from a nurse. I had not heard of this as an alternative to treating autoimmune conditions. The book shares how "low dose naltrexone (LDN) modifies the disease processes of MS at the cellular level, as well as decreases the symptoms. It can be used to improve sleep, balance hormones, improve the body's ability to detoxify, help stabilize epigenetic changes, improve the health in the gut, and modulate the immune response, changing immune pathways to heal healthier ones." Since I was learning about changing the mind at a cellular level through meditation, I wanted to explore this option. I asked my functional medicine doctor if he would write a prescription for me, and he agreed. I got it filled at a compound pharmacy, and from my research, the results looked to be successful. Unfortunately, my neurologist will not prescribe it because there is not substantial research. I share this for those who are curious about the book and if it resonates to find a doctor who will help you get on this alternative medication. I believe you can also get it online at a reasonable price.

It is important to note at the time of publication that I had been on LDN for only a few months. I am unsure how long I will be taking it. I have noticed that I am sleeping better. Because I have not taken prescribed medication for a long time, I will reevaluate how I feel after six months. As always, I let my body tell me what it needs, and it always leads me in the right direction. The way I do this is by sitting still, placing my hand on my heart, another on my gut, and talking to my body, asking what is best.

I was so focused on using food as medicine and detox protocols to solve my health problems that I just wasn't ready to do the trauma work. It was just too much, and I had to do things in stages. Once I had cleaned up my body, I began to work with a therapist and process everything that happened that dreadful day. I had to learn how to integrate and release the sadness and anger instead of running away from it. It was then that I realized how learning emotional regulation could have made things different. However, I also learned that this was the path I needed to walk, even if I was handicapped. Now, I can teach others through my story, as a survivor of addiction, verbal and physical abuse, and abandonment. I want them to know that trauma survivors can heal and reclaim their lives by learning to love themselves again. I did this by reclaiming my innate value, worth, and putting myself first by building good boundaries. To make this happen, I had to take an active role to not disassociate from the trauma but to be with it and resolve it, so it could be released from my body. I was extremely controlling and had to release that pattern, amongst many others. We are human and soak up patterns like a sponge. As I began to heal and balance my body, it started to regenerate and thrive. Allowing the energy to flow freely was crucial, as pent-up emotions had wreaked havoc on my systems for decades. When the energy is blocked, organs and systems can break down. By LEARNING HOW TO RELEASE and allow emotions to flow, my health improved significantly.

My FREEDOM came from telling a NEW STORY.

In my previous life, claiming the diagnosis of "MS", I went on Copaxone, Tecfidera, Tysabri. It wasn't until I decided to take a stand against the abusive relationship I had with the pharmaceutical industry that I found freedom. I made the bold decision to discontinue the long list of medications I had been taking for almost a decade, and that's when I finally experienced a sense of liberation.

As I reflect on both diet lifestyles, I've come to realize that the true path to freedom was not through what I ate but working through and integrating healthy ways of being and learning to love myself from the inside out. Instead of constantly striving and putting energy into diets, I found that focusing on telling myself a new story that I CAN heal. My inner healing was the key to genuine transformation and self-acceptance. It was time for ALICE to change and TRANSFORM herself. There was no diet that was going to save me, no magic pill. I was going to have to go down the rabbit hole and make peace with it ALL and FORGIVE. I could not bypass this—I HAD TO WORK ON ME!

I now eat a balanced diet, VERY LOW SUGAR, and focus on healing my gut on the candida diet lifestyle to combat the yeast and bacteria which have not yet healed. I work with the meridians and energy centers (chakras) in the body, and I know when the energy is stuck, and I am not in flow. I have learned practices that I do on myself, such as Reiki, Donna Eden's energy routine, and several forms of meditation to clear energy from the body and organs.

All of the symptoms I once had are no longer part of my day-to-day experience. The only thing that reminds me I even have a health condition is the fact that I am not able to walk freely and balance for long distances, which is improving every day. I do a daily practice of crawling with knee pads to help with core strength, and I walk up and down steps every day. In addition to eating better, my big things I have liked doing and gotten positive results from were heavy metal chelation, vitamin C infusions, saunas, parasite cleanses, coffee enemas, colonics, castor oil packs, and many other things to detox toxins out of the body. As a result, I no longer feel severe brain fog, fatigue, and my mind is sharper. I go over all of these on my YouTube channel *Style Your Glow with Alice*. I understand it is expensive and some may not want to pay out-of-pocket. I did a GoFundMe to raise the funds to pay for these costs and found scholarships from the MS Society listed in resources below. By the grace of God, everything I have needed on my healing path was covered, from juicers, to a Vitamix, water filters, saunas, organic food expenses, etc. I receive my energy from food and supplements and have been free from the pharmaceuticals my neurologist prescribed for seven years. I now use plant tinctures and homeopathy to help balance my nervous system, such as ALA (support the brain barrier), vitamin D, B12 and B complex, liquid zinc, CoQ10, and others, which my doctor suggests for me according to my lab tests. I am hopeful to add in more sugar eventually and eat even more of a balanced diet, but for now, I'm focusing on my gut and intuition. Every morning, I dedicate time to connecting with my body and listening to its needs.

I have come to the conclusion that the root cause of my body's troubles was a cytokine storm, triggered by severe stress, which brought forth deeply held, unprocessed trauma. This stress, combined with the buildup of heavy metals from having mercury fillings taken out and put back in, exposure to toxins in a closed-down college dorm with asbestos, parasites from a near-death experience due to food poisoning in Paris, mold deep in my cells, along with fungicides, yeast, and bacteria running rampant in my body—all of it began to make sense.

I learned how to release the past and move through the trauma, forgiving myself along the way. Establishing a healthy relationship with my body and setting boundaries became part of my journey (though I'm still a work-in-progress). As I started to develop deep self-love and gratitude towards my body, my perspective on my illness began to shift.

I leaned into understanding how and why my life spun out of control. Instead of searching for external reasons, I began looking within myself for the answers.

I began to FORGIVE IT ALL!

I have been walking with a cane (or what I call the crutch) for nine years. I am trying my best to rehabilitate my body, walking freely without the crutch in my home. When I am out in public, I practice not using it to retrain my brain. I am not where I want to be yet; it takes time, and I'm hopeful.

If you are reading this and have received the devastating diagnosis of MS or know someone who has, I want to offer hope that healing and freedom are possible. It's essential to remember that everyone's journey is unique, and finding answers within yourself is crucial. I'm not suggesting that you have to go off your medication; that decision is yours to make. The most important thing is to believe in the possibility of healing and never lose hope.

In summary, my healing journey has taken me from Fear (False Evidence Appearing Real), to Flow, and finally, to FREEDOM! I switched the narrative I tell myself to "I AM" healing verses, staying in the mentality of "There is nothing to be done". I feel this experience unfolded to happen FOR me, not TO me. Now, I am healthier, truly in love with my body, and I've learned to embrace more patience, kindness, and compassion towards myself and others. Most importantly, I feel a deep connection to spirit and a newfound appreciation for the small things in life.

MS for me means "Mindset Shift", and I work daily on my mindset and hope to share how I do this with others on my social media.

This journey has transformed me in ways I could never have imagined. I am still not where I want to be after the tragic day in the hospital, and I still have forgiveness work to do. I walk with the cane when I need it. Each day, I practice "free walking", and I am more flexible now. I also work on my mood and my thoughts. I have come a long way in learning how to reverse my victim mentality by speaking to myself differently. I no longer talk like I "have" MS; instead, I speak of it as a result of a manifestation of who I once was. I have compassion and love for the girl I was back when I received my diagnosis. Now, I have an entirely new outlook! I hope sharing my journey helps to inspire others to make small changes in their lives and proves that MS is possible to overcome. I now know and understand that my body has my back. I am no longer defined by this illness. It's in my past, and I have stopped talking about it like I have something wrong with me.

At this point, I reflect on the past nine years of my healing journey. I've worked on detoxing drugs from my body, learned the power of healing herbs and foods, and prioritized putting myself first. I've let go of the bullshit, limiting beliefs, and outdated patterns I inherited from my parents—patterns that no longer serve me. Now, I am paving a new life, filled with balance, joy, fun, excitement, gratitude, and love. Being on the other side of it feels exhilarating, and I hold onto the hope of walking completely free someday. Taking one day at a time, I recognize my limits and put myself first above all else, setting solid boundaries.

Witnessing the regeneration in my own body every day on this journey to wellness is remarkable. It's essential to remember how far I have come and that I am someone's inspiration and goal. This keeps me motivated and driven to move forward. I want you to know that wherever you are on your own journey, there is always a light at the end of the tunnel. I'm here holding the torch of freedom for YOU! Remember, healing is possible, and there's hope for a brighter and healthier future ahead.

The light in ME loves the light in YOU!
Xoxo, Alice

If you want to learn how I manage my health and wellness, you can follow me at www.styleyourglow.com and on social @styleyourglow369 on YouTube, Instagram, TikTok, Linked in, & Pinterest.

Check out your local food share resources in your city to help you with free, organic food. For example, I was a volunteer in St. Louis for the St. Louis Food Share Network, and in Minneapolis called Sisters Camelot, where I was able to get organic food for free to help me in my healing.

I have also benefited from grants from the following programs. Hopefully, they can help you, too:

MS Society 1-800-344-4867 (canes, equipment, help with mental health) MS Association of America 1-800-532-7667 (equipment, MRI reimbursement)

MS Foundation also MS Focus 1-888-673-6287 (rent, utilities, eyeglasses, transportation, cooling program, etc.)

United Way 211

Modest Needs 1-844-667-3776

37

Story by

MARIA INDERMÜHLE

Diagnosed in 2012
Currently 45 years old
Lives in Switzerland (from Scotland)
Instagram: @first_food_first
www.firstfoodfirst.com

My body was in lockdown before lockdown ever happened. The diagnosis of multiple sclerosis (MS) helped me navigate COVID's lockdown because it all felt so strangely familiar. A few years earlier, I couldn't leave my home when my body went into "lockdown". During that period, I had no feeling from my chin down, and my husband was spoon-feeding me. However, this time was slightly different. The world might have gone into lockdown, but my body did not.

As people's mental health plummeted and anxiety heightened, I felt a deep, indescribable, inner peace wash over me, which I felt guilty for having when so many people were struggling to grasp this new reality that hit us all like a tornado. I chose to focus on hope—not fear.

In 2012, when I was given the diagnosis of MS, I asked the neurologists lots of questions: What causes MS, and why did I have it? Only to be met with shrugged shoulders and a shaking of heads. So, I made it my mission to find out. And find out I did. Everything makes perfect sense to me now. Numerous factors led to my MS diagnosis, with some of these factors manifesting many years before any symptoms appeared.

I strongly believe that the story of our life is the story of our health. It was through understanding and making sense of my own life and the events that took place beforehand that I was able to do something positive about the diagnosis, changing the trajectory of the disease. I still live with MS, but MS doesn't run or ruin my life like it once did.

When I was told I had multiple sclerosis, which was described to me as a "progressive disease", which meant "progressive decline", I was sent away to rearrange my home to accommodate a wheelchair. Despite the negativity conveyed to me, I remained hopeful. It's sad to say that my hope was met by a very annoyed neurologist. I was mocked and laughed at for having such hope. I understand why he reacted like this because daily he was seeing such destructive and debilitating symptoms of MS destroying people's lives. In his mind, why would I be any different?

Over these past eleven years since my diagnosis, I have not stopped clinging to hope. Health starts with hope. Take away hope, and what do we have—a pretty sad existence.

Let me tell you a little about my life before MS.
I was a Retail Sales Manager back home in Inverness in the Highlands of Scotland, pouring all my time and energy into driving sales and smashing weekly targets, providing excellent customer service skills, and motivating a sales team. I was barely making enough money for myself to pay the rent for my flat, run a car, and eat. It was becoming overwhelming, and I was stressed. Then, I was invited to go to Switzerland for the weekend. Little did I know my life was about to change!

That weekend, I fell in love at first sight. This man, who is now my husband, opened the door and smiled, and I knew in that very instant that he was the man I would marry! During that weekend, in May 2010, the volcano erupted in Iceland, cancelling many flights all over the world, including mine from Geneva to Edinburgh. It allowed me to have more time in the country which would soon become "home".

It was a whirlwind romance. Within six months, we were engaged. We were married four months later, saying our vows on April Fool's Day (but in the afternoon—anything you do in the morning on April Fool's Day can be classified as a joke).

Now, Switzerland is not known for being the cheapest of countries, and it was because of this that my husband suggested I get any dental treatment done before I leave the Highlands of Scotland. It made sense, so that's what I did. One week before our big day, I had my appointment with the dentist which required me to have four fillings put in my mouth. These fillings were what's known as "silver fillings". What I now realize is that these fillings actually contain more mercury than silver. The World Health Organization (WHO) considers mercury to be one of the top ten most toxic substances to human health. Yet, that day when I innocently sat in the dentist's chair, not only was I being exposed to one of the world's most toxic substances, but I gave permission for it to be put in my mouth, not knowing what I know now. Certainly, my MS diagnosis wasn't the result of a single factor but rather an accumulation of various factors, with mercury exposure being just one of them.

After the fillings were completed, I distinctly remember tasting metal in my mouth. It didn't go away for about two weeks. It was so bad that I couldn't even taste the food on our wedding day. I brought this up to the dentist who dismissed me, informing me that it was normal, and it would go away. This marked the beginning of medical professionals dismissing my health concerns when things felt off in my body.

Now that I am practicing functional medicine in my online clinic, I consider it crucial for me to understand a client's timeline (the events that have taken place in their life before they fell sick). The questions that are the most beneficial in providing that "ah-ha" moment for me, as well as the client, are:
"When was the last time you felt well?
"You have never felt well since when?"
"What was happening at that time?"

Had I been asked those questions, I would have replied: "I have not felt well since the day I went to the dentist and got four silver fillings put in my mouth."

Immediately after getting married, we went to Switzerland. French was spoken in the part we were going to live in, so my husband enrolled me in an Intensive French Class. I was quite excited about embracing this new skill; however, nothing prepared me for how difficult I was going to find it to retain anything I was being taught. On top of struggling to remember all the new vocabulary, I was now experiencing what felt like thousands of ants running up and down my spinal cord, and I could hardly breathe. It was as if someone was sitting on my chest.

I did what most people would and visited the doctor, but he promptly dismissed my symptoms. Without even taking my blood pressure, he suggested I take some antidepressants. According to him, I was too young to have anything seriously wrong with me; it was probably homesickness. I knew I wasn't depressed—far from it! I had just gotten married to the man I loved and was extremely happy. Despite feeling something was wrong in my body, he wouldn't listen, and it was frustrating not to be taken seriously.

As the summer progressed, so did my symptoms. My right leg became weak; I felt like it was dragging. And the vision in my right eye was going blurry. It felt like my body was shutting down on me at a rapid rate.

I began spending my days researching my symptoms on the computer. One day, I came across an article that made my symptoms sound very similar to what is known as multiple sclerosis. I returned to the same doctor who had dismissed me a few months earlier and asked him if he could refer me to see a neurologist because of my discovery. With some hesitation, he agreed to refer me to the Neurology Department at the nearest hospital.

The hospital visits for additional tests were already unpleasant (I underwent a lumbar puncture, MRI, and blood tests), but what made the experience even more challenging was the way they delivered the diagnosis and prognosis. I recall a female neurologist, around my husband's and my age, casually announcing the multiple sclerosis diagnosis. It was evident that this was just routine for her, as she had likely delivered such news to countless others before us.

Although I had researched a little about MS, I was still unaware of what it would really mean, and the course of action that conventional medicine would advise me to take. I wasn't even aware that there was "no cure". So, when I was informed that I needed to start medication immediately, I honestly thought I would be on it for ten days, and then I would be fine. All the symptoms would disappear, and I would move on with my life as normal. But it didn't work like that. This medication was Copaxone (an injection I needed to give myself every day), and it was to become my new life.

I remember the neurologist excitedly revealing to us a box of syringes that I could choose from, depending on what color I'd like. We were sitting there like dazzled rabbits in front of a car's headlights, unable to make sense of the current situation, yet this woman was eager for us to choose a color of the syringe before she saw her next patient. And I was expected to inject myself every day for the rest of my life. It really was like a horror movie. I just wanted to wake up!

"My husband and I want to start a family," I said.
"You can't start a family while you're on this medication. If that is what you want, then you should start it now before you go on the medication," said the female neurologist, with a framed photo of her two beautiful children on her desk. I felt like I had just been punched in the stomach. I was already struggling to keep myself on my feet and go to the bathroom alone without being pregnant. I couldn't possibly imagine carrying a baby while feeling like this. I knew in my heart it wouldn't be sensible. Honestly, it was all quite difficult to process. This was when I was sent home to rearrange my house to accommodate a wheelchair.

I had now been given a diagnosis of multiple sclerosis, and the picture being portrayed to me was not pretty. The diagnosis told me what I had, but it didn't tell me why I had it. No hope was offered to me—only medication, and that wasn't going to cure me. It was only going to slow down the progression of the disease. There must be something I could do. "This truly can't be it!" I thought.

I now had a new passion and purpose in life: to get answers as to why I had MS! This soon consumed my every waking second. My questions weren't answered in conventional medicine. These questions were not taught in traditional, western medical schools. For them, the solution was: "Just take the medication." Today's medical model consists of "name it, blame it, tame it", and that was exactly what they were offering me. Then, I realized that I had been asking all the right questions to the wrong people. At this point, I wanted to get to the root cause of these horrific symptoms, and nothing was going to stop me.

One day, I found something on the internet that transformed my perspective on MS forever. I stumbled across a story of a man who had fallen sick after going to the dentist and having silver fillings put in his mouth, which resulted in an MS diagnosis. It was a light-bulb moment for me! I, too, had fallen sick just after a visit to the dentist. What material were my fillings made from? It was silver, right? Turns out, not entirely. Silver fillings are 50% mercury; only 35% is silver. Mercury is a neuron toxic. Could it be responsible for my neurological symptoms? I needed to find out.

I now realize that toxins can interfere with bodily functions. When the body begins to lose function, investigating toxins becomes crucial. Unfortunately, this investigation didn't take place within the Neurology Department at the hospital because it's not their focus when a patient exhibits nervous system problems. Another thing I've learned is that the sicker you are, the more toxins you may have in your body, including mold, heavy metals like mercury and lead, and so on. But back then, this was all new to me, a revelation that led me down a whole new rabbit hole - one that excited me, and I had no desire to come out of anytime soon.

After discovering all this about mercury and the neurological symptoms it can cause, I had convinced myself that I didn't have MS after all, but I actually had mercury poisoning. I just knew I had to get all this mercury out of my mouth.

There are many things I'd like to highlight here about the removal of "silver" (mercury) amalgam fillings. Removing mercury fillings is not for the faint hearted. You need to be super careful to make sure that the safe, appropriate precautions are taken when removed. Finding a certified International Academy of Oral Medicine and Toxicology (IAOMT) dentist will guarantee you are protected, using the "SMART protocol".

Prior to any dental procedures aimed at removing mercury fillings, it's crucial that the client maintains regular and daily bowel movements, ensuring they are not constipated. Addressing nutrient deficiencies should be a priority also, making it highly advisable to collaborate with a qualified nutritional therapist or Functional Medicine Practitioner several months in advance. The good stuff needs to be put in the body first before you take any of the bad stuff out. Removing mercury fillings from your mouth does not mean you're cured of MS. I've had all my silver fillings removed from my mouth, and I still live with MS. However, my health has significantly improved after having had them removed. As I stated before, if the dentist does not remove mercury correctly, you can become even sicker—this is what happened to me.

Now, here's the thing which fascinates me. Toxins like fat. Mercury loves fat. What are our brains made out of? What is the myelin sheath that is being destroyed in MS made out of? Yes—fat. If Mercury loves fat, and I had mercury in my mouth, it makes perfect sense to me that this toxin may well be a contributing factor to my health problems. The mouth is located quite close to our brain. We have what's called the blood brain barrier, and this usually keeps things out that shouldn't be there. However, mercury is a toxic substance that can cross over quite easily, and when it does, it is keen to nestle quite comfortably in our brain. What I would like to better understand is this: we are told that in MS, the immune system is attacking itself and destroying the myelin sheath of the nerve. But why is it doing this? Is it because it detects a foreign invader in the body (like mercury) and reacts by attacking it? I prefer to think of my immune system as a defender, so I struggle to comprehend why it would attack me without a clear reason. If it's attacking me to protect me, then I can understand that. Or is it actually mercury or other toxins that are physically damaging the nerve networks and potentially responsible for destroying the fatty tissue called myelin? I had an unwelcome 'guest' in my brain, and this intruder was ruining my life.

Once mercury has reached the brain, it is not easy to remove. With the support of a naturopath, I started removing mercury. At one point, I removed too much mercury too quickly, and it was this that left me paralyzed from the chin down for several weeks. This took me to a dark place I never thought I would find myself. I remember one evening when everything had really gotten to me. I couldn't even feel my husband's hand touching my body. I could only feel it when he touched my face. I'd had enough; I just couldn't take any more. I didn't want to die, but I also didn't want to live like this.

That evening, I told my husband that in the morning, I wanted to contact EXIT. EXIT provides assisted suicide here in Switzerland. My mind was made up. I didn't want my gorgeous, dashing husband to be my carer. He didn't sign up for this! I remember that evening as if it were yesterday. We cried and cried as we clung to each other.. I couldn't feel his touch, but I could feel his love. That night, we prayed. I learned something that evening about prayer that I didn't know before: True prayer requires no words; it's something words cannot express. We prayed as we clung together, tears streaming down our faces.

The next morning when we woke up, I rubbed my fingertips together like I often did, expecting to feel nothing. That morning was different; I felt something! I could actually FEEL my fingertips! Words could not express the pure joy I felt. I didn't just experience joy; I also regained hope.

I abandoned the thought of Assisted Suicide immediately. I felt such an inner strength and purpose that my health would improve. I would have to do the work, but I would get all that mercury out of me, and my health would be better than it's ever been. I remember being on the seat at the kitchen table and saying to my husband with so much conviction and determination, which I know every cell in my body heard: "I WILL get better! And when I get better, I'm going to go on and help other people, too." I had an even greater purpose and passion. This was going to be my source of motivation in the months ahead and continues to be so today.

I know mercury is extremely good at what it does in that it fills a cavity really well and isn't expensive. However, every time you drink a hot cup of tea, a vapor is released that crosses over our blood brain barrier, causing havoc to the nervous system. There's a good video available online on this topic explaining how mercury vapor is released during chewing, removal, or placement. You can watch the video by looking up the title called "SMOKING TEETH = POISON GAS" on YouTube.

Over the years, dentists' health has raised concerns due to their close association with mercury. Dentistry has historically had high suicide rates (source: https://onlinelibrary.wiley.com/doi/full/10.1111/bcpt.13199). Recent research suggests that dentists' suicide rates have improved, likely linked to reduced use of mercury amalgam fillings. Since 2018, the European Union banned amalgam fillings for children under fifteen and pregnant or breastfeeding women. Despite its high toxicity, some dental procedures still use this material. Several European countries, like Germany, Denmark, Norway, and Sweden, have already banned its use, with others in the process. The UK is now planning to phase out mercury amalgam fillings for environmental reasons.

Remember the Mad Hatter in Alice in Wonderland? He made hats. In that century, they used mercury to stiffen the felt. Many people with this occupation developed tremors, distorted vision, confused speech, and even psychosis. Mercury is known to affect the nervous, digestive, and immune system. Later on, I discovered that not only did I have high levels of mercury in my body, but I also had lead.

I believe, and I've personally demonstrated, that reducing the toxic load in my body helped improve my health and restore its balanced state. You've probably heard the saying: "We are what we eat." I prefer to think of it another way: "We are what we eat, drink, breathe, touch, and can't eliminate." What can't you currently eliminate from your body that may be keeping you sick? For me, it was mercury.

But what is mercury? Mercury is a natural substance found in the earth's crust. It can be released into the environment when there's a volcano eruption. Human activity is often the cause of mercury release. Why is it so dangerous? Because of its fumes. You can't see its vapors, but they can travel far and wide. A broken thermometer would expose you to hazardous vapors of mercury. These levels that are released can be absorbed by the lungs and are known to have negative effects on the kidneys and brain. They have also been shown to accumulate in certain tissues of the body. Mercury can be found in various sources, including thermometers, fluorescent lights, batteries, light bulbs, dental fillings, cosmetics, pharmaceuticals, coal, large fish (such as tuna and swordfish), jewelry, paint, blood pressure gauges, and contact lens solution.

The APO-E 4 gene is a known major risk factor for neurodegenerative diseases, including Alzheimer's disease. This gene has demonstrated a reduced ability to eliminate and detoxify mercury. Research has indicated that individuals with the APO-E 4 gene may be more susceptible to various diseases linked to mercury exposure. If Alzheimer's disease is prevalent in your family, there's a potential risk of carrying the APO-E4 gene, which could decrease your capacity to eliminate mercury. Alzheimer's is in my family.

I am not a doctor, but I consider it disappointing, saddening, and terribly worrying that mercury exposure is not investigated after an MS diagnosis in our current medical model within Western Medicine, especially when we have studies to show a potential link with neurodegenerative diseases. Thankfully, within functional medicine, this link is known, and it is taken very seriously. We ask the important questions to understand the client and their health journey: What has happened in this person's life to make them so sick? What toxins have they been exposed to? Could their occupation be exposing them to toxins?

In 1989, the Swedish Journal of Biological Medicine suggested an association between multiple sclerosis and high amounts of mercury. It reported that people with MS showed higher levels of mercury in their spinal fluid than the average person. https://www.iomcworld.org/open-access/a-hypothesis-and-additional-evidence-that-mercury-may-be-an-etiological-factor-in-multiple-sclerosis.pdf

In the *Journal of Multiple Sclerosis 2020*, Vol. 7, Issue 3, Robert Siblerud & Joachim Mutter wrote, "Studies have found a correlation between MS and dental cavities and dental amalgams. The greatest source of mercury comes from dental amalgams, according to the WHO. Previous studies have shown MS symptoms and physiological changes improve, following dental amalgam removal." The study concluded that "mercury is possibly an etiological factor in multiple sclerosis".

Below are some other studies of interest:
Other study 2012 PMID: 22068727
https://pubmed.ncbi.nlm.nih.gov/22068727/

Study in 2018 PMID: 29959651
https://pubmed.ncbi.nlm.nih.gov/29959651/

A Study in 2023 'Potentially toxic elements in the brains of people with Multiple Sclerosis'
https://pubmed.ncbi.nlm.nih.gov/36635465/
PMID: 36635465

A person's reaction to mercury will depend on that person's individual health status and their genetic predisposition and environmental factors, although I personally do not believe that there is any safe level of this toxin for the human body. People can live with mercury fillings their entire life and never receive an MS diagnosis. I know plenty of people who have a mouth full of silver fillings, and they are currently living well.

There are many factors to consider, and a "one-size-fits-all approach" does not work. No two people are the same. I know that drug modifying therapies (DMT's) are often given to people diagnosed with MS, and they can certainly slow down the progression of the disease. But, if a toxin remains in the person's body, no DMT is ever going to make it better in the long term.

Although it was eleven years ago, I remember the day well when I shared the link I had discovered between mercury and neurological symptoms with the neurologist, only to be laughed at. He told me that I was talking bulls**t! Had I not asked these questions and sought the right help, I would still be sick.

I remember this particular neurologist turning to my husband and saying to him, "Your wife is in serious denial of her diagnosis." In other words, he just wanted me to take the medication, accept everything he said, and stop asking questions he clearly couldn't answer. If I had listened to everything he had said and accepted it all, I know I wouldn't be walking up the Swiss mountains, as I do every day now while living with MS.

After detoxing from heavy metals, I became firmly convinced that I didn't have MS despite the diagnosis. I was living a healthy life and wanted to maintain it. So, I committed to a three-year nutrition study, commuting every other weekend from Geneva, Switzerland to Edinburgh, Scotland. This was a time long before Zoom calls!

This entire challenging experience allowed me to see that my health was MY responsibility—no one else's, not my husband's, not my siblings', not my parents'. It's not even my doctors' responsibility. It's the action I take daily to go in the direction of health and not disease—from the thoughts I think, to the foods I buy (which enter my body, telling it how to feel and function), to the company I keep, to the hours I sleep, to what I put on and in my body. There's a lot to consider, but it's all possible, and extremely important when prioritizing progressive health. It's about creating a new lifestyle that fits well for you and your body. It's not a diet; it's a lifestyle.

I have chosen never to claim MS; instead, I say, "I was given the diagnosis of MS," and there's a lot I can do about it. I consider that way of viewing the diagnosis to be way more empowering for me. Many people have expressed the need to come to terms with the diagnosis and to "accept" it. If that works for them, then that's wonderful; I respect that. Personally, I have no desire to accept MS. I don't see why I should accept something I would rather not have. I had to accept way too much in other areas of my life where I had no choice in the matter. But with MS, I can choose how I view it, and how I deal with it.

When I discovered the connection not only between mercury and MS, but also feeling the HUGE improvement in my health after my mercury fillings were removed, a lot of anger surged within me. Anger that I allowed the dental professionals to put such a toxic substance in my mouth, which I believe triggered some of the most horrendous neurological symptoms.

Wayne Dryer once said, "All blame is a waste of time." And so it is.
I needed to let all the hurt and anger go. There was a lot of stuff that I had to work through. This is where journaling and having a coach helped me.

I was living so well for years without any symptoms until last summer—August 2022—and boom! A huge MS flare literally floored me, leaving me unable to walk for six weeks. It came as a shock. I had become complacent. I wasn't eating the way I knew I should be.

During lockdown, I became slightly obsessed with sourdough bread. Sourdough is known for its health benefits, but it still contains some gluten, if it is not gluten-free. MS and gluten are not friends. I should have known better. It was an extremely hot summer here in Switzerland, and I had experienced a huge emotional stress. One morning at the beginning of August 2022, I woke up to a lack of feeling on the left side of my face—completely numb. This got worse over the next few days, and within the week, I was no longer able to walk. It was scary but not like before. This time it was different. This time, I knew why I had the flare and what I could do about it. I had been here before. Again, I felt that deep, quiet inner peace.

A couple of months earlier, I was in Edinburgh, and I attended a talk by Dr. Rangan Chatterjee, who is a doctor for the National Health Service (NHS) in England, UK, but he is also a Functional Medicine Practitioner. His talk was incredibly helpful, but one thing he said that evening, as it rained torrentially outside, was that emotions are real.
When he uttered those words, I felt like he was speaking directly to me, as if no one else was in the room. Gosh....he was so right. Emotions ARE real. They can have a huge, negative impact on our bodies when living with multiple sclerosis. And here I was, two months later, proving the truth of those words. It was a shocker.

So, what did I do about it? I contacted the people close to me and told them my decision to switch off my phone for the month of August. I needed no distractions and no electrical devices. After all, it was the communication relayed down through this little object that contributed to my now flare. I turned it right off and put it in a drawer, away from my view. I felt a sigh of relief immediately after. Everything's going to be okay…

The most frustrating thing about that flare in August is I know I could have prevented it. I lost the function of my legs and my left hand for several weeks, but thankfully, function was restored again within a few weeks. Within conventional medicine when function is lost, patients are often told that it will not return. I have proved that it can, and it has, but it took a lot of work on my part. It was anything but easy. I didn't take any pharmaceutical medicine, and I still don't. I am not against medication. It has its place. I might have to take it later on, who knows? But right now, I have chosen not to. One of the great things about life is that we get to choose and decide what is best for us as individuals.

I have learned that our bodies can repair themselves when given the right environment to do so. What are those conditions? Well, I think this is where individual, personalized nutrition is key. I also think this is where the Wahls Protocol® fits in beautifully; eating foods that your body recognizes and knows what to do with. Within a few weeks, I was back on my feet again. Now that the heavy metals have been removed from my body which was most certainly driving the progression of MS for me, I don't experience MS symptoms when I eat well. I consider that hugely empowering; the power that lies on my fork.

I recall moments when I couldn't feel anything from my chin down, and my husband had to feed me with a spoon. During those times, it truly felt like the world was collapsing around me, and all I wanted was to die. Strangely, I was more worried about how this diagnosis was affecting my dear husband more than myself. That's the reality, a diagnosis touches the lives of more than just the person receiving it.

The MS diagnosis can be just the beginning of a whole new, rather wonderful world, like it was for me. I see it as an extraordinary invitation to live life differently from how you lived before and from the people around you. You start to see things, people, places, and situations very differently. To me, MS stands for "Multiple Strengths". I always knew I was strong, but MS has pushed me to my limits. I am way stronger than I ever knew I was.

I know there are some terrific neurologists out there, but unfortunately, I didn't meet one until very recently when I discovered a prestigious specialist in the field. I was pleasantly surprised at how interested he was in me and my story. He didn't speak down to me or swear at me, and he certainly did not dismiss anything I shared. He was not like any of the other medical professionals I had previously seen. I now have a truly fabulous neurologist whom I trust, respect, and admire. Having a yearly appointment with him has become crucial to me. However, it took time —ten years—to find the right one for me. Seek out a neurologist who truly listens and understands you.

"Disease is an imbalance. You have too many things that you don't need and not enough of what you do need."–Dr. Sydney Baker. I certainly can relate to that.

MS—no one gets it, unless they've got it. Not everyone will understand your journey. That's fine. It's not their journey to make sense of; it's yours. The most important thing is that YOU understand why you've got it, why you've arrived at this place with compromised health, and what you can do about it. This is where functional medicine comes in and shines!

We can be grateful for medical intervention. Conventional Medicine is fantastic for acute health issues. If I break a leg, I am going to the

Accident and Emergency (A&E), and I will be so grateful that they are able to put it back together again! It's incredible. However, when it comes to chronic health conditions, autoimmune conditions, multiple sclerosis—there is no medication that can cure them. It may help slow down the progression of the disease, but it will continue to advance until dietary and lifestyle changes are implemented, and the underlying cause is identified and addressed. Nothing changes if nothing changes.

After my diagnosis, I was seeking support. I thought by writing an open, honest letter to the people I considered close to me, telling everyone at the same time what the doctors had announced to me, I'd be supported. I read so many amazing accounts of people who shared their health concerns and diagnoses and were met with incredible support. However, this was not my experience. The reality was people didn't know what to do with what I had just told them. I was often met with silence. It's like they were scared of it—scared that they themselves would "catch it", as if it were contagious. I longed to make sense of my alarming health situation as my body progressively shut down with each passing day. I was desperate for support but was struggling to find it. However, the whole experience taught me that I don't need lots of people in my life. I just need the right people. I have that now. It's important you have that, too. It's not the quantity, it's the quality.

Any experience that allows us to understand and enter another person's experience is worth going through. It's a true blessing to connect with people who have and are experiencing similar health challenges. I often have people say to me with tears streaming down their cheeks, "You're the first person I've spoken to that gets it." Having that said to me makes everything I've experienced worth it. I only get it because I've got it. It's a real privilege to be that "first person". MS has provided a unique opportunity for me to cultivate deep and meaningful relationships, and it's also been an effective filter for the people in my life.

If you don't believe your health is going to improve, I guarantee it won't. It won't because you won't be doing anything to change it. However, if you have hope, and health begins with hope, there is a heck of a good chance that your life will change for the better.

I have huge respect for the Medical Profession, but I've learned that you don't have to believe everything the neurologist says. What my neurologist was telling me was not on my vision board! Why would I want to attach a wheelchair to it just because he said so?

Within functional medicine, we dig deep into what's causing and driving the symptoms and creating DIS-ease in the body. This is so unique and individual. What may be causing and driving your symptoms, won't be what was driving mine. A personalized, individual approach is key here. MS isn't going anywhere. If you have been diagnosed with it, currently, there is no cure, so it's going to accompany you throughout your life.

For me, I prefer it to be more like a silent partner rather than the CEO. I thrive despite MS; I'm not confined to a wheelchair as I was once told I would be. The future remains uncertain, but that's true for everyone, isn't it? My focus is on living a life today that my future self will be grateful for.

What has enabled me to be the CEO of my life is identifying my personal antecedents, triggers, and mediators (ATM's). These will all differ from person to person. I invite you to go to my website and download my free workbook, "Surviving to Thriving: 3 Simple Steps that have transformed my life living with MS". It will describe to you in more detail the benefits of knowing your personal ATM's and what you can do about them.

I owe so much to the incredible, selfless individual Dr. Terry Wahls, who was ridiculed and dismissed by other health professionals and fellow neurologists for bringing to everyone's attention that food really does matter. After she changed her diet and lifestyle, she was able to get out of a tilt-reclining wheelchair! Truly transformational! I now live my life on a Wahls Paleo™ Level 2. I have no desire to ever put gluten, dairy, or eggs past my lips again! When I do, I FEEL it and suffer for it. This was why I had my flare last year.

It hasn't been easy, but nothing worthwhile in life ever is. This applies to changing your diet and lifestyle. The taste of health tastes way better than any cake or cheese ever could! But it's a choice. And I can now easily choose the choice that gives me good results because I am super clear on my personal "why" and "what" I need my health for. Without knowing those things, I don't think I would be as committed as I am.

My health relies on me making the best decisions I can. If I don't, there will be consequences for me, and those consequences are not something I want. Just after getting married, I expected my husband to lead me to the bedroom. Instead, he was leading me to the bathroom! I had no strength in my legs to get there myself. I really have no desire to ever go back there. To achieve that, there are things I need to do and things I must avoid on a daily basis. My health depends on it.

Something I consider extremely important is checking in with myself more than I check my phone. I actually have a love/hate relationship with the mobile phone. Yes, I enjoy it. It keeps me connected to friends and family back home in Scotland, and I use it for my business, connecting with my Instagram followers. But sometimes I feel I could quite easily live without one. Anytime I have experienced dry eyes or broken sleep, you can be sure the fault lies with technology!

MS has really changed me. The thing is, I had to change. Before the arrival of MS, I was living a life that I didn't necessarily choose, but it was all I knew. MS allowed me to stop, reflect, and really consider how I was living. MS changed how I saw the world around me and the people in it. I began seeing things differently and started listening more to what people didn't say, and started to see what people didn't do. I became more discerning. I quickly discovered that people show us what we need to see, and it wasn't always easy to accept this new reality.

Another way in which MS has changed me is I don't go along with things I don't want. If that means being misunderstood, then so be it. There were very few people there for me after my MS diagnosis. It's important to me that I listen to my gut and live in alignment with my values. I'm not interested in living my life for the approval of other people.

When I was training to become a Wahls Health Protocol Practitioner, I remember a module where she encouraged us to think of the gifts of our circumstances—gifts that MS has brought to us. I really do believe that Dr. Wahls's diagnosis of MS has been a gift to the world. What she's done and continues to do for neurology is impressive. This would never have happened if she had not gone through what she did. Her grit is to be admired and applauded.

MS has given me many gifts. It forced me to come out of the fast lane. For the first time in my life, at thirty-four years of age, I discovered that there was a slow lane. You know the hard shoulder at the side of the motorway? Well, that's where I ended up. My body just stopped. However, those signs were there when I was belting along the highway with my foot on the gas. Living life in the slow lane serves me much better. I don't see the point of trying to get anywhere fast; I just enjoy the journey. The view is way better, too! You see way more. You don't see very much when your foot is on the gas.

MS has also given me a passion. I discovered what my strengths were as MS put me in a position where I automatically used them without even realizing I had them. Knowing your personal strengths is important. When you attach your values to your goals, you can get to where you want to be. That's what I've done, and I believe anyone can do that, too. Our bodies want us to be well. They've been created to function in a certain way, but sadly, life and its stressors can disrupt things. Often, it leaves us in a place where we have to unlearn a few things, embrace, and learn some new things.

One thing I realize when I look over the previous years and the many events of my life, MS didn't just happen, and it didn't happen overnight. I think of the mold exposure crawling up my bedroom wall when I was a kid, the lack of vegetables in my diet, the lack of sleep from working night shifts in a bakery, the childhood stresses that had a huge negative impact on my nervous system at such a young age, the lack of vitamin D due to living in Scotland, Epstein Barr Virus which I had at age twenty-two, and what tipped me was the exposure to mercury when I allowed a dentist to put four silver fillings in my mouth.

My bucket was already full of stressors and toxins, but this exposure, along with the stress of closing a shop, arranging our marriage, and moving to a foreign country just tipped the toxic bucket. I find the bucket analogy very helpful to understand how I came to arrive at the diagnosis of multiple sclerosis. This bucket represents our life, and it gets filled with things that are toxic. Once it gets full, it spills over, often displaying symptoms of disease. It's time to empty that bucket. I am a big believer in having to look back before we can move forward. It has helped me to make sense of the diagnosis and why I was given it. I also know what I can do about it, and I do that well.

I have read many books over the years, but the one that made a huge impression on me was recommended by my acupuncturist. It's called *The Biology of Belief*, written by Bruce Lipton. What a read! I strongly believe that this book helped me change the trajectory of the disease, not be defined by MS, and embrace the knowledge that MS happened for me, not to me. It also helped me to be crystal clear as to what meaning I gave the diagnosis. In one chapter, the author speaks about the importance of what we think and believe about a health challenge. He writes in this book about a man who was diagnosed with cancer of the esophagus. He was treated for it, but the doctors said that it would return. The man died shortly after his diagnosis. The discovery that was made after his death has had a huge impact on me. When they performed the autopsy on him, they found very little cancer. There wasn't even enough cancer to kill him. It's written that "he died with cancer, but not from cancer". The reason the man died was because he believed he was going to die. Since I read that chapter in the book, I came to realize the importance of my thoughts. I needed to be careful with what I thought, what I said to myself about my diagnosis, and what meaning I gave it.

Immediately after my MS diagnosis was given to me, I decided NOT to believe what the neurologists were trying to convince me. One day, I discharged myself from the hospital. I really didn't want to hear any more of their negativity. It wasn't healthy, and it wasn't benefiting my brain in any way!

Gandhi said: "Your beliefs become your thoughts. Your thoughts become your words. Your words become your actions. Your actions become your habits. Your habits become your values. Your values become your destiny." I know I have been given the diagnosis of MS, but I don't believe what I was told would be the prognosis. Why do I have to believe that? It doesn't do me any good! I believe I can live well with MS, and I have, and I am, and I will continue to, so long as I focus on prioritizing progressive health using the principles of functional medicine.

In the same book, Lipton mentions the Placebo Effect, but he also makes mention of the Nocebo. He describes the Placebo Effect as a "positive suggestion that improves health". The opposite to this is what's called the "Nocebo Effect", and this is when a negative suggestion damages health. Everything I was told eleven years ago had the HUGE potential to negatively affect me and cause damage. Therefore, I choose to focus only on the positive suggestions! Have you ever considered that maybe your MS symptoms have worsened because you were told by your neurologist that they were only going to get worse? Everything the mind says, the body hears. You cannot separate the mind from the body.

Conventional medicine dismissed me. They listened only to reply. It was all about them and what they could do for me by providing medication to slow down the progression of the disease. Functional medicine, on the other hand, provided me with an abundance of hope. They listened with the intent to understand my unique needs, looking beyond symptoms and addressing the root cause. It was all about me. They encouraged me to explore everything I could do to support my health, emphasizing the importance of diet and lifestyle to create health.

I'm now a Wahls Protocol® Health Practitioner, and I'm thrilled to be joining Dr. Wahls and her tribe of Health Practitioners in creating an epidemic of health! I recently did an allergy test confirming an allergy to eggs, which really surprised me. While undergoing the Wahls Protocol® training, I learned that eggs rank as the third most common allergen, and interestingly, they are excluded from the Wahls Protocol. We know that eggs can be a powerhouse of nutrition, and many people benefit from them, but many people can react to them too. I used to eat a lot of eggs, but since removing them completely from my diet, I feel better because of it.

In the summer, breakfast often consists of chia seed pudding with berries or a green smoothie. In the winter, I often enjoy a hot vegetable soup in the morning or some salmon and vegetables. Anytime I eat, I will have some protein to balance my blood sugar. I eat nine to twelve vegetables a day. It's not as difficult as it may sound when you can hide them in soups and smoothies. I try to eat within an eight-hour window.

These past eleven years have been hard. People look at my beautiful, post-card images that I take and share on Instagram and my life here in the picturesque Switzerland, but they don't see the half! The journey, the heartache, and the work I had to put in to get where I am now...and the work continues. Getting to where I am with my health has been distressing, as well as fulfilling. While people my age were getting married and starting families, I was endeavoring to navigate a new life with MS and educating myself about functional medicine to slow down the progression of the disease.

When I couldn't walk, I promised myself that when I could walk again, I would never stop walking! I have kept that promise to myself, and I aim to walk 10,000 steps every day. Sometimes I can walk all 10,000 steps at once with my husband, up in the Swiss Alps where I live. Sometimes I just do 5,000 steps in the morning and 5,000 steps in the afternoon. Walking is non-negotiable for me.

I've recently returned from a visit to my home country, Scotland, where, one day, I walked an incredible 25,000 steps by Loch Ness. Just eight months prior, I couldn't walk at all. So, whoever you are reading this, perhaps you are also experiencing a loss of function in your body and struggling to walk. I believe that with the right support, your health can improve, just as mine has.

YOU have to do the hard work to live well with MS—and it IS hard work. It really is. I'm not going to sugar coat it. Change is hard, but change can be worth it. You don't need to do it alone. Get yourself a Nutritional Therapist or Functional Medicine Practitioner who knows and understands what's going on in the body with MS, understands how environmental toxins affect the body, and what needs to be considered. Get yourself a neurologist who fills you with hope—not fear. Look at the people who are living well with MS. Look at the recent research studies being done. Look at Dr. Terry Wahls and read her books. There's so much hope all around you if you choose to see it, focus on it, and be inspired by it.

What do you need your health for?
What does your health mean to you?
What is your WHY?
These questions are key when prioritizing progressive health. It will take work. It's hard not to be eating or living like everyone else around you. But I think life in a wheelchair would be even harder. I know what I would rather choose. As Simon Alexander Ong wrote in his book Energize: "Choose your hard." That's what I'm doing, and that's what I encourage you to do, too. Your hard may become phenomenally great. I hope it will.

FINAL NOTE

"Before you heal someone, ask him if he is willing to give up the things that made him sick." -Hippocrates

As we reach the end of this book, I hope these stories have not only inspired you but also encouraged you to take a moment to reflect on your own life. The purpose of this book has been to shine a light on aspects that deserve recognition and change. It's not just about MS or autoimmune diseases; it's a call to awareness, an invitation to slow down and reevaluate our lives.

Our ancestors had wisdom we can learn from, and with today's technology and knowledge, we can create a healthier, more harmonious world, instead of heading down a destructive path. It's as simple as pausing to take a deep breath, enjoying the smell of flowers, and appreciating the beauty that surrounds us.

We hope you've found this book to be a valuable guide. In closing, remember that while healing isn't guaranteed, it's always within reach. The life you choose to lead is firmly in your hands. Join us on **www.BeatingMultipleSclerosis.com** to explore all the limitless possibilities together.

Printed in Great Britain
by Amazon

28576068R00229